MANAGEMENT OF ACUTE PULMONARY EMBOLISM

CONTEMPORARY CARDIOLOGY

CHRISTOPHER P. CANNON, MD
SERIES EDITOR
ANNEMARIE M. ARMANI, MD
EXECUTIVE EDITOR

MANAGEMENT OF ACUTE PULMONARY EMBOLISM

Edited by

STAVROS V. KONSTANTINIDES, MD

Professor of Medicine
Department of Cardiology and Pulmonology
Georg August University
Goettingen, Germany

Foreword by

Samuel Z. Goldhaber, MD

Professor of Medicine
Harvard Medical School
Staff Cardiologist
Brigham and Women's Hospital
Boston, MA

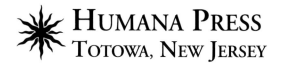

HUMANA PRESS
TOTOWA, NEW JERSEY

© 2007 Humana Press Inc.
999 Riverview Drive, Suite 208
Totowa, New Jersey 07512
www.humanapress.com

All rights reserved. No part of this book may be reproduced, stored in a retrieval system, or transmitted in any form or by any means, electronic, mechanical, photocopying, microfilming, recording, or otherwise without written permission from the Publisher.

The content and opinions expressed in this book are the sole work of the authors and editors, who have warranted due diligence in the creation and issuance of their work. The publisher, editors, and authors are not responsible for errors or omissions or for any consequences arising from the information or opinions presented in this book and make no warranty, express or implied, with respect to its contents.

Due diligence has been taken by the publishers, editors, and authors of this book to assure the accuracy of the information published and to describe generally accepted practices. The contributors herein have carefully checked to ensure that the drug selections and dosages set forth in this text are accurate and in accord with the standards accepted at the time of publication. Notwithstanding, as new research, changes in government regulations, and knowledge from clinical experience relating to drug therapy and drug reactions constantly occurs, the reader is advised to check the product information provided by the manufacturer of each drug for any change in dosages or for additional warnings and contraindications. This is of utmost importance when the recommended drug herein is a new or infrequently used drug. It is the responsibility of the treating physician to determine dosages and treatment strategies for individual patients. Further it is the responsibility of the health care provider to ascertain the Food and Drug Administration status of each drug or device used in their clinical practice. The publisher, editors, and authors are not responsible for errors or omissions or for any consequences from the application of the information presented in this book and make no warranty, express or implied, with respect to the contents in this publication.

Production Editor: Rhukea J. Hussain

Cover illustrations: Inset *(left to right)*: Figs. 8 and 12 from Chapter 2.

For additional copies, pricing for bulk purchases, and/or information about other Humana titles, contact Humana at the above address or at any of the following numbers: Tel.: 973-256-1699; Fax: 973-256-8341, E-mail: orders@humanapr.com; or visit our Website: www.humanapress.com

This publication is printed on acid-free paper. ∞

ANSI Z39.48-1984 (American National Standards Institute) Permanence of Paper for Printed Library Materials.

Photocopy Authorization Policy:

Authorization to photocopy items for internal or personal use, or the internal or personal use of specific clients, is granted by Humana Press Inc., provided that the base fee of US $30.00 is paid directly to the Copyright Clearance Center at 222 Rosewood Drive, Danvers, MA 01923. For those organizations that have been granted a photocopy license from the CCC, a separate system of payment has been arranged and is acceptable to Humana Press Inc. The fee code for users of the Transactional Reporting Service is: [978-1-58829-644-3 • 1-58829-644-X/07 $30.00].

Printed in the United States of America. 10 9 8 7 6 5 4 3 2 1

eISBN 1-59745-287-4

ISBN-13: 978-1-58829-644-3

Library of Congress Cataloging-in-Publication Data

Management of acute pulmonary embolism / edited by Stavros V. Konstantinides.
    p. ; cm. -- (Contemporary cardiology)
  Includes bibliographical references and index.
    ISBN-10: 1-58829-644-X (alk. paper)
  1. Pulmonary embolism. 2. Pulmonary embolism--Treatment.
I. Konstantinides, Stavros. II. Series: Contemporary cardiology
(Totowa, N.J. : Unnumbered)
  [DNLM: 1. Pulmonary Embolism--diagnosis. 2. Pulmonary Embolism--therapy. 3. Acute Disease--therapy.   WG 420 M266 2007]
  RC776.P85M362 2007
  616.2'49--dc22

                                                                                            2006008250

FOREWORD

Acute pulmonary embolism causes dread among physicians and patients. The diagnosis is often difficult to establish, and the cause is often unclear. Management is controversial, because advice from specialists may be based more upon bias than upon evidence.

Pulmonary embolism is receiving more attention now than ever before. The National Quality Forum is writing guidelines to ensure "best practices" in acute care hospitals. The Joint Commission that accredits US hospitals is planning to issue directives within the next few years to optimize prevention and treatment of pulmonary embolism. In March 2006, the National Comprehensive Cancer Network issued guidelines on treatment of cancer patients with pulmonary embolism. The US Surgeon General's Office held an unprecedented 2-day symposium in May 2006 on pulmonary embolism. New patient advocacy and self-help groups are emerging throughout the United States. Public service announcements are educating laypersons about pulmonary embolism with respect to risk factors and warning signs. A new nonprofit organization, the North American Thrombosis Forum (www.NATFonline.org) has been established to focus on research, clinical, and public policy issues related to thrombosis. The topic of "clot" has become "hot."

Pulmonary embolism as a discipline does not "belong" to any single group. It requires collaboration among emergency medicine, internal medicine, cardiology, pulmonary, hematology, and radiology physicians as well as interventional radiologists and cardiologists and cardiac surgeons. Websites provide useful information but are not sufficiently detailed or nuanced to guide complex management decisions. Because of the disparate disciplines involved in the study of pulmonary embolism, coupled with exponentially increasing advances in our understanding of this disease, a scientifically rigorous and contemporary textbook fills an unmet need.

Stavros Konstantinides, MD, is a leader in the field of acute pulmonary embolism. As a cardiologist, he has carried out pioneering work in echocardiography, biomarker elucidation, and thrombolysis of pulmonary embolism. Through the multicenter registries and trials that he has organized, Professor Konstantinides has established a personal connection to a global network of pulmonary embolism specialists. Using his considerable persuasive skills, he has enlisted key experts to take time from their busy schedules to contribute to this outstanding textbook.

Management of Acute Pulmonary Embolism is not a book that will rest for long on the bookshelf. With its recent references, clear-cut tables, and beautiful illustrations, it will serve as a practical compendium for use in daily clinical practice. I plan to take it with me when I am summoned to the Emergency Department, Intensive Care Unit, or when I consult on outpatients with pulmonary embolism. Armed with this textbook, I will have at my fingertips all of the information I need, compiled in 19 superb chapters, to manage any aspect of this illness.

Management of Acute Pulmonary Embolism is organized in three sections: diagnosis, treatment, and special topics. The diagnosis section has up-to-date chapters on clinical evaluation; cardiac biomarkers, including troponin, BNP, and pro-BNP; and imaging, including the latest technological developments in chest CT scanning and venous ultra-sound examination. Importantly, these timely advances are synthesized in two summary chapters. Perrier "puts it all together" for clinically stable patients, and the Editor himself writes a masterpiece chapter with diagnostic algorithms for hemodynamically unstable patients.

The therapy section updates our use of heparin, low-molecular-weight heparin, fondaparinux, warfarin, and thrombolysis, but goes far beyond the usual topics to include novel approaches such as pulmonary embolectomy (now modified to achieve survival rates that exceed 90%) and new devices for suction catheter embolectomy. A controversial chapter in this section more or less advocates thrombolysis for pulmonary embolism patients undergoing cardiopulmonary resuscitation. Although we need not necessarily agree with this philosophy, the author makes his case elegantly and provides "food for thought."

The final section on special topics will be especially useful in the outpatient setting. How extensive a thrombophilia workup should be undertaken? What are the special considerations for cancer patients who have pulmonary embolism? How should pulmonary embolism be managed during pregnancy? What should we do to prevent a patient from being the 1 in 1 million who boards a long-haul air flight and collapses and dies from pulmonary embolism upon deplaning 6–18 h later? Finally, for the 4% of patients who develop chronic thromboembolic pulmonary hypertension after acute pulmonary embolism, how can we optimize their management?

Management of Acute Pulmonary Embolism will receive magnificent reviews and become a best-seller among specialty textbooks. For the medical student or investigator, it is the starting point for future study. For the practicing physician, it is indispensable. I feel privileged to know Professor Konstantinides personally. I congratulate him and express my admiration and gratitude for the strides he has made in the field of acute pulmonary embolism by compiling and editing this important new text.

Samuel Z. Goldhaber, MD
Professor of Medicine
Harvard Medical School
Staff Cardiologist
Brigham and Women's Hospital
Boston, MA

PREFACE

Management of venous thromboembolism has long been characterized by a high degree of complexity and a disappointing lack of both efficacy and efficiency. The clinical symptoms and signs of acute pulmonary embolism (PE) are notoriously nonspecific, and ubiquitously available bedside tests such as the ECG, chest X-ray, and clinical chemistry can offer little assistance apart from strengthening or weakening the clinical suspicion. Thus, for almost 30 years, confirmation of the diagnosis relied on ventilation-perfusion lung scan and/or pulmonary angiography. However, scintigraphy frequently yields nondiagnostic findings, and pulmonary angiography is an invasive procedure that may place the patient at risk of life-threatening complications besides requiring local expertise and sophisticated logistics to be readily available on an around-the-clock basis. These risks and limitations of individual tests led to the development of complex multistep diagnostic algorithms, which were successfully tested in well-designed management studies but have proven extremely difficult to implement in clinical practice. As a result, the diagnosis of potentially life-threatening PE was frequently missed in many patients who subsequently died of the disease without receiving appropriate treatment, while other patients unnecessarily underwent a battery of potentially hazardous, time-consuming, and costly procedures because of a vague, poorly documented clinical suspicion.

Luckily, things are now beginning to look better for patients with PE, and for the physicians caring for them. The recent development of structured models for assessment of clinical pretest probability, the widespread use of D-dimer testing in the hospital and the outpatient setting, and the enormous technical advances of multidetector-row CT scan, are radically changing our approach to patients with suspected PE. These modalities form the basis for contemporary diagnostic algorithms that are not only efficient and reliable, but also simple, fast, noninvasive, and "user-friendly." Furthermore, the prognostic importance of right ventricular (RV) dysfunction has been recognized, and a number of studies have demonstrated the value of echocardiography and laboratory biomarkers for risk stratification of PE. Simplified treatment regimens using low-molecular-weight heparins are now available for hemodynamically stable patients with PE, while early thrombolysis and technical advances in surgical and interventional treatment permit successful removal of thrombus in massive PE.

Pulmonary embolism is of interest (and importance) to physicians of almost all disciplines, being encountered across the entire spectrum of clinical medicine. In *Management of Acute Pulmonary Embolism*, traditional, novel, and evolving aspects related to the diagnosis and treatment of PE are highlighted by an international team of experts who have significantly contributed to the advances in this exciting field. The book is divided into three parts. The first part focuses on the contemporary diagnostic approach to the patient with suspected PE and begins with a critical review of currently used models for assessing clinical probability, and the utility of D-dimer testing. Next, the imaging procedures for visualizing pulmonary thromboemboli are presented, placing emphasis on the emerging role of spiral CT as the new diagnostic gold standard, but also emphasizing the importance and practicability of an early noninvasive ultrasound evaluation of the leg veins. Risk stratification of pulmonary embolism is, as mentioned above, evolving into an important determinant of successful PE management, and three chapters are devoted to biochemical and imaging tests allowing detection of right ventricular dysfunction, and of a patent foramen ovale. Finally, in Chapters 7 and 8, our current state of knowledge is summarized in up-to-date diagnostic algorithms. These are aimed at helping the clinician walk through the individual tests and find the fastest and most efficient pathway for confirmation or exclusion of PE both in hemodynamically stable and in unstable patients, always considering the logistics and expertise available on site.

The second part provides an update of the therapeutic options for patients with PE. Contemporary regimens of anticoagulation with unfractionated and low-molecular-weight heparins are presented and discussed, as is the intensity and optimal duration of oral anticoagulation for secondary prophylaxis, the controversial topic of thrombolysis in PE, and the advantages of early surgical embolectomy provided that the appropriate setup is available. In this section, emphasis is also placed on the management of patients with fulminant PE undergoing cardiopulmonary resuscitation, explaining the scientific background favoring aggressive use of thrombolysis in this setting and the potential to save lives in a seemingly desparate situation. Furthermore, the recent technical advances in interventional (catheter-based) thrombus aspiration are presented, a therapeutic option that may yield impressive results at the hands of a skilled interventionalist.

The third part of the book deals with those specific aspects which make venous thromboembolism such a unique disease requiring multidisciplinary management strategies. A number of highly relevant and controversial topics are critically discussed, including the need for thrombophilia screening after diagnosis of PE, the association between PE and cancer, and the true magnitude of PE-related risk in "economy-class" passengers. A detailed chapter is devoted to the care of pregnant patients with acute PE and to secondary prophylaxis of PE in pregnancy, a particularly sensitive area of research and clinical practice for which little direct evidence and no formal guidelines exist. Finally, a comprehensive review focuses on the management of chronic thromboembolic pulmonary hypertension, the feared long-term complication of PE that may not be as rare and elusive as previously thought.

Writing a book on a rapidly evolving field poses a tremendous challenge, since such an effort bears the risk of providing outdated, overhauled information if the book cannot be completed within a relatively short period of time. I am therefore particularly thankful to each one of the authors who took every effort not only to present and discuss their topic in the best possible manner but also to meet the publication deadline, which makes it possible to present a really *contemporary* overview of PE management. I hope that the reader will find *Management of Acute Pulmonary Embolism* as informative and enjoyable as I did throughout this exciting process.

Stavros V. Konstantinides, MD

CONTENTS

CONTRIBUTORS

FRÉDÉRIC ADNET, MD, PhD • *Hôpital Avicenne, Bobigny, France*

GIANCARLO AGNELLI, MD • *Division of Internal and Cardiovascular Medicine—Stroke Unit, Department of Internal Medicine, University of Perugia, Perugia, Italy*

LISHAN AKLOG, MD • *Department of Cardiothoracic Surgery, Mount Sinai School of Medicine, New York, NY*

ANI C. ANYANWU, MD • *Department of Cardiothoracic Surgery, Mount Sinai Medical Center, New York, NY*

SHANNON M. BATES, MDCM, MSc • *Department of Medicine, McMaster University, Hamilton, Ontario, Canada*

CECILIA BECATTINI, MD • *Division of Internal and Cardiovascular Medicine—Stroke Unit, Department of Internal Medicine, University of Perugia, Perugia, Italy*

JAN BEYER, MD • *Division of Vascular Medicine, Carl Gustav Carus University Clinic, Technical University of Dresden, Dresden, Germany*

BERND W. BÖTTIGER, MD, DEAA • *European Resuscitation Council; and Department of Anesthesiology, Ruprecht Karls University, Heidelberg, Germany*

JEAN CATINEAU, MD • *Hôpital Avicenne, Bobigny, France*

ANNA FALANGA, MD • *Hematology Division, Department of Hematology-Oncology, Ospedali Riuniti, Bergamo, Italy*

ANNETTE GEIBEL, MD • *Department of Cardiology and Angiology, Albert Ludwig University, Freiburg, Germany*

EVANGELOS GIANNITSIS, MD • *Department of Cardiology, Angiology, and Pulmonology, Ruprecht-Karls University, Heidelberg, Germany*

RUSSELL D. HULL, MBBS, MSc, FRCPC, FACP • *Thrombosis Research Unit, Foothills Hospital, University of Calgary, Calgary, Alberta, Canada*

WOLFGANG KASPER, MD • *St. Josef's Hospital, Wiesbaden, Germany*

HUGO A. KATUS, MD • *Department of Cardiology, Angiology and Pulmonology, Ruprecht-Karls University, Heidelberg, Germany*

WALTER KLEPETKO, MD • *Department of Cardiothoracic Surgery, Medical University of Vienna, Austria*

STAVROS V. KONSTANTINIDES, MD • *Department of Cardiology and Pulmonology, Georg August University, Goettingen, Germany*

NILS KUCHER, MD • *Cardiovascular Division, Interventional Cardiology, University Hospital, Zurich, Switzerland*

IRENE M. LANG, MD • *Department of Cardiology, Medical University of Vienna, Austria*

CLAUDE LAPANDRY, MD • *Hôpital Avicenne, Bobigny, France*

FRÉDÉRIC LAPOSTOLLE MD • *Hôpital Avicenne, Bobigny, France*

SIMON J. MCRAE, MBBS • *Department of Haematology, The Queen Elizabeth Hospital, Adelaide, South Australia, Australia*

GUY MEYER, MD • *Faculté de Médecine, Université Paris-Descartes, and Assistance Publique Hôpitaux de Paris, Hôpital Européen Georges Pompidou, Paris, France*

ARNAUD PERRIER, MD • *Division of General Internal Medicine, Department of Medicine, Geneva University Hospital and Geneva Faculty of Medicine, Geneva, Switzerland*

ANDREA PICCIOLI, MD • *Department of Medical and Surgical Sciences, and Internal Medicine, University of Padua, Padua, Italy*

GRAHAM F. PINEO, MD, FRCPC, FACP • *Thrombosis Research Unit, Foothills Hospital, University of Calgary, Calgary, Alberta, Canada*

PAOLO PRANDONI, MD • *Department of Medical and Surgical Sciences, and Internal Medicine, University of Padua, Padua, Italy*

JAMES G. RAVENEL, MD • *Department of Radiology, Medical University of South Carolina, Charleston, SC*

HANNO RIESS, MD • *Department of Hematology and Oncology, University Clinic Charité, Campus Virchow Hospital, University Medicine, Berlin, Germany*

SEBASTIAN M. SCHELLONG, MD • *Carl Gustav Carus University Clinic, Division of Vascular Medicine, Technical University of Dresden, Dresden, Germany*

U. JOSEPH SCHOEPF, MD • *Department of Radiology, Medical University of South Carolina, Charleston, SC*

FABIAN SPÖHR, MD • *Department of Anesthesiology, Ruprecht Karls University, Heidelberg, Germany*

PHILIP S. WELLS, MD, FRCPC, MSc • *Department of Medicine, Ottawa Hospital, University of Ottawa, and the Ottawa Health Research Institute,Ottawa, Ontario, Canada*

MANFRED ZEHENDER, MD • *Department of Cardiology and Angiology, Albert Ludwig University, Freiburg, Germany*

I

DIAGNOSTIC APPROACH TO THE PATIENT
WITH SUSPECTED PULMONARY EMBOLISM

1

Clinical Probability and D-Dimer Testing

Philip S. Wells, MD

CONTENTS

SUMMARY

In order to address the well-known inadequacies in diagnostic imaging for pulmonary embolism (PE), health care providers can utilize pretest probability estimates in conjunction with the likelihood ratios of diagnostic tests. This approach helps define more accurately the posttest probability of a disease with a given imaging result. In the case of PE, we have the benefit of proven clinical prediction rules to help assess the pretest probability. Furthermore, the D-dimer test, which measures the degradation product of a cross-linked fibrin blood clot, can also be employed in diagnostic algorithms. It is, however, important to keep in mind that although all D-dimer tests lie on the same receiver operating characteristic curve, some have higher sensitivity than others. Thus, when patients are clinically classified as low-probability, moderate-sensitivity D-dimer tests can be performed next, and a negative result will suffice to rule out PE. Because the negative likelihood ratio with these tests is approx 0.20, the patient's pretest probability of PE must be less than 10% to rule out PE with a negative D-dimer. If, on the other hand, a high-sensitivity D-dimer test is used in patients who have a low or moderate probability of PE, are PE-unlikely by the Wells model, or low- to moderate-probability by the Wicki clinical model, the physician can avoid the need for diagnostic imaging when the D-dimer is negative. In this latter case, the likelihood ratio of 0.06 with the high-sensitivity D-dimer implies that, if patients have a pretest probability of no more than 22%, a negative D-dimer will negate the need for diagnostic imaging. Importantly, combining D-dimer and pretest probability not only allows selection of patients appropriate for diagnostic testing, but also helps interpret the imaging test result as potentially false-negative or false-positive, and thus allows for standardization of the diagnostic workup of PE.

From: *Contemporary Cardiology: Management of Acute Pulmonary Embolism*
Edited by: S. Konstantinides © Humana Press Inc., Totowa, NJ

Key Words: Pulmonary embolism; diagnosis; pretest probability; D-dimer; clinical prediction.

INTRODUCTION

In the past, mismanagement of pulmonary embolism (PE) used to be a frequent problem *(1)*, but the diagnostic workup for suspected PE has now evolved to include ultrasound imaging, clinical pretest probability assessment, D-dimer testing, computerized tomographic pulmonary angiography (CTPA), and magnetic resonance angiography. In fact, we are currently observing an encouraging decrease in mortality from PE, which may reflect both more accurate diagnosis and the use of algorithms to decrease the number of unproven cases *(2,3)*. This chapter will focus on studies that have evaluated clinical assessment and D-dimer testing, and describe how they can be employed in diagnostic algorithms for the investigation of patients with suspected PE.

IMAGING PROCEDURES FOR PULMONARY EMBOLISM

Pulmonary angiography has long been regarded as the gold standard test for the diagnosis of PE, but pulmonary angiography is an invasive procedure requiring a skilled radiologist and a cooperative patient. Although the procedure is usually well tolerated, arrhythmias, hypotension, and other adverse reactions to contrast dye may be observed *(4)*. In many centers, pulmonary angiography is unavailable, and in others it is simply not practical to use this procedure routinely to exclude PE. In addition, a negative pulmonary angiogram does not exclude the future development of thromboembolic complications. For example, in the PIOPED study, 1.6% of patients with normal pulmonary angiograms developed PE over the 1-yr follow-up period. Most of these events occurred within 1 mo of the procedure *(5,6)*.

Ventilation-perfusion (V/Q) lung scanning has been the imaging procedure of choice in patients with suspected PE for almost two decades. A normal perfusion lung scan essentially excludes the diagnosis of PE, and a high-probability lung scan has an 85–90% predictive value for PE *(6,7)*. Unfortunately, most lung scans fit into a nondiagnostic category (neither normal nor high-probability), in which the incidence of PE varies from 10 to 30% and further investigation is necessary. Limitations with V/Q scans have recently led to CTPA as the first imaging test in many centers for the investigation of patients with suspected PE. However, this test also has certain limitations, many of which are not appreciated by clinicians. CTPA is an evolving technology, with early single-slice detectors unable to sufficiently visualize subsegmental arteries *(8)*. In 2000, a pooled analysis of comparative studies using single-slice detector CT scans compared to pulmonary angiography as the gold standard determined that CTPA had a sensitivity between 53 and 100% and a specificity between 81 and 100% for the diagnosis of PE *(9)*. In an earlier meta-analysis, Forgie et al. had reported the pooled sensitivity to be 72% (95% confidence interval [CI], 59–83%) and the specificity 95% (95% CI, 89–98%), except for central PE (i.e., involving the main, lobar, or segmental pulmonary arteries), in which the sensitivity increased to 94% (95% CI, 86–98%) whereas the specificity remained high (94%; 95% CI, 88–98%) *(10)*. Because pulmonary angiography studies have shown that up to 36% of PEs may be limited to the subsegmental arteries, and small emboli may be harbingers for subsequent thromboembolic complications, management studies including use of CTPA were needed. As discussed below (*see* in "Approach to Patients With

Suspected Pulmonary Embolisms") and in Chapter 7, management studies have now been performed, and the initial fears that CT would miss PE seem to be unfounded, provided that CT is used in conjunction with ultrasound, clinical assessment, or D-dimer. Moreover, with current multidetector-row scanners, diagnostic sensitivity is becoming better (Chapter 2), although falsely detecting PE may still be an issue. A more recent meta-analysis suggested that CTPA has greater discriminatory power than V/Q scanning with regard to the normal and/or near-normal threshold for excluding PE, but CTPA and V/Q scan with high probability threshold were similar for the diagnosis of PE. The pooled sensitivity and the specificity of CTPA were 86% and 93.7%, respectively [11]. However, a recent study suggests use of a multidetector row CTPA is likely to have a higher sensitivity [12].

CT may also be used in conjunction with V/Q scanning. For example, Mayo et al. demonstrated that patients with nondiagnostic V/Q scans who are investigated by CT will have a definitive diagnosis in 80% of cases [13]. Furthermore, CT may identify alternative causes for symptoms in patients with suspected PE, although it needs to be kept in mind that several parenchymal and pleural changes, including wedge-shaped pleural opacities, are nonspecific and can be found both in patients with and without PE [14].

The following chapters in this book will elaborate more on imaging procedures in the diagnostic workup of PE.

CLINICAL SUSPICION
AND PRETEST LIKELIHOOD OF PULMONARY EMBOLISM

Clinical Symptoms and Signs

PE is suspected in many patients with respiratory or chest complaints because of the nonspecific nature of the presenting signs and symptoms. As such, it is worthwhile to explore the value of these signs and symptoms when considered individually.

There are several reports on the sensitivity and specificity of individual signs and symptoms [15–18]. Patient age is consistently a statistically significant univariate predictor of PE, a fact consistent with population-based epidemiological data demonstrating an increased incidence of PE with age [19]. On the other hand, individual presenting symptoms generally do not reliably differentiate between patients with and without PE. Possible exceptions include pleuritic chest pain, sudden dyspnea, and symptoms suggestive of lower-extremity DVT, all of which are consistently more frequent in patients with PE. Moreover, although hemoptysis is overall an unusual presenting symptom in suspected PE, in many studies hemoptysis was consistently more common in patients with confirmed PE than in those without the disease. Risk factors predisposing to venous thromboembolic disease have also been well characterized in the literature [20]. In a review of 1231 patients treated for confirmed venous thromboembolic disease, one or more risk factors were present in more than 96% of the cases [21]. Immobilization, recent surgery, malignancy, and previous venous thromboembolic disease are more common in patients with PE.

Intuitively, patients with PE would be more likely to have tachypnea and tachycardia than patients without PE, but these differences are usually not significant [15]. There appear to be no differences in blood pressure, the presence of pleural rub on auscultation, or body temperature between patients with confirmed and those with (only) suspected PE [18]. Furthermore, one commonly held misconception is that the presence of chest wall tenderness in patients with pleuritic chest pain excludes PE *(23)*. Finally, the presence of a fourth heart sound (S4), a loud second pulmonary heart sound (P2), and inspiratory crackles on chest auscultation were all more common in patients with PE than patients without in one study *(16)*.

ECG Findings and Blood Gas Analysis

A variety of electrocardiographic (ECG) changes have been suggested to have diagnostic value in patients with PE *(15,16,24,25)*. However, the majority of these investigations only studied patients with confirmed PE, whereas few authors reported on the prevalence of ECG changes in patients with suspected PE. We studied unselected patients with suspected PE using standard outcome measures. Our findings showed that only tachycardia and incomplete right bundle branch block were significantly more frequent in PE patients *(26)*. Finally, neither normal nor abnormal alveolar-arterial (A-a) oxygen tension gradient assist in the diagnosis of PE, and blood gas analysis is generally of little value in the diagnostic workup *(27–30)*.

Overall Assessment of Clinical Probability

Despite the limitations of the individual clinical predictors previously described, the PIOPED investigators demonstrated that the overall clinical assessment (i.e., the clinicians' overall diagnostic impression) could be useful in diagnostic management. Experienced clinicians were able to separate a cohort of patients with suspected PE into high-, moderate-, and low-probability groups, using clinical assessment alone *(31)*. More recently, Perrier and colleagues also were able to stratify patients into different risk categories using clinical assessment *(32)*. In both of these studies, patients were stratified into risk categories using the clinical judgment of individual clinicians, which was based on the overall diagnostic impression without using a predefined clinical decision tool. However, with such empiric assessment, the exact methods used by each clinician to estimate pretest probably are difficult to measure or reproduce *(33)*. In addition to considering explicit information such as vital signs and risk factors, clinicians incorporate many implicit methods to decide whether or not PE is present; including, for example, the degree of discomfort exhibited by the patient, whether or not the patient has a convincing history of symptoms that the particular clinician associates with PE, and whether or not another diagnosis can explain the patient's complaints. The problems with empiric assessment are: (1) clinicians often disagree (even for broad categories) on the pretest probability of PE *(34)*; (2) the clinician's experience level appears to influence the accuracy of his or her pretest assessment *(35)*; and (3) probability estimates often tend to follow a middle road, so that fewer patients are categorized by the clinicians into the more useful low- or high-probability groups. Thus, the empiric method has drawbacks, but it is the easiest method to use, as there is no requirement to memorize criteria.

A few years ago, we published our experience with an explicit clinical model to determine pretest probability for PE using clinical findings, ECG, and chest X-ray *(22)*. Another author group questioned the usefulness of this model, but it needs to be mentioned that (1) their study did not use the model prospectively or for clinical decisions; (2) the study had a very high overall PE rate; (3) many patients suspected of PE did not complete the study; and (4) physician gestalt assessments were poor, in contrast to other studies *(36)*.

We subsequently performed a logistic regression analysis of the clinical data collected in our earlier *(22)* study to derive a simplified explicit clinical model *(37)* (Table 1). A

Table 1
Variables Used to Determine Patient Pretest Probability for Pulmonary Embolism (PE)

- Clinical signs and symptoms of deep vein thrombosis (DVT)   [3.0 points]
  (minimum of leg swelling and pain with palpation of the deep veins)
- PE as / more likely than an alternative diagnosis   [3.0 points]
- Heart rate greater than 100/min   [1.5 points]
- Immobilization or surgery in the previous 4 weeks   [1.5 points]
- Previous DVT/PE   [1.5 points]
- Hemoptysis   [1.0 points]
- Malignancy (on treatment, treated in the last 6 mo, or palliative)   [1.0 points]

> Low probability < 2.0
> Moderate probability 2.0–6.0
> High probability > 6.0
> PE unlikely ≤ 4.0
> PE likely > 4.0

validation study revealed that the simplified explicit clinical model was capable of separating patients into low-, moderate-, and high-risk subgroups, although emergency physicians had a lower threshold for suspecting PE, so that the overall PE rates were lower than the original study *(38,22)*. We currently use the same model, but prefer to classify patients as PE-unlikely (score of 4 or less) or PE-likely (score >4). The main limitation of this model is the need for the physician to consider an alternative diagnosis, and this may be dependent on the physician's experience and expertise. However, the κ for interobserver variability was reasonable (0.60; unpublished data), despite performing the repeat assessment up to 18 h after the first assessment. In a further study, Wolf et al. demonstrated moderate to substantial interrater agreement and reproducibility of the Wells et al. model *(39)*. Reproducibility was also demonstrated in low risk patients *(40)*. Of note, no other prediction rule has evaluated interrater agreement and reproducibility.

Selection of patients with a relatively low pretest probability comprises the single most important factor in the derivation of a protocol to safely rule out PE. Bosson et al. recently published their unique evaluation of more than 1500 patients with suspected PE *(40)*. They confirmed that the model published by our group accurately categorized patients as having low (5.5%), moderate (26.7%), or high (49.6%) probability for PE, and they also demonstrated that quantitative D-dimer values can further assist in the diagnostic approach (discussed later).

Other clinical assessment/prediction rules have also been reported. Miniati and colleagues reported that their combination of clinical predictors (symptoms, ECG findings, and chest X-ray findings) had a negative predictive value of 94%, and PE could be excluded in 42% of patients in their validation set *(41)*. However, this study enrolled a high-prevalence population, did not perform logistic regression to develop a simple rule, had a high PE rate of 10% in the low-risk group, and the described criteria for the low-risk group could apply to any patient with even minimal chest symptoms.

Wicki et al. devised a model in emergency room patients that could be performed by nonclinicians (Table 2) *(42,43)*. In fact, comparisons with the model developed by our own group have demonstrated both rules to be effective *(44)*. Potential disadvantages of the Wicki model are that (1) it is difficult to memorize; (2) it has not been tested or derived in hospitalized patients; (3) the PE rate in the low-probability group was 10% (which may

Table 2
Clinical Model Described by Wicki et al.
for Assessment of Pretest Probability for Pulmonary Embolism (PE)

Criteria	Points
Age 60–79 yr	1
Age >79 yr	2
Prior deep vein thrombosis/PE	2
Recent surgery	3
Heart rate >100 min^{-1}	1
PaCO$_2$, mmHg	
<36	2
36–39	1
PaO$_2$, mmHg	
<49	4
49–60	3
>60–71	2
>71–82	1
Chest X-ray	
Plate-like atelectasis	1
Elevation of hemidiaphragm	1

Score range	Mean probability of PE	Patients with this score	Interpretation of risk
0–4	10%	49%	Low
5–8	38%	44%	Moderate
9–12	81%	6%	High

be too high for use with certain D-dimer assays; discussed later); (4) there is no consideration of other diagnoses and most of the points given to a patient are nonspecific; and (5) it has only been tested in one center.

Kline et al. have studied the issue of PE diagnosis in the emergency department, where the need to rule out PE generally results in screening many patients with a low prevalence of PE (45). Their strategy doubled the rate of screening for PE, had a false negative rate of less than 1%, and did not increase the pulmonary vascular imaging rate. Their decision rule was: "a patient aged 50 yr or older, or any (patient with) a pulse rate greater than the systolic blood pressure, *and* either (1) unexplained hypoxemia (SaO$_2$ on pulse oximetry <95% while breathing room air) or (2) unilateral leg swelling or recent surgery or hemoptysis" was "unsafe" and required a V/Q scan or CTPA. If the physician felt that their unstructured estimate of PE was high regardless of the decision rule, patients underwent imaging. In a further study, they suggested that if all the previous factors are negative *and* the patient has no prior venous thromboembolic event *and* is not on oral hormone therapy, the patient is at low risk for PE (46).Unfortunately, this rule has proved less useful in very low-risk patients in the emergency room, and as such physicians must be careful not to screen all emergency room patients with dyspnea for PE. Finally, a further rule published by Hyers et al. has demonstrated utility in a management study (47,48).

In summary, there are several prediction rules to choose from, and not much evidence exists to advise one over the other. But the use of these rules appears to improve the diagnostic process for PE, as outlined in the next section.

D-DIMER TESTING

D-dimer is a degradation product of a cross-linked fibrin blood clot. D-dimer levels may also be increased by a variety of nonthrombotic disorders including recent major surgery, hemorrhage, trauma, pregnancy, cancer, sepsis, or acute arterial thrombosis. D-dimer assays are, in general, sensitive but nonspecific markers for venous thromboembolism, and therefore a positive D-dimer result is *not* useful to "rule in" the diagnosis of venous thromboembolism. Rather, the potential value is for a negative test result to exclude the diagnosis. The negative predictive value of the D-dimer depends on the sensitivity of the assay and is inversely related to the prevalence of venous thromboembolism in the population under study. On the other hand, the specificity of the particular D-dimer assay and the particular population under study influence the utility of the assay to exclude the diagnosis of venous thromboembolism. For instance, use of a very nonspecific assay or the testing of very ill hospitalized patients would be predicted to be of limited value because of the expected high number of positive results, many of which would be false positives. D-dimer levels have also been demonstrated to increase with age, and some advocate that D-dimer should not be performed in patients more than 80 yr old *(49–51)*.

There are qualitative and quantitative D-dimer assays. Visual inspection is employed with qualitative D-dimer assays and the results are interpreted as positive or negative. The first tests developed were latex agglutination assays including the D-dimer test (Diagnostica Stago), the Dimertest and Dimertest II (Agen Biomedical), Minutex® (Biopool), Nephelotex (Biopool), and Accuclot™ (Sigma Diagnostics). In one study of 600 patients, the Accuclot had a sensitivity of 90% and specificity of 72% *(52)*. In general, however, although the sensitivity of the latex agglutination assays has indeed been in the previous range, their specificity is likely to be much lower, in the order of 45%.

The second type of qualitative assays is a whole blood agglutination assay (SimpliRED™, Agen Biomedical). The SimpliRED is the qualitative test with the largest body of clinical evidence to date. The sensitivity and specificity of the SimpliRED D-dimer in clinical trials has been similar to that of the other visual inspection assays, with Stein reporting a sensitivity ranging from 78 to 83% and specificity from 64 to 74% *(53)*. Overall, qualitative D-dimer assays offer the advantage that they are simple to perform, have a rapid turnaround time, and are inexpensive. Interobserver reliability has been questioned in at least three studies *(54–56)*, although a fourth study found excellent interobserver reliability *(57)*. Regardless, it is advisable that only trained observers perform and interpret these assays. Second-generation latex assays are quantitative (IL-test, Tinaquant®, Liatest, and so on) and are generally of higher sensitivity, consistently demonstrating sensitivity in the low 90% range and specificity in the mid 40% range.

Rapid, automated enzyme-linked immunosorbent assays (ELISAs) such as the VIDAS (Biomerieux) have demonstrated the highest sensitivity, at an average of 97 to 98%. The membrane ELISAs such as the Instant IA (Diagnostica Stago) have demonstrated a sensitivity of approx 92% and a specificity of approx 50%.

In summary, the existing data suggest that most D-dimer assays lie on the same Receiver Operating Characteristic curve, although one meta-analysis suggests that the Dimertest, Nycocard®, and Turbiquant® were significantly worse then the other assays *(53,58,59)*. In other words, as sensitivity increases, specificity decreases. Overall, the data suggest that the accuracy of specific D-dimer tests is similar regardless of whether suspected DVT or PE is evaluated *(53)*.

APPROACH TO PATIENTS
WITH SUSPECTED PULMONARY EMBOLISM

My recommended approach to diagnosis in patients with suspected PE involves the use of clinical probability and D-dimer to guide interpretation and need for imaging tests. The safety of a protocol for the diagnosis of PE is primarily defined by the rate of eventually detected PE in patients in whom the protocol excluded the diagnosis, i.e., the false-negative rate. Because protocols are very unlikely to result in a 0% posttest probability, a low threshold of approx 1 to 2% is targeted. This threshold is comparable to the rate of PE or DVT at follow-up after a normal (negative) result of pulmonary angiography as the traditional reference standard. This threshold is also justified because a further accepted method to rule out PE is a normal result on a V/Q scan, which has been demonstrated to be associated with a PE rate of approx 1% during follow-up *(60–63)*. Trying to achieve an even lower PE rate with a negative result seems unrealistic, because the rate of PE discovered in a composite population of hospitalized patients and outpatients without recognized signs or symptoms of PE but who underwent contrast-enhanced CT scanning of the chest ranged from 1.5 to 3.4% *(64,65)*. Finally, if a posttest probability less than 1% is sought, this would lead to an unacceptable trade-off in increased pulmonary vascular imaging, and increased false-positive diagnosis of PE.

The Need for D-Dimer Testing

Several studies have evaluated V/Q scanning and CTPA without concomitant use of the D-dimer. Our group has validated approaches combining either V/Q scanning with clinical probability or CTPA with clinical probability *(37,66)*. The largest prospective CTPA study to date combined clinical probability and ultrasound imaging with CTPA *(48)*. Patients with a negative CTPA, negative ultrasound, and low or moderate pretest probability had PE excluded and the follow-up event rates were 1.8%. Importantly, 15% of patients had a negative CTPA but a positive ultrasound study. A recent meta-analysis suggested that a negative CT rules out PE, but, as the authors pointed out, only one study employed CT alone and all the others used various combinations of lower extremity ultrasound imaging for DVT, clinical probability, and D-dimer *(67)*.

The D-dimer assay can be the first objective test used in addition to clinical assessment with the goal of determining which patients require diagnostic imaging. Clinicians must appreciate that the choice of the D-dimer test depends both on its sensitivity and its specificity. Although sensitivity is important, a safe protocol must also have reasonably high specificity for two reasons: (1) if the specificity is very poor, PE will ultimately be ruled-out without imaging tests in only a small subset of the patients, because low specificity implies that fewer patients with suspected PE will have negative D-dimer results; and (2) a test with low specificity will lead to increased use of imaging tests in relatively low-risk patients and may thus result in more frequent false-positive imaging tests. In fact, if CTPA and V/Q scans were performed without the consideration of clinical probability or the D-dimer, there would be evidence of a diagnostic "positive" result in approx 5 and 10% of patients without PE, respectively *(68–71)*. These rates are even higher in low clinical-probability patients. Low-probability patients with a negative D-dimer can have PE excluded, but low-probability patients with a positive D-dimer will have a PE probability of approx 15%. Application of Bayes' theorem to this latter group of low-probability patients indicates that the posttest probability of PE with a positive CTPA is

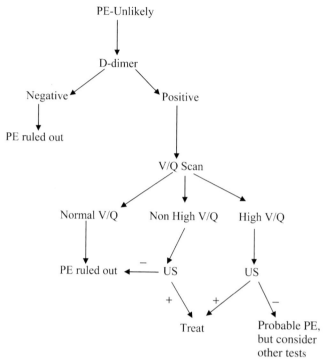

Fig. 1. Strategy for diagnosis of pulmonary embolism (PE) using ventilation-perfusion in patients who are PE-unlikely.

only in the order of 72%, and as such, one must consider that the CTPA result may be a false positive *(72)*.

Clinical Probability and Qualitative D-Dimer Testing

I recommend that physicians use our clinical model to categorize patients' pretest probabilities as low, moderate, or high. Alternatively, our model can also be used to score patients as "PE-likely" or "PE-unlikely." When patients are clinically classified as having low probability for PE, the SimpliRED, IL test, or another qualitative D-dimer test can be performed next, and a negative result will rule out PE. Because the negative likelihood ratio with the IL test and SimpliRED is approx 0.20, the patient's pretest probability of PE must be less than 10% to rule out PE with a negative D-dimer. For example, if the pretest probability is 5% or less, the posttest probability will be approx 1%; and if the pretest probability is 10%, the posttest probability will be just over 2% *(72)*.

Patients who are PE-unlikely based on the clinical model but have a positive D-dimer test, and those who are PE-likely on clinical grounds, should undergo V/Q scans or CTPA as outlined in Figs. 1–3. Bilateral deep vein ultrasound may be performed in PE-likely patients if the V/Q scan is nondiagnostic or the CTPA is normal (Fig. 3). On the other hand, high-probability V/Q scans or positive results on CT should be considered diagnostic of PE (Fig. 3), unless the pretest clinical probability is low (Figs. 1 and 2). In this latter case, the results should be reviewed with the radiologist to exclude a false-positive result. Confirmatory venous ultrasound or conventional pulmonary angiography may also have to be performed because, given the relatively high false-positive rate of imaging tests in the

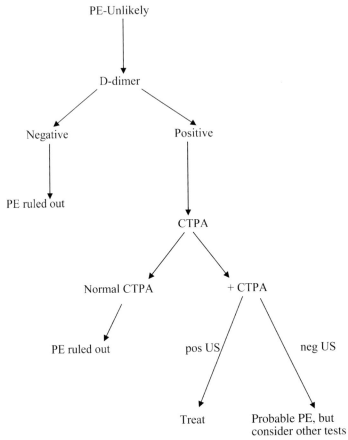

Fig. 2. Strategy for diagnosis of pulmonary embolism (PE) using computerized tomographic pulmonary angiography in patients who are PE-unlikely.

low-probability population, many of these patients could be subjected to unnecessary oral anticoagulation therapy with risk of major hemorrhage. Other possible consequences of unnecessary anticoagulation due to a false-positive imaging test may include increased expenditure on health and life insurance, lifestyle changes, and even psychological effects, but none of these have been quantified.

In general, negative D-dimer and negative imaging results in moderate- and perhaps high-probability patients negate the need for either serial ultrasound testing or angiography (Fig. 3). This strategy should result in less than 1% of patients with "excluded" PE experiencing venous thromboembolic events during 3-mo follow-up.

Clinical Probability and Quantitative (ELISA) D-Dimer Testing

The proposed algorithms may be slightly different if ELISA D-dimer assays are used instead of qualitative tests. Thus, if the VIDAS D-dimer is used in patients who have low or moderate probability of PE, are PE-unlikely by our model (Table 1), or have low or moderate probability by the Wicki clinical model (Table 2), the physician can avoid the need for diagnostic imaging when the D-dimer is negative. The likelihood ratio of 0.06 with the VIDAS test implies that even if these patients can have a pretest probability of 22%, a negative D-dimer will still negate the need for diagnostic imaging. As mentioned,

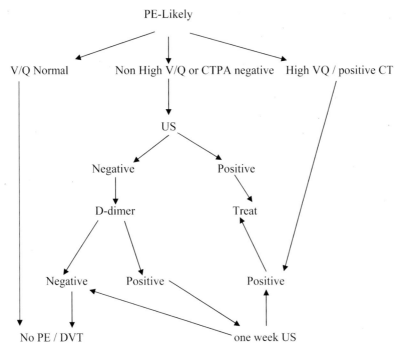

Fig. 3. Strategy for diagnosis of pulmonary embolism (PE) using computerized tomographic pulmonary angiography or ventilation-perfusion in patients who are PE-likely.

the VIDAS is limited by its very low specificity in the elderly and hospitalized patients, and thus imaging tests would often be required in these groups. Although Perrier et al. have suggested that a negative VIDAS D-dimer may negate the need for diagnostic imaging irrespective of pretest probability, I personally am reluctant to adopt this strategy *(73,74)*.

Are Diagnostic Algorithms an Overkill?

It is possible that the use of diagnostic algorithms will increase the number of patients in whom a diagnosis of PE is considered, as, with implementation of an algorithm, physicians may "screen" patients for PE. Our recent study suggests this possibility, because PE was detected in only 8% of patients in whom the diagnosis was considered *(37)*. The increase in the number of patients considered for possible diagnosis of PE can increase the overall number of imaging tests performed. Goldstein et al. implemented a D-dimer-based screening system for hospitalized patients and found a 40% increase in the rate of V/Q scanning *(75)*. This may create the sense that algorithms will not improve efficiency, but I am convinced that algorithms do have a positive effect. It can be calculated, for example, that the implementation of the screening system makes it possible to definitely confirm the diagnosis of PE in more patients. In fact, in the study by Goldstein et al., although the D-dimer protocol led to an increase in the rate of V/Q scanning of inpatients, the percentage of V/Q scans that were ultimately read as positive for PE actually increased. Furthermore, the number of patients in whom PE was diagnosed almost doubled in the centers using a D-dimer algorithm. Additionally, at hospitals in which pulmonary vascular imaging is not available at night, algorithms may offer a rational method to decide which patients should receive temporary anticoagulation until pulmonary vascular imaging is available. Emergency physicians faced with a requirement to understand so many diseases welcome protocols that safely simplify care.

SUMMARY AND CONCLUSIONS

Recent advances in the management of patients with suspected PE have both improved diagnostic accuracy and made management algorithms safer and more accessible. Ongoing clinical trials are evaluating whether these diagnostic processes can be made even simpler and less expensive. Patients at low risk with a negative D-dimer can avoid imaging tests and those at moderate risk with a negative quantitative D-dimer can have the diagnosis excluded without the need for imaging tests. Diagnostic strategies should include pretest clinical probability, D-dimer assays and noninvasive imaging tests.

ACKNOWLEDGMENTS

Dr. Wells is the recipient of a Canada Research Chair in Thromboembolic Diseases.

REFERENCES

1. Schluger N, Henschke C, King T, et al. Diagnosis of pulmonary embolism at a large teaching hospital. J Thorac Imaging 1994;9:180–184.
2. Berghout A, Oudkerk M, Hicks SG, Teng TH, Pillay M, Buller HR. Active implementation of a con-senus strategy improves diagnosis and management in suspected pulmonary embolism. Q J Med 2000; 93:335–340.
3. Horlander KT, Mannino DM, Leeper KV. Pulmonary embolism mortality in the United States, 1979–1998. An analysis using multiple-cause mortality data. Arch Intern Med 2003;163:1711–1717.
4. Stein PD, Athanasoulis C, Alavi A, et al. Complications and validity of pulmonary angiography in acute pulmonary embolism. Circulation 1992;85:462–468.
5. PIOPED Investigators. Value of the ventilation/perfusion scan in acute pulmonary embolism. Results of the prospective investigation of pulmonary embolism diagnosis (PIOPED). JAMA 1990;263:2753–2759.
6. Henry JW, Relyea B, Stein PD. Continuing risk of thromboemboli among patients with normal pulmo-nary angiograms. Chest 1995;107:1375–1378.
7. Hull RD, Hirsh J, Carter CJ, et al. Pulmonary angiography, ventilation lung scanning, and venography for clinically suspected pulmonary embolism with abnormal perfusion lung scan. Ann Intern Med 1983; 98:891–899.
8. Remy-Jardin M, Remy J, Artraud D, Fribourg M, Beregi JP. Spiral CT of pulmonary embolism: diag-nostic approach, interpretive pitfalls and current indications. Eur Radiol 1998;8:1376–1390.
9. Rathbun SW, Raskob G, Whitsett TL. Sensitivity and specificity of helical computed tomography in the diagnosis of pulmonary embolism: a systematic review. Ann Intern Med 2000;132:227–232.
10. Forgie MA, Wells PS, Wells G, Millward S. A systematic review of the accuracy of helical CT in the diagnosis of acute pulmonary embolism. Blood 1997;90:3223.
11. Hayashino Y, Goto M, Noguchi Y, Fukui T. Ventilation-perfusion scanning and helical CT in suspected pulmonary embolism: meta-analysis of diagnostic performance. Radiology 2005;234:740–748.
12. Perrier A, Roy PM, Sanchez O, et al. Multidetector-row computed tomography in suspected pulmonary embolism. N Engl J Med 2005;352:1760–1768.
13. Mayo JR, Remy-Jardin M, Muller NL, et al. Pulmonary embolism: prospective comparison of spiral CT with ventilation-perfusion scintigraphy. Radiology 1997;205:447–452.
14. Shah AA, Davis SD, Gamsu G, Intriere L. Parenchymal and pleural findings in patients with and patients without acute pulmonary embolism detected at spiral CT. Radiology 1999;211:147–153.
15. Stein PD, Saltzman HA, Weg JG. Clinical characteristics of patients with acute pulmonary embolism. Am J Cardiol 1991;68:1723–1724.
16. Stein PD, Terrin ML, Hales CA, et al. Clinical, laboratory, roentgenographic, and electrocardiographic findings in patients with acute pulmonary embolism and no pre-existing cardiac or pulmonary disease. Chest 1991;100:598–603.

17. Susec O, Boudrow D, Kline JA. The clinical features of acute pulmonary embolism in ambulatory patients. Acad Emerg Med 1997;4:891–897.
18. Manganelli D, Palla A, Donnamaria V, Giuntini C. Clinical features of pulmonary embolism. Doubts and certainties. Chest 1996;107(1 Suppl):25S–32S.
19. Anderson FA Jr, Wheeler HB, Goldberg RJ, et al. A population-based perspective of the hospital incidence and case-fatality rates of deep vein thrombosis and pulmonary embolism. The Worcester study. Arch Intern Med 1991;151:933–938.
20. Anderson FA Jr, Wheeler HB. Venous thromboembolism. Risk factors and prophylaxis. Clin Chest Med 1995;16:235–251.
21. Anderson FA Jr, Wheeler HB. Physician practices in the management of venous thromboembolism: a community-wide survey. J Vasc Surg 1992;15:707–714.
22. Wells PS, Ginsberg JS, Anderson DR, et al. Use of a clinical model for safe management of patients with suspected pulmonary embolism. Ann Intern Med 1998;129:997–1005.
23. Hull RD, Raskob G, Carter CJ, et al. Pulmonary embolism in outpatients with pleuritic chest pain. Arch Intern Med 1988;148:838–844.
24. Stein PD, Dalen JE, McIntyre KM, Sasahara AA, Wenger NK, Willis PW III. The electrocardiogram in acute pulmonary embolism. Prog Cardiovasc Dis 1975;17:247–257.
25. Ferrari E, Imbert A, Chevalier T, Mihoubi A, Morand P, Baudouy M. The ECG in pulmonary embolism. Predictive value of negative T waves in precordial leads—80 case reports. Chest 1997;111:537–543.
26. Rodger MA, Makropoulos D, Turek M, et al. Diagnostic value of the electrocardiogram in suspected pulmonary embolism. Am J Cardiol 2000;86:807–809.
27. McFarlane MJ, Imperiale TF. Use of the alveolar-arterial oxygen gradient in the diagnosis of pulmonary embolism. Am J Med 1994;96:57–62.
28. Stein PD, Goldhaber SZ, Henry JW. Alveolar-arterial oxygen gradient in the assessment of acute pulmonary embolism. Chest 1995;107:139–143.
29. Stein PD, Goldhaber SZ, Henry JW, Miller AC. Arterial blood gas analysis in the assessment of suspected acute pulmonary embolism. Chest 1996;109:78–81.
30. Rodger MA, Carrier MC, Jones GN, et al. Diagnostic value of arterial blood gas measurement in suspected pulmonary embolism. Am J Respir Crit Care Med 2000;162:2105–2108.
31. PIOPED Investigators. Value of the ventilation/perfusion scan in acute pulmonary embolism. Results of the prospective investigation of pulmonary embolism diagnosis (PIOPED). JAMA 1990;263:2753–2759.
32. Perrier A, Desmarais S, Miron MJ, et al. Non-invasive diagnosis of venous thromboembolism in outpatients. Lancet 1999;353:190–195.
33. Richardson WS. Where do pretest probabilities come from? ACP J Club 1999;4:68–69.
34. Jackson RE, Rudoni RR, Pascual R. Emergency physician assessment of the pretest probability of pulmonary embolism. Acad Emerg Med 1999;4:891–897.
35. Rosen MP, Sands DZ, Morris J, Drake W, Davis RB. Does a physician's ability to accurately assess the likelihood of pulmonary embolism increase with training? Acad Med 2000;75:1199–1205.
36. Sanson BJ, Lijmer JG, MacGillavry MRM, Turkstra F, Prins MH, Buller HR. Comparison of a clinical probability estimate and two clinical models in patients with suspected pulmonary embolism. Thromb Haemost 2000;83:199–203.
37. Wells PS, Anderson DR, Rodger MA, et al. Excluding pulmonary embolism at the bedside without diagnostic imaging: management of patients with suspected pulmonary embolism presenting to the emergency department by using a simple clinical model and D-dimer. Ann Intern Med 2001;135:98–107.
38. Wells PS, Anderson DR, Rodger MA, et al. Derivation of a simple clinical model to categorize patients probability of pulmonary embolism: increasing the models utility with the SimpliRED D-dimer. Thromb Haemost 2000;83:416–420.
39. Wolf SJ, McCubbin TR, Feldhaus KM, Faragher JP, Adcock DM. Prospective validation of Wells criteria in the evaluation of patients with suspected pulmonary embolism. Ann Emerg Med 2004;44:503–510.
40. Bosson JL, Barro C, Satger B, Carpentier PH, Polack B, Pernod G. Quantitative high D-dimer value is predictive of pulmonary embolism occurrence independently of clinical score in a well-defined low risk factor population. J Thromb Haemost 2005;3:93–99.
41. Miniati M, Prediletto R, Formichi B, et al. Accuracy of clinical assessment in the diagnosis of pulmonary embolism. Am J Respir Crit Care Med 1999;159:864–871.
42. Wicki J, Perneger TV, Junod AF, Bounameaux H, Perrier A. Assessing clinical probability of pulmonary embolism in the emergency ward: a simple score. Arch Intern Med 2001;161:92–97.

43. Wicki J, Perrier A, Perneger TV, Bounameaux H, Junod AF. Predicting adverse outcome in patients with acute pulmonary embolism: a risk score. Thromb Haemost 2000;84:548–552

44. Chagnon I, Bounameaux H, Aujesky D, et al. Comparison of two clinical prediction rules and implicit assessment among patients with suspected pulmonary embolism. Am J Med 2002;113:269–275.

45. Kline JA, Webb WB, Jones AE, Hernandez-Nino J. Impact of a rapid rule-out protocol for pulmonary embolism on the rate of screening, missed cases, and pulmonary vascular imaging in an urban US emergency department. Ann Emerg Med 2004;44:490–502.

46. Kline JA, Mitchell AM, Kabrhel C, Richman PB, Courtney DM. Clinical criteria to prevent unnecessary diagnostic testing in emergency department patients with suspected pulmonary embolism. J Thromb Haemost 2004;2:1247–1255.

47. Hyers TM. Venous thromboembolism. Am J Respir Crit Care Med 1999;159:1–14.

48. Musset D, Parent F, Meyer G, et al. Diagnostic strategy for patients with suspected pulmonary embolism: a prospective multicentre outcome study. Lancet 2002;360:1914–1920.

49. Bosson JL, Barro C, Satger B, Carpentier PH, Polack B, Pernod G. Quantitative high D-dimer value is predictive of pulmonary embolism occurrence independently of clinical score in a well-defined low risk factor population. J Thromb Haemost 2005;3:93–99.

50. Bosson JL, Labarere J, Sevestre MA, et al. Deep vein thrombosis in elderly patients hospitalized in subacute care facilities. A multicenter cross-sectional study of risk factors, prophylaxis and prevalence. Arch Intern Med 2003;163:2613–2618.

51. Righini M, Goehring C, Bounameaux H, Perrier A. Effects of age on the performance of common diagnostic tests for pulmonary embolism. Am J Med 2000;109:357–361.

52. Kovacs MJ, MacKinnon KM, Anderson DR, et al. A comparison of three rapid D-dimer methods for the diagnosis of venous thromboembolism. Br J Haematol 2001;115:140–144.

53. Stein PD, Hull RD, Patel KC, et al. D-Dimer for the exclusion of acute venous thrombosis and pulmonary embolism. A systematic review. Ann Intern Med 2004;140:589–602.

54. Perzanowski C, Dellweg D, Eiger G. Limited use of the SimpliRED assay in confirming pulmonary embolism. Thromb Haemost 2004;91:633–635.

55. Meyer G, Fischer AM, Collignon MA, et al. Diagnostic value of two rapid and individual D-dimer assays in patients with clinically suspected pulmonary embolism: comparison with microplate enzyme-linked immunosorbent assay. Blood Coagul Fibrinolysis 1998;9:603–608.

56. de Monye W, Huisman MV, Pattynama PMT. Observer dependency of the Simplired D-Dimer assay in 81 consecutive patients with suspected pulmonary embolism. Thromb Res 1999;96:293–298.

57. Turkstra F, van Beek EJR, Buller HR. Observer and biological variation of a rapid whole blood d-dimer test. Thromb Haemost 1998;79:1–3.

58. Kraaijenhagen RA, Lijmer JG, Bossuyt PMM, Prins MH, Heisterkamp SH, Buller HR. The accuracy of D-dimer in the diagnosis of venous thromboembolism : a meta-analysis. In: Kraaijenhagen RA, ed. *The Etiology, Diagnosis and Treatment of Venous Thromboembolism.* Repro Deventer, Deventer, The Netherlands; 2000, pp. 159–183.

59. Heim SW, Schectman JM, Siadaty MS, Philbrick JT. D-dimer testing for deep venous thrombosis: a metaanalysis. Clin Chem 2004;50:1136–1147.

60. Henry JW, Relyea B, Stein PD. Continuing risk of thromboemboli among patients with normal pulmonary angiograms. Chest 1995;107:1375–1378.

61. Hull RD, Raskob GE, Coates G, Panju AA. Clinical validity of a normal perfusion lung scan on patients with suspected pulmonary embolism. Chest 1990;97:23–26.

62. van Beek EJ, Kuyer PMM, Schenk BE, Brandjes DPM, ten Cate JW, Buller HR. A normal perfusion lung scan in patients with clinically suspected pulmonary embolism: frequency and clinical validity. Chest 1995;108:170–173.

63. Kipper MS, Moser KM, Kortman KE, Ashburn WL. Longterm follow-up of patients with suspected pulmonary embolism and a normal lung scan. Perfusion scans in embolic suspects. Chest 1982;82:411–415.

64. Gosselin MV, Rubin GD, Leung AN, Huang J, Rizk NW. Unsuspected pulmonary embolism: prospective detection on routine helical CT scans. Radiology 1998;208:209–215.

65. Storto ML, Di Credico A, Guido F, Larici AR, Bonomo L. Incidental detection of pulmonary emboli on routine MDCT of the chest. AJR Am J Roentgenol 2005;184:264–267.

66. Anderson DR, Kovacs MJ, Dennie C, et al. Use of spiral computerized tomography contrast angiography and ultrasonography to exclude the diagnosis of pulmonary embolism in the emergency department. (Accepted for publication J Emerg Med 2005;29:399–404.)

67. Moores LK, Jackson WL Jr, Shorr AF, Jackson JL. Meta-analysis: outcomes in patients with suspected pulmonary embolism managed with computed tomographic pulmonary angiography. Ann Intern Med 2004;141:866–874.
68. Rathbun SW, Raskob G, Whitsett TL. Sensitivity and specificity of helical computed tomography in the diagnosis of pulmonary embolism: a systematic review. Ann Intern Med 2000;132:227–232.
69. Worsley DF, Alavi A. Comprehensive analysis of the results of the PIOPED study. Prospective Investigation of Pulmonary Embolism Diagnosis Study. J Nucl Med 1995;36:2380–2387.
70. Mullins MD, Becker DM, Hagspiel KD, Philbrick JT. The role of spiral volumetric computed tomography in the diagnosis of pulmonary embolism. Arch Intern Med 2000;160:293–298.
71. Cohen J. *Statistical Power Analysis for the Behavioural Sciences, 2nd ed.* Lawrence Erlbaum Associates: Hillsdale; 1988.
72. Bayes T. An essay towards solving a problem in the doctrine of chances. Philos Trans R Soc Lon 1763; 53:370–418.
73. Perrier A, Roy P-M, Aujesky D, et al. Diagnosing pulmonary embolism in outpatients with clinical assessment, D-Dimer measurement, venous ultrasound, and helical computed tomography: a multicenter management study. Am J Med 2004;116:291–299.
74. Perrier A, Desmarais S, Miron MJ, et al. Non-invasive diagnosis of venous thromboembolism in outpatients. Lancet 1999;353:190–195.
75. Goldstein NM, Kollef MH, Ward S, Gage BF. The impact of the introduction of a rapid D-dimer assay on the diagnostic evaluation of suspected pulmonary embolism. Arch Intern Med 2001;161:567–571.

2 Imaging of Acute Pulmonary Embolism

James G. Ravenel, MD
and U. Joseph Schoepf, MD

CONTENTS

SUMMARY

The past decade has seen a shift in the imaging paradigm for acute pulmonary embolism (PE) from a combination of clinical acumen, ventilation-perfusion scintigraphy, and conventional pulmonary angiography to computed tomographic pulmonary angiography (CTPA). The ability to perform CT rapidly with direct visualization of thrombi allows for rapid and reliable diagnosis or exclusion of PE in the vast majority of cases. In the same setting, CT can provide information on right heart function, offer an evaluation of the deep venous system through indirect CT venography, as well as allow for the detection of alternative diagnoses that may account for the patient's symptoms. Published experience with CTPA has established that a negative result reliably excludes clinically significant PE in more than 98% of cases. As a result, CT has become the preferred first-line imaging test in the evaluation of suspected acute PE.

Key Words: Computed tomography; pulmonary angiography; ventilation-perfusion scintigraphy.

INTRODUCTION

Acute pulmonary embolism (PE) is a relatively common event with a wide spectrum of clinical presentations that range from small asymptomatic and incidentally detected

From: *Contemporary Cardiology: Management of Acute Pulmonary Embolism*
Edited by: S. Konstantinides © Humana Press Inc., Totowa, NJ

subsegmental PE to life-threatening central PE causing hypotension, myocardial infarction, and cardiogenic shock. The overall incidence has been estimated at approx 1 per 1000 population in the United States *(1)*, and 3-mo mortality may be higher than 15% *(2)*. Thus, because of the relatively high mortality of PE and the treatable nature of the disease, the diagnosis is often sought in the evaluation of acute dyspnea and hypoxia. Imaging studies remain a critical step for establishing the diagnosis.

CHEST X-RAY

The chest radiograph is rarely, if ever, diagnostic of PE, and thus the main role of chest radiography is to identify important alternative diagnoses such as congestive heart failure and pneumonia. In the latter case, the diagnosis of PE can be dismissed early and the need for further, advanced imaging studies may be obviated. On the other hand, chest radiographs may aid in triaging patients suspected of having PE to the next imaging test. For instance, if the chest radiograph is normal, there is a high likelihood of a diagnostic result from ventilation-perfusion (V/Q) scintigraphy. If, however, the chest radiographs are abnormal, V/Q scanning is likely to be nondiagnostic and cross-sectional imaging, particularly computed tomographic pulmonary angiography (CTPA), would be the preferred strategy. This is of particular value when weighing the risks and benefits of performing these tests, particularly in consideration of radiation dose and intravenous contrast.

In the setting of acute PE, chest radiographs are often normal or show minor abnormalities such as subsegmental atelectasis and small pleural effusion *(3)*. The presence of segmental or lobar atelectasis as well as large pleural effusion should suggest a diagnosis other than PE, although, unfortunately, the two coexist on occasion. Pulmonary infarcts are uncommonly visualized on chest radiographs (Fig. 1), but, when present, are seen as wedge shaped air-space opacities typically located at the costophrenic sulci (also known as Hampton's hump). With extensive PEs and large central clots, regional hypoperfusion may be evident as areas of decreased lung attenuation with an associated paucity of vascular markings (Westermark's sign).

IMAGING THE DEEP VENOUS SYSTEM

This diagnostic test is discussed in more detail in the following chapter (Chapter 3). Because duplex venous ultrasound is a relatively easy study to perform and interpret, some authors have advocated bilateral lower extremity studies early in the algorithm for the work-up of PE. The rationale is that deep venous thrombosis (DVT) and PE are treated in essentially the same manner and that a positive result would thus obviate the need for further imaging. As explained in Chapter 7, this may indeed be a reasonable consideration in many patients suspected of having PE. It should be noted, however, as a limitation of this strategy, that failure to diagnose PE in the setting of venous thromboembolism may result in incorrect (over)diagnosis of PE recurrence during follow-up, particularly with the use of V/Q scintigraphy *(4,5)*.

V/Q SCINTIGRAPHY
Validation

Prior to widespread usage of CT, V/Q scintigraphy was the test of choice to screen for PE. The most recent source of knowledge comes from the Prospective Investigation of Pulmonary Embolism Diagnosis (PIOPED), a large multi-institutional study to deter-

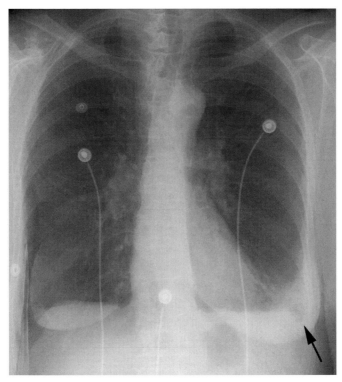

Fig. 1. Pulmonary infarct. Frontal chest radiograph reveals wedge-shaped area of air-space disease in left costophrenic sulcus (arrow), also known as Hampton's Hump.

mine the utility of V/Q scintigraphy with conventional angiography as the reference standard *(6)*. Rather than the traditional interpretation of the test as "positive" or "negative," the results of the study were used to stratify the chance of PE based on the scintigraphic pattern (Table 1). As the intent of the study was to promote V/Q scintigraphy as a screening test, the results were presented to maximize sensitivity. In order to accomplish this task, however, all but the normal scans had to be grouped together as an abnormal result, raising the sensitivity to 98% *(6)*. Unfortunately, this also resulted in a very low specificity of 10% *(6)*. Based on the results of this study as well as the prior work by Hull *(7,8)*, venous ultrasound followed by conventional angiography and/or venography (if the ultrasound was negative) was recommended to follow all but normal lung scans *(9)*.

Using clinical suspicion as a guide (*see* Chapter 1), the accuracy of V/Q scintigraphy can be improved. For instance, combining a clinical probability of less than 20% with a low-probability scan indicated a mere 4% likelihood of PE *(6)*. Further refinements of the data were also used to modify low-probability studies *(10)* and then create a "very low-probability" category with the risk of PE being less than 10% *(11,12)*. It should be noted, however, that current evidence supports withholding anticoagulation only in the setting of a normal V/Q scan *and* negative DVT evaluation *(6,13)*.

Despite the available data and recommendations, it is clear that the results of V/Q scintigraphy are frequently misapplied *(14–16)*. Interpreting physicians may use their own "gestalt" approach rather than following the established criteria *(17)*. Patients with low or intermediate probability studies often do not undergo further testing despite the published recommendations *(15,16)*, perhaps owing to a lack of understanding of V/Q scintigraphy's

Table 1
Modified PIOPED Criteria for Pulmonary Embolism (PE) *(10)*

Category	% Posttest probability of PE
Normal	<2
– No perfusion abnormalities	
Very low probability *(11)*	<10
– Nonsegmental perfusion defect	
– Perfusion defect smaller than chest X-ray finding	
– Stripe sign	
– Triple match mid/upper lung	
– Less than three small segmental defects	
Low probability	<15
– Multiple matched defects	
– Defect with larger chest X-ray abnormality	
– Less than three small segmental defects	
– Nonsegmental defects	
Intermediate probability	~33
– One moderate or less than two large defects	
– Corresponding lower lung zone defect and chest X-ray abnormality	
– Ventilation-perfusion defects and small effusion	
– Difficult to categorize as high or low probability	
High probability	>85
– Two large segmental perfusion defects without ventilation or chest X-ray abnormality	
– One large and two moderate perfusion defects	
– Four moderate perfusion defects	

role as a screening rather than a diagnostic test. Based on the rapid advances of CT technology and the limitations of V/Q scintigraphy, utilization of this test is decreasing *(18)*.

Interpretation

Besides the published PIOPED criteria (*see* Table 1), other criteria proposed earlier by McNiel *(19)*, Biello *(20)*, and Hull *(8)* can be used to assess the probability of PE. Although these sets of criteria have (subtle) differences, none is clearly superior to the rest *(21)*. Moreover, despite the wealth of information, interpretation remains a subjective process in clinical practice and, at the end of the analysis, the category (probability of PE) may be assigned on a "gut feeling" rather than objective use of fixed criteria. This leads to intraobserver variations that may not disappear even with fixed training *(22,23)*. It appears that the Hull criteria have the least intraobserver variability when compared with the PIOPED criteria or the gestalt approach *(17)*. Despite conventional wisdom, it does not appear that the presence of underlying disease or critical illness affects the overall reliability of V/Q scintigraphy *(24,25)*.

The rationale of V/Q scintigraphy lies in the fact that portions of lung subtended by a vessel will remain ventilated when perfusion is interrupted by an embolus, resulting in V/Q mismatch. This appears as a wedge-shaped defect in the perfusion scan with normal ventilation. The probability is then based on the size and number of mismatched segments and subsegments (Fig. 2). In the presence of underlying lung disease or disordered ventilation, interpretation can be more difficult. A matched segment may occur as a result

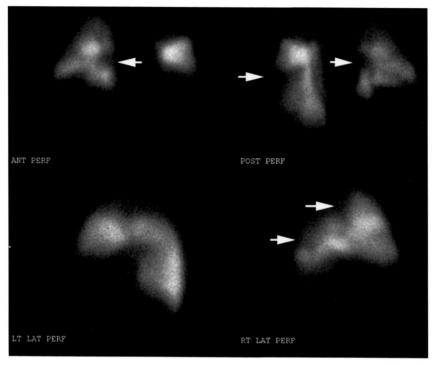

Fig. 2. Acute pulmonary embolism. Perfusion scan reveals multiple wedge-shaped perfusion defects (arrows). High-probability scan in setting of normal ventilation.

of shunting of blood flow away from nonventilated segments, embolic disease to poorly ventilated lung tissue, or pulmonary infarction. When a triple match (abnormal chest radiograph, ventilation, and perfusion in the same region) occurs in the upper lobe, it is generally considered to be due to shunting of blood, whereas a triple match occuring in the lower lobe may be due to pulmonary infarction.

CONVENTIONAL PULMONARY ANGIOGRAPHY

Validation

The technique of conventional angiography dates back to the 1950s. It gained increasing popularity over the next two decades and was validated by negative outcome studies. Still, the early data were somewhat limited and did not necessarily reflect today's imaging patterns. In the largest original cohort of 247 patients (imaged over a 6-yr period), the rate of definitive diagnosis, positive or negative, was 74% and subsequent development of PE was not reported (26). In the PIOPED study, the rate of subsequent PE after 1 yr of follow-up was 1.6% for 380 negative angiograms (27). When the results of the PIOPED trial and the three other outcome trials performed at that time are analyzed together, 15/733 (2.0%) subjects had subsequent PE after a negative pulmonary angiogram (7,27–29). Primarily based on these studies and the lack of other imaging options, catheter pulmonary angiography was regarded as gold standard for imaging PE.

Although relatively invasive compared to other imaging modalities (30,31), catheter angiography is a rather safe procedure. Major complications including hematoma, renal failure, respiratory distress, and death occur in less than 1% of the patients, and the death

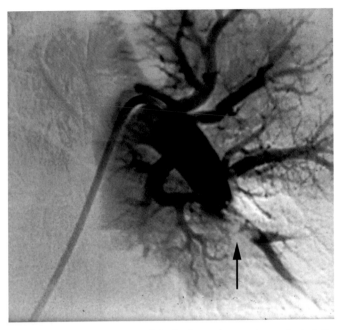

Fig. 3. Acute pulmonary embolism. Selective digital subtraction angiography in left pulmonary artery reveals segmental branch filling defect (arrow) diagnostic of pulmonary embolism.

rate across several studies was less than 0.5% *(30)*. Despite the safety record, many physicians are reluctant to order this study, particularly in patients in whom thrombolytic treatment is either planned or already being administered.

Although negative outcome studies establish the safety of withholding anticoagulation in a negative study, they cannot *per se* establish accuracy. Attempts to determine the reproducibility of conventional angiogram interpretations amongst different observers has met with mixed success. In the PIOPED study, observer agreement overall was 81% (98% for lobar, 90% for segmental, and 66% for subsegmental embolus), and the agreement on negative results became significantly less as the quality of the study decreased *(30)*. Clearly, interobserver variability at the subsegmental level is a significant problem ranging from 40–66% for two observers *(30,32–34)*. Given that the use of catheter angiography is in decline *(35,36)*, the overall reliability in the hands of relatively inexperienced angiographers may be significant and should be considered a major limitation at this time.

Interpretation

Four basic patterns of abnormality have been described: (1) intraluminal filling defects; (2) vascular cut-offs; (3) regional oligemia; and (4) asymmetric flow *(26,37)*. The first two are considered to be the most specific findings of PE. Intraluminal filling defects usually result from incomplete occlusion of a vessel and can sometimes be difficult to detect because of flow around the thrombus. Vascular cut-offs result from complete occlusion and are also difficult to detect in peripheral vessels (Fig. 3). Generally, the lack of perfusion distal to a vascular cut-off is considered secondary evidence of thrombus. Other pathophysiologic factors may lead to regional oligemia and flow asymmetry, and thus detection of such abnormalities requires a careful search for definitive signs of emboli. By themselves, oligemia and flow asymmetry are rather nonspecific findings.

MAGNETIC RESONANCE IMAGING

MRI may become a valid tool to evaluate patients with suspected PE and absolute or relative contraindications to computed tomography (CT) such as renal failure or pregnancy. Unfortunately, there are few well designed clinical trials of MRI. A recent meta-analysis found that only 3 of 28 studies performed met stringent criteria for the evaluation of a diagnostic imaging technique *(38)*. This study also revealed that gadolinium-based MRI has good diagnostic sensitivity (77–87%) and specificity (95–98%) *(39–41)*. The major disadvantages are long examination times, the need for a relatively long breath hold (a crucial problem in patients with acute PE), and the inappropriateness of the method for imaging critically ill patients. However, as technology advances and breath-hold techniques are refined, MRI is likely to emerge as a viable alternative for patients with contraindications to contrast-enhanced CT. An example of this is magnetic resonance angiography using gradient-recalled echo techniques with sensitivity encoding. In a preliminary study *(42)*, the breath hold for this technique was approx 36 s with a per-patient sensitivity and specificity of 92 and 94%, respectively, when compared to conventional angiography. Although sensitivity dropped to 70% in peripheral lung zones, the results overall compared favorably to multidetector CT.

COMPUTED TOMOGRAPHY

With rapid improvements in technology, the current generation of multidetector CT scanners allows an acquisition of the entire thorax with submillimeter resolution within a comfortable breath hold of less than 10 s *(43)*. Improvements in temporal resolution with rotation times of 0.5 s and less reduce the number of nondiagnostic CT scans, particularly in patients with underlying lung disease *(44)*. Although 1.0- to 1.25-mm slice thickness may not be necessary to detect large PE, it clearly provides a better depiction of subsegmental vessels and improves interobserver agreement *(45,46)*.

To obtain a diagnostic study, a rapid contrast bolus (3–5 ccs per second) and accurate bolus tracking are critical. A secure intravenous catheter is necessary, preferably 18–20 gauge in the antecubital fossa. A saline chaser helps to reduce artifacts from dense contrast in the superior vena cava, but is not universally available at this time.

Validation

CT has become the method of choice for imaging PE in clinical routine in most institutions. Although meta-analyses have suggested that CT has not been adequately evaluated compared to the "gold" standard *(47–49)*, these reports focused on only earlier studies. The most recent comparison of four-row multidetector CT (MDCT) and digital subtraction angiography showed 100% sensitivity and 89% specificity for CT with three "false-positives", which were, however, considered as true-positive CT and false-negative conventional angiography at review *(50)*. Direct comparison of CT to conventional angiography may not be appropriate for other reasons as well. The interobserver reproducibility for a confident diagnosis of PE with MDCT exceeds the correlation with selective pulmonary angiography *(34,46,51)*. Because of the reluctance to perform routine conventional angiography, and perhaps as important, a declining experience in the interpretation of conventional pulmonary angiograms, the validity of conventional angiography as a diagnostic standard is no longer certain. PIOPED II, a large multicenter study to assess the accuracy of CT, used a composite diagnostic standard rather than performing

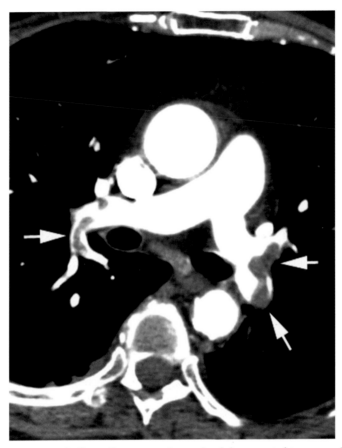

Fig. 4. Acute pulmonary embolism. Contrast-enhanced axial computed tomography reveals low-attenuation emboli in the right and left pulmonary arteries (arrows).

conventional angiography in all cases *(52)*. The preferable means for validation of CT is therefore the performance of negative outcome studies, the same scientific investigations used to establish conventional angiography as the reference standard.

Negative predictive value of CT has consistently been shown to surpass 96% both with single detector *(53–59)* and multidetector techniques *(60–68)*. Underlying lung disease *(59)*, inpatient status *(54)*, and results of V/Q scan *(56,58)* did not appear to have appreciable effects on the negative predictive value. Thus, if the CT study is interpreted as negative for PE with acceptable image quality, anticoagulation can possibly be safely withheld without adversely affecting patient outcome *(see also* Chapter 7). It should be noted in this regard that CT has undergone much more rigorous evaluation in far greater numbers of patients than conventional angiography to be established as the "gold" standard in the diagnosis of PE *(69)*.

Interpretation

The diagnosis of PE is usually straightforward, relying on the direct observation of a central filling defect surrounded by a rim of contrast in a pulmonary artery (Figs. 4 and 5). Often emboli lodge at bifurcation points and continue into both branch vessels. A sharp vessel cut-off or absence of vessel filling also provides evidence of PE, but may be more

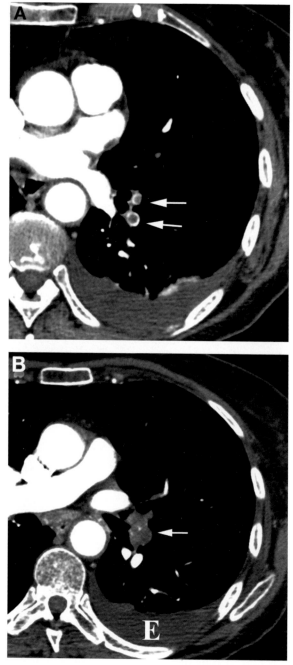

Fig. 5. Appearances of acute pulmonary embolism on computed tomography. (**A**) Filling defect surrounded by rim of contrast (arrows). (**B**) Complete vascular cut-off (arrow) with absent distal flow. Note also left pleural effusion (**E**).

difficult to perceive. Vessels that run parallel to the axial plane, particularly right middle lobe and lingular branches, are often better evaluated with coronal, sagittal, or off-axis oblique reformations, which can be performed rapidly at a number of advanced viewing work stations (Figs. 6–8). Reformations allow these vessels to be viewed in cross-section

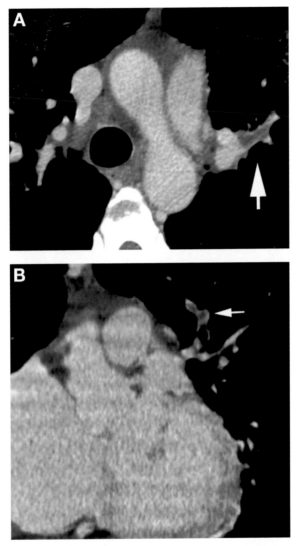

Fig. 6. Value of reformatted images. (**A**) Axial image reveals apparent filling defect in anterior segmental branch of left upper lobe (arrow). Appearance can be mistaken for volume averaging with adjacent structures. (**B**) Oblique coronal reformatted image reveals typical appearance of filling defect surrounded by rim of contrast (arrow).

similar to upper and lower lobe vessels and increase diagnostic confidence, as well as reduce false-positive studies due to artifacts *(70)*.

Secondary findings may also be present to suggest the diagnosis. Infarcts present as peripheral wedge-shaped areas of ground-glass opacity or consolidation (Fig. 9), and in one study occurred in 25% of cases with PE *(71)*. Localized oligemia (Fig. 10) may also be seen (CT Westermarks's sign), although in most cases the embolus causing hypoperfusion is easily identifiable. Nonspecific abnormalities such as subsegmental atelectasis and small pleural effusions are often encountered both in patients with and without PE. Often, these findings are helpful in alerting the study interpreter to carefully evaluate the relevant vascular supply. A clear benefit of CT is the depiction of alternative diagnoses not otherwise suspected when PE is absent *(71,72)*.

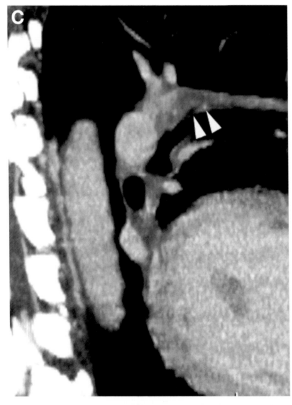

Fig. 6. (C) Oblique sagittal reformatted image defines extent of embolus within the vessel (arrowheads).

Pitfalls and Artifacts

Difficulties in interpreting CT images may be the result of problems with contrast enhancement, image reconstruction, and patient cooperation. Although usually not a problem in clinical practice, dense opacification of the superior vena cava can occasionally cause beam-hardening artifacts to obscure the pulmonary arteries in the medial right upper lobe. On the other hand, a poor bolus is a limitation often difficult to overcome, as contrast differences between an embolus and vessel lumen are difficult to detect. Occasionally, narrowing the window and level setting will allow for more confident interpretation, but in most cases either a repeat bolus of contrast or an alternative imaging technique should be performed.

Stair-step artifacts can mimic PE by simulating filling defects on axial images. They can usually be identified by alternating images of increased and decreased vascular attenuation and confirmed by bands of low and high attenuation on multiplanar reformations (Fig. 11).

Despite scan times approaching 5–10 s, dyspneic patients still may not be able to adequately suspend respiration. The motion from respiration can blur vessels making it impossible to detect emboli. Respiratory motion is best confirmed by viewing at lung window settings. Motion artifacts due to transmitted cardiac pulsation particularly affect the right middle lobe and the lingual and medial lower lobes. Electrocardiogram-gating of chest CT scans reduces artifacts caused by cardiac pulsation and improves the evaluation of adherent thoracic structures *(73,74)*; however, this technique also lengthens the breath

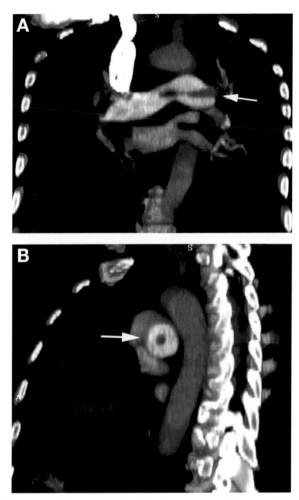

Fig. 7. Using three-dimensional images to define the extent of disease. **(A)** Coronal thick-slab volume rendered image reveals saddle embolus extending into both right and left pulmonary arteries (arrow). **(B)** Sagittal thick-slab volume rendered image allows for better analysis of the degree of occlusion by saddle embolus (arrow).

hold (potentially substituting breathing artifact for pulsation artifact) and increases the radiation dose.

Subsegmental Emboli

Subsegmental emboli are a vexing imaging and clinical problem (Fig. 12). One of the leading criticisms of CT is the inconsistent depiction of subsegmental vessels in earlier studies. This is a flawed argument, as V/Q scans would most likely be interpreted as low- or very low-probability in the setting of isolated subsegmental emboli. Such findings generally do not lead to further testing (75,76), and the interobserver variability of conventional angiography is also poor at the subsegmental level (30,34). Thus, there is no good standard for assessment of subsegmental emboli. Perhaps the greatest advantage of multidetector CT is the improved and more consistent visualization of subsegmental pulmonary arteries up to sixth and seventh order branches (77). At 1-mm collimation, optimal analysis of subsegmental vessels is possible and there is a higher detection rate of small

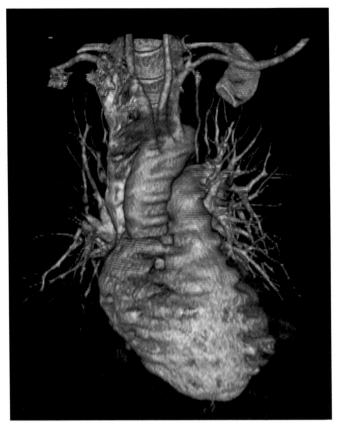

Fig. 8. Using three-dimensional images to define the extent of disease. Frontal projection of three-dimensional volume rendering reveals markedly diminished flow to right lung evidenced by asymmetry of pulmonary vessels.

emboli than with thicker collimation *(46,78)*. However, although there may be no doubt among the interpreting radiologists as to the absence or presence of small isolated emboli based on a good-quality MDCT scan, such findings may be difficult to "prove" in correlation studies.

It has also been suggested that CT may be too sensitive. In one study, 37% of subjects with a CT diagnosis of isolated subsegmental PE did not receive anticoagulation and had no adverse outcome *(79)*. It may be that, in the absence of DVT as indicated by compression ultrasound or indirect CT venography, patients with adequate cardiopulmonary reserve who are otherwise at low risk may not need treatment *(80)*. Unfortunately, there is no good evidence to suggest when it is safe or advantageous to withhold anticoagulation.

CT Assessment of Severity and Right Ventricular Dysfunction

Right heart failure remains a major cause of mortality in patients with acute PE *(81)*. Because of increased pulmonary vascular resistance and hypoxic vasoconstriction, the pressure in the right ventricle rises and, in massive PE, may result in dilation and hypokinesis of the right ventricular myocardium. Traditionally, echocardiography has been utilized to make this determination *(82)* (*see* Chapter 4). However, information about right ventricular dysfunction can also be gleaned from CT. In response to major PE, there is relative

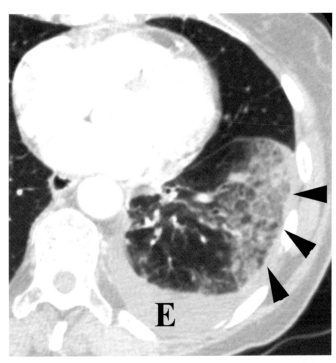

Fig. 9. Pulmonary infarct on computed tomography. Axial image reveals wedge-shaped area of mixed ground glass opacity and consolidation (arrowheads) with associated pleural effusion (**E**).

enlargement of the right ventricle compared to the left ventricle, although evidence suggests that this may be more a function of left ventricular collapse than right ventricular dilation *(83)*. Nonetheless, the right ventricular/left ventricular ratio (RV_D/LV_D) corre-lates relatively well with clinical severity, and a ratio greater than 1.5 appears to be suf-ficiently diagnostic of "massive" PE *(84,85)*. Indeed, in patients with a (RV_D/LV_D) greater than 0.9, significantly more adverse events were observed. Increases in RV_D/LV_D and bowing of the intraventricular septum (Fig. 13) to the left have been associated with the need for admission to an intensive care unit. The major limitation of CT in severity assess-ment, particularly compared to echocardiography, is the inability to obtain dynamic infor-mation including wall motion abnormalities and tricuspid valve regurgitation *(86)*.

A second means of assessing severity can be derived from the degree of vascular obstruction noted at CT. Scoring systems based on conventional angiography such as the Miller index *(87)* have been adapted for use in CT. The most commonly used system assigns a value of 0, 1, or 2 to each segmental artery indicating no obstruction, partial obstruction, or complete occlusion *(88)*. More proximal emboli are scored based on the total of segmental vessels in the affected vascular territory. This results in a maximum score of 40 and the degree of obstruction is presented as a percentage. An obstruction index of 40% or greater has been correlated with right ventricular dilation at echocardiography *(88)* and, in one small study, five of six subjects who died of PE had an obstruction index of greater than 60% *(89)*. Still, as evidenced by retrospective studies, there is clearly overlap between "severe" and "nonsevere" PE when relying on the obstruction index *(83)*. From a variety of studies, it appears that at an obstruction index threshold greater than 40% cor-relates with severity and need for aggressive therapy, but does not act as an independent

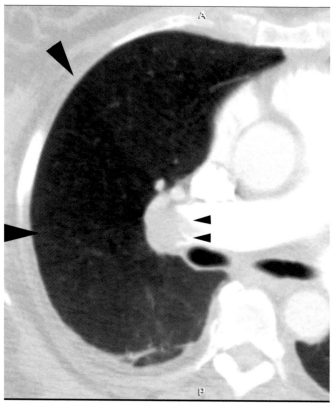

Fig. 10. Computed tomography Westermark sign. Thin-slab axial minimum intensity projection image reveals wedge-shaped region of hypoperfusion (large arrowheads) relative to normal parenchyma due to central pulmonary embolism (small arrowheads).

predictor of mortality *(83,86,90)*. In clinical practice, using this form of severity assessment is more cumbersome than RV_D/LV_D ratio.

RADIATION DOSE CONSIDERATIONS

The effective dose for the typical CT for PE ranges from 3–6 mSv and the absorbed dose in breast tissue is approx 21 mGy, depending on the tube current *(91)*. By way of comparison, screening mammography has an approximate breast dose of 2.5 mGy *(91)*. In the vast majority of cases, the risk-benefit ratio for imaging clearly favors performing the examination, two clinical scenarios warranting particular attention. In young women with normal chest radiographs, there is a high likelihood of a diagnostic V/Q scan and a lower breast-absorbed dose. In pregnant patients (*see* Chapter 17), because of the excretion of radiopharmaceutical via the urinary bladder, the absorbed radiation dose to the developing embryo is higher, 1–2 mGy, for V/Q scan vs 0.1–0.2 mGy for chest CT, and thus CT is favored *(92,93)*, although the radiation dosage in both imaging procedures is well below the fetal threshold of 50 mSv.

With V/Q scanning, radiation dose can be lowered in two ways. Under certain circumstances it is possible to perform the exam without ventilation images, e.g., in an otherwise healthy young patient with normal chest radiograph. Similarly, the radio-labeled macroaggregated albumin particles can be reduced to half for perfusion imaging. For CT, new

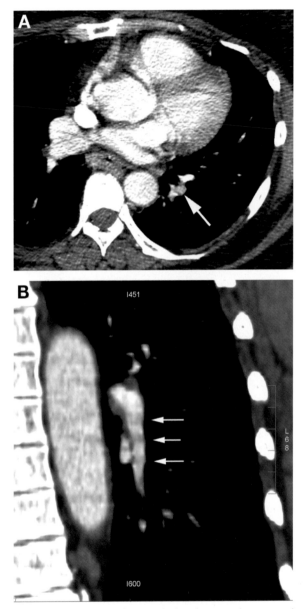

Fig. 11. Stair-step artifact. (**A**) Axial image shows relative decrease in attenuation in basilar segmental vessel (arrow), an appearance that may be mistaken for pulmonary embolism. (**B**) Coronal reformatted image reveals typical stair step appearance at multiple levels (arrows). Embolus would appear as extending along the long axis of the vessel.

techniques such as tube current modulation (available on all new multidetector scanners) as well as manually lowering tube current mA and tube rotation time will decrease radiation dose *(94)*. If these parameters are lowered too much, however, the result can be excessive quantum mottle and a nondiagnostic CT exam. Thus, CT exams require a careful balancing of dose and image quality. The specific effect of low-dose techniques on the detection of PE has not been scientifically evaluated to date.

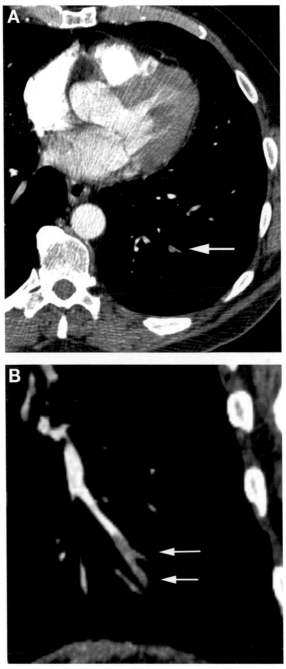

Fig. 12. Subsegmental embolus. (**A**) Axial image reveals tiny filling defect in small basilar pulmonary artery (arrow). (**B**) Oblique coronal reformatted image along vessels long axis confirms presence and documents extent of embolus (arrows).

COST-EFFECTIVE IMAGING

Because of the wide array of studies available for the diagnosis of PE, cost-efficacy analysis becomes a complex undertaking and depends on the sensitivity assigned to CT compared to the other competing strategies, and the pretest clinical probability. Several

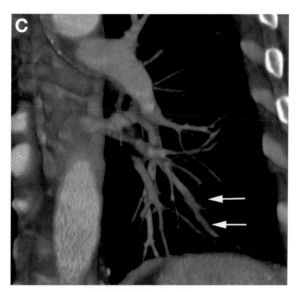

Fig. 12. (C) Coronal thick slab volume rendered image shows embolus (arrows) in relationship to adjacent normal arteries. The defect that would be produced at ventilation-perfusion scan would be expected to be read as very low probability for pulmonary embolism.

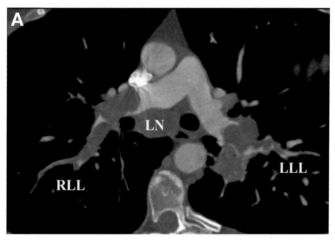

Fig. 13. Assessment of right ventricular dysfunction. **(A)** Curved reformatted image created to display main and lower lobe arteries reveals extensive emboli with extensive vascular occlusion. LN, subcarinal lymph node related to known primary lung malignancy.

analyses have been performed, based primarily on data from single-detector CT *(95–97)*. Assuming an 85% diagnostic sensitivity, CT strategies become more cost-effective than V/Q strategies *(95,96)*, although it should be emphasized that these strategies also require the use of ultrasound and D-dimer testing (*see* Chapter 7). Unfortunately, these analyses omit an important factor for the use of CT, i.e., the ability to rapidly indicate alternative diagnoses that would also favor CT over any one of the competing strategies *(98)*. When the clinical probability of DVT is high, strategies that include lower extremity ultrasound followed by CT appear to be the most efficacious use of imaging, with a cost-effectiveness ratio below $20,000 (US dollars) per life saved *(99)*. Whether indirect CT venog-

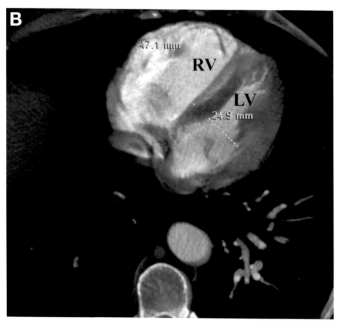

Fig. 13. (B) Axial image through heart reveals bowing of the interventricular septum to left and $RV_D/LV_D = 1.9$, both signs of right ventricular strain.

raphy in the setting of CT for PE will result in lower costs through the elimination of ultrasound studies is not clear.

CONCLUSION

Although many options remain for the diagnosis of PE, the preferred strategy is to use CT as a first-line diagnostic test in the vast majority of circumstances.

REFERENCES

1. Goldhaber SZ, Elliott CG. Acute pulmonary embolism: part I: epidemiology, pathophysiology, and diagnosis. Circulation 2003;108(22):2726–2729.
2. Carson JL, Kelley MA, Duff A, et al. The clinical course of pulmonary embolism. N Engl J Med 1992; 326(19):1240–1245.
3. Elliott CG, Goldhaber SZ, Visani L, DeRosa M. Chest radiographs in acute pulmonary embolism. Results from the International Cooperative Pulmonary Embolism Registry. Chest 2000;118(1):33–38.
4. Monreal M, Ruiz J, Fraile M, et al. Prospective study on the usefulness of lung scan in patients with deep vein thrombosis of the lower limbs. Thromb Haemost 2001;85(5):771–774.
5. Lopez-Beret P, Pinto JM, Romero A, Orgaz A, Fontcuberta J, Oblas M. Systematic study of occult pulmonary thromboembolism in patients with deep venous thrombosis. J Vasc Surg 2001;33(3):515–521.
6. Value of the ventilation/perfusion scan in acute pulmonary embolism. Results of the prospective investigation of pulmonary embolism diagnosis (PIOPED). The PIOPED Investigators. JAMA 1990;263(20): 2753–2759.
7. Hull RD, Hirsh J, Carter CJ, et al. Pulmonary angiography, ventilation lung scanning, and venography for clinically suspected pulmonary embolism with abnormal perfusion lung scan. Ann Intern Med 1983; 98(6):891–899.
8. Hull RD, Hirsh J, Carter CJ, et al. Diagnostic value of ventilation-perfusion lung scanning in patients with suspected pulmonary embolism. Chest 1985;88(6):819–828.
9. Bone RC. Ventilation/perfusion scan in pulmonary embolism. 'The Emperor is incompletely attired'. JAMA 1990;263(20):2794–2795.

10. Freitas JE, Sarosi MG, Nagle CC, Yeomans ME, Freitas AE, Juni JE. Modified PIOPED criteria used in clinical practice. J Nucl Med 1995;36(9):1573–1578.
11. Stein PD, Gottschalk A. Review of criteria appropriate for a very low probability of pulmonary embolism on ventilation-perfusion lung scans: a position paper. Radiographics 2000;20(1):99–105.
12. Stein PD, Relyea B, Gottschalk A. Evaluation of individual criteria for low probability interpretation of ventilation-perfusion lung scans. J Nucl Med 1996;37(4):577–581.
13. Hull RD, Raskob GE, Coates G, Panju AA. Clinical validity of a normal perfusion lung scan in patients with suspected pulmonary embolism. Chest 1990;97(1):23–26.
14. Chan WL, McLean R, Carolan MG. What happens after a lung scan? Management and outcome of patients in a regional hospital. Australas Radiol 2002;46(4):375–380.
15. Hull RD, Raskob GE. Low-probability lung scan findings: a need for change. Ann Intern Med 1991; 114(2):142–143.
16. Schluger N, Henschke C, King T, et al. Diagnosis of pulmonary embolism at a large teaching hospital. J Thorac Imaging 1994;9(3):180–184.
17. Hagen PJ, Hartmann IJ, Hoekstra OS, Stokkel MP, Postmus PE, Prins MH. Comparison of observer variability and accuracy of different criteria for lung scan interpretation. J Nucl Med 2003;44(5):739–744.
18. Stein PD, Kayali F, Olson RE. Trends in the use of diagnostic imaging in patients hospitalized with acute pulmonary embolism. Am J Cardiol 2004;93(10):1316–1317.
19. McNeil BJ. A diagnostic strategy using ventilation-perfusion studies in patients suspect for pulmonary embolism. J Nucl Med 1976;17(7):613–616.
20. Biello DR, Mattar AG, McKnight RC, Siegel BA. Ventilation-perfusion studies in suspected pulmonary embolism. AJR Am J Roentgenol 1979;133(6):1033–1037.
21. Webber MM, Gomes AS, Roe D, La Fontaine RL, Hawkins RA. Comparison of Biello, McNeil, and PIOPED criteria for the diagnosis of pulmonary emboli on lung scans. AJR Am J Roentgenol 1990;154(5): 975–981.
22. Christiansen F, Andersson T, Rydman H, Qvarner N, Mare K. Rater agreement in lung scintigraphy. Acta Radiol 1996;37(5):754–758.
23. Christiansen F, Andersson T, Rydman H, Mare K. Rater agreement at lung scintigraphy after consensus training. Acta Radiol 1997;38(1):92–94.
24. Henry JW, Stein PD, Gottschalk A, Relyea B, Leeper KV Jr. Scintigraphic lung scans and clinical assessment in critically ill patients with suspected acute pulmonary embolism. Chest 1996;109(2):462–426.
25. Worsley DF, Alavi A, Palevsky HI, Kundel HL. Comparison of diagnostic performance with ventilation-perfusion lung imaging in different patient populations. Radiology 1996;199(2):481–483.
26. Dalen JE, Brooks HL, Johnson LW, Meister SG, Szucs MM Jr, Dexter L. Pulmonary angiography in acute pulmonary embolism: indications, techniques, and results in 367 patients. Am Heart J 1971;81(2): 175–185.
27. Henry JW, Relyea B, Stein PD. Continuing risk of thromboemboli among patients with normal pulmonary angiograms. Chest 1995;107(5):1375–1378.
28. Cheely R, McCartney WH, Perry JR, et al. The role of noninvasive tests versus pulmonary angiography in the diagnosis of pulmonary embolism. Am J Med 1981;70(1):17–22.
29. Novelline RA, Baltarowich OH, Athanasoulis CA, Waltman AC, Greenfield AJ, McKusick KA. The clinical course of patients with suspected pulmonary embolism and a negative pulmonary arteriogram. Radiology 1978;126(3):561–567.
30. Stein PD, Athanasoulis C, Alavi A, et al. Complications and validity of pulmonary angiography in acute pulmonary embolism. Circulation 1992;85(2):462–468.
31. Zuckerman DA, Sterling KM, Oser RF. Safety of pulmonary angiography in the 1990s. J Vasc Interv Radiol 1996;7(2):199–205.
32. Quinn MF, Lundell CJ, Klotz TA, et al. Reliability of selective pulmonary arteriography in the diagnosis of pulmonary embolism. AJR Am J Roentgenol 1987;149(3):469–471.
33. van Beek EJ, Brouwerst EM, Song B, Stein PD, Oudkerk M. Clinical validity of a normal pulmonary angiogram in patients with suspected pulmonary embolism—a critical review. Clin Radiol 2001;56(10): 838–842.
34. Diffin DC, Leyendecker JR, Johnson SP, Zucker RJ, Grebe PJ. Effect of anatomic distribution of pulmonary emboli on interobserver agreement in the interpretation of pulmonary angiography. AJR Am J Roentgenol 1998;171(4):1085–1089.
35. Trowbridge RL, Araoz PA, Gotway MB, Bailey RA, Auerbach AD. The effect of helical computed tomography on diagnostic and treatment strategies in patients with suspected pulmonary embolism. Am J Med 2004;116(2):84–90.

36. Rubboli A, Leonardi G, de Castro U, Bracchetti D. Diagnostic approach to acute pulmonary embolism in a general hospital. A two-year analysis. G Ital Cardiol 1998;28(2):123–130.

37. Dalen JE, Mathur VS, Evans H, et al. Pulmonary angiography in experimental pulmonary embolism. Am Heart J 1966;72(4):509–520.

38. Stein PD, Woodard PK, Hull RD, et al. Gadolinium-enhanced magnetic resonance angiography for detection of acute pulmonary embolism: an in-depth review. Chest 2003;124(6):2324–2328.

39. Meaney JF, Weg JG, Chenevert TL, Stafford-Johnson D, Hamilton BH, Prince MR. Diagnosis of pulmonary embolism with magnetic resonance angiography. N Engl J Med 1997;336(20):1422–1427.

40. Gupta A, Frazer CK, Ferguson JM, et al. Acute pulmonary embolism: diagnosis with MR angiography. Radiology 1999;210(2):353–359.

41. Oudkerk M, van Beek EJ, Wielopolski P, et al. Comparison of contrast-enhanced magnetic resonance angiography and conventional pulmonary angiography for the diagnosis of pulmonary embolism: a prospective study. Lancet 2002;359(9318):1643–1647.

42. Ohno Y, Higashino T, Takenaka D, et al. MR angiography with sensitivity encoding (SENSE) for suspected pulmonary embolism: comparison with MDCT and ventilation-perfusion scintigraphy. AJR Am J Roentgenol 2004;183(1):91–98.

43. Schoepf UJ, Costello P. CT angiography for diagnosis of pulmonary embolism: state of the art. Radiology 2004;230(2):329–337.

44. Remy-Jardin M, Tillie-Leblond I, Szapiro D, et al. CT angiography of pulmonary embolism in patients with underlying respiratory disease: impact of multislice CT on image quality and negative predictive value. Eur Radiol 2002;12(8):1971–1978. Epub 2002 Jun 26.

45. Patel S, Kazerooni EA, Cascade PN. Pulmonary embolism: optimization of small pulmonary artery visualization at multi-detector row CT. Radiology 2003;227(2):455–460.

46. Schoepf UJ, Holzknecht N, Helmberger TK, et al. Subsegmental pulmonary emboli: improved detection with thin-collimation multi-detector row spiral CT. Radiology 2002;222(2):483–490.

47. Eng J, Krishnan JA, Segal JB, et al. Accuracy of CT in the diagnosis of pulmonary embolism: a systematic literature review. AJR Am J Roentgenol 2004;183(6):1819–1827.

48. Mullins MD, Becker DM, Hagspiel KD, Philbrick JT. The role of spiral volumetric computed tomography in the diagnosis of pulmonary embolism. Arch Intern Med 2000;160(3):293–298.

49. Rathbun SW, Raskob GE, Whitsett TL. Sensitivity and specificity of helical computed tomography in the diagnosis of pulmonary embolism: a systematic review. Ann Intern Med 2000;132(3):227–232.

50. Winer-Muram HT, Rydberg J, Johnson MS, et al. Suspected acute pulmonary embolism: evaluation with multi-detector row CT versus digital subtraction pulmonary arteriography. Radiology 2004;233(3):806–815.

51. Stein PD, Henry JW, Gottschalk A. Reassessment of pulmonary angiography for the diagnosis of pulmonary embolism: relation of interpreter agreement to the order of the involved pulmonary arterial branch. Radiology 1999;210(3):689–691.

52. Gottschalk A, Stein PD, Goodman LR, Sostman HD. Overview of Prospective Investigation of Pulmonary Embolism Diagnosis II. Semin Nucl Med 2002;32(3):173–182.

53. Blachere H, Latrabe V, Montaudon M, et al. Pulmonary embolism revealed on helical CT angiography: comparison with ventilation-perfusion radionuclide lung scanning. AJR Am J Roentgenol 2000;174(4):1041–1047.

54. Bourriot K, Couffinhal T, Bernard V, Montaudon M, Bonnet J, Laurent F. Clinical outcome after a negative spiral CT pulmonary angiographic finding in an inpatient population from cardiology and pneumology wards. Chest 2003;123(2):359–365.

55. Garg K, Sieler H, Welsh CH, Johnston RJ, Russ PD. Clinical validity of helical CT being interpreted as negative for pulmonary embolism: implications for patient treatment. AJR Am J Roentgenol 1999;172(6):1627–1631.

56. Goodman LR, Lipchik RJ, Kuzo RS, Liu Y, McAuliffe TL, O'Brien DJ. Subsequent pulmonary embolism: risk after a negative helical CT pulmonary angiogram—prospective comparison with scintigraphy. Radiology 2000;215(2):535–542.

57. Lomis NN, Yoon HC, Moran AG, Miller FJ. Clinical outcomes of patients after a negative spiral CT pulmonary arteriogram in the evaluation of acute pulmonary embolism. J Vasc Interv Radiol 1999;10(6):707–712.

58. Ost D, Rozenshtein A, Saffran L, Snider A. The negative predictive value of spiral computed tomography for the diagnosis of pulmonary embolism in patients with nondiagnostic ventilation-perfusion scans. Am J Med 2001;110(1):16–21.

59. Tillie-Leblond I, Mastora I, Radenne F, et al. Risk of pulmonary embolism after a negative spiral CT angiogram in patients with pulmonary disease: 1-year clinical follow-up study. Radiology 2002;223(2):461–467.

60. Coche E, Verschuren F, Keyeux A, et al. Diagnosis of acute pulmonary embolism in outpatients: comparison of thin-collimation multi-detector row spiral CT and planar ventilation-perfusion scintigraphy. Radiology 2003;229(3):757–765.

61. Kavanagh EC, O'Hare A, Hargaden G, Murray JG. Risk of pulmonary embolism after negative MDCT pulmonary angiography findings. AJR Am J Roentgenol 2004;182(2):499–504.

62. Musset D, Parent F, Meyer G, et al. Diagnostic strategy for patients with suspected pulmonary embolism: a prospective multicentre outcome study. Lancet 2002;360(9349):1914–1920.

63. Perrier A, Roy PM, Sanchez O, et al. Multidetector-row computed tomography in suspected pulmonary embolism. N Engl J Med 2005;352(17):1760–1768.

64. Qanadli SD, Hajjam ME, Mesurolle B, et al. Pulmonary embolism detection: prospective evaluation of dual-section helical CT versus selective pulmonary arteriography in 157 patients. Radiology 2000;217(2):447–455.

65. Swensen SJ, Sheedy PF II, Ryu JH, et al. Outcomes after withholding anticoagulation from patients with suspected acute pulmonary embolism and negative computed tomographic findings: a cohort study. Mayo Clin Proc 2002;77(2):130–138.

66. Nilsson T, Olausson A, Johnsson H, Nyman U, Aspelin P. Negative spiral CT in acute pulmonary embolism. Acta Radiol 2002;43(5):486–491.

67. Krestan CR, Klein N, Fleischmann D, et al. Value of negative spiral CT angiography in patients with suspected acute PE: analysis of PE occurrence and outcome. Eur Radiol 2004;14(1):93–98. Epub 2003 Aug 26.

68. Gottsater A, Berg A, Centergard J, Frennby B, Nirhov N, Nyman U. Clinically suspected pulmonary embolism: is it safe to withhold anticoagulation after a negative spiral CT? Eur Radiol 2001;11(1):65–72.

69. Quiroz R, Kucher N, Zou KH, et al. Clinical validity of a negative computed tomography scan in patients with suspected pulmonary embolism: a systematic review. JAMA 2005;293(16):2012–2017.

70. Remy-Jardin M, Remy J, Cauvain O, Petyt L, Wannebroucq J, Beregi JP. Diagnosis of central pulmonary embolism with helical CT: role of two-dimensional multiplanar reformations. AJR Am J Roentgenol 1995;165(5):1131–1138.

71. Shah AA, Davis SD, Gamsu G, Intriere L. Parenchymal and pleural findings in patients with and patients without acute pulmonary embolism detected at spiral CT. Radiology 1999;211(1):147–153.

72. van Rossum AB, Pattynama PM, Mallens WM, Hermans J, Heijerman HG. Can helical CT replace scintigraphy in the diagnostic process in suspected pulmonary embolism? A retrolective-prolective cohort study focusing on total diagnostic yield. Eur Radiol 1998;8(1):90–96.

73. Flohr T, Prokop M, Becker C, et al. A retrospectively ECG-gated multislice spiral CT scan and reconstruction technique with suppression of heart pulsation artifacts for cardio-thoracic imaging with extended volume coverage. Eur Radiol 2002;12(6):1497–1503. Epub 2002 Apr 25.

74. Schoepf UJ, Becker CR, Bruening RD, et al. Electrocardiographically gated thin-section CT of the lung. Radiology 1999;212(3):649–654.

75. Sostman HD, Ravin CE, Sullivan DC, Mills SR, Glickman MG, Dorfman GS. Use of pulmonary angiography for suspected pulmonary embolism: influence of scintigraphic diagnosis. AJR Am J Roentgenol 1982;139(4):673–677.

76. Henschke CI, Mateescu I, Yankelevitz DF. Changing practice patterns in the workup of pulmonary embolism. Chest 1995;107(4):940–945.

77. Remy-Jardin M, Remy J, Artaud D, Deschildre F, Duhamel A. Peripheral pulmonary arteries: optimization of the spiral CT acquisition protocol. Radiology 1997;204(1):157–163.

78. Ghaye B, Szapiro D, Mastora I, et al. Peripheral pulmonary arteries: how far in the lung does multidetector row spiral CT allow analysis? Radiology 2001;219(3):629–636.

79. Eyer BA, Goodman LR, Washington L. Clinicians' response to radiologists' reports of isolated subsegmental pulmonary embolism or inconclusive interpretation of pulmonary embolism using MDCT. AJR Am J Roentgenol 2005;184(2):623–628.

80. Goodman LR. Small pulmonary emboli: what do we know? Radiology 2005;234(3):654–658.

81. Mansencal N, Redheuil A, Joseph T, et al. Use of transthoracic echocardiography combined with venous ultrasonography in patients with pulmonary embolism. Int J Cardiol 2004;96(1):59–63.

82. Kasper W, Geibel A, Tiede N, et al. Distinguishing between acute and subacute massive pulmonary embolism by conventional and Doppler echocardiography. Br Heart J 1993;70(4):352–356.

83. Collomb D, Paramelle PJ, Calaque O, et al. Severity assessment of acute pulmonary embolism: evaluation using helical CT. Eur Radiol 2003;13(7):1508–1514. Epub 2003 Feb 7.

84. Quiroz R, Kucher N, Schoepf UJ, et al. Right ventricular enlargement on chest computed tomography: prognostic role in acute pulmonary embolism. Circulation 2004;109(20):2401–2404. Epub 2004 May 17.

85. Reid JH, Murchison JT. Acute right ventricular dilatation: a new helical CT sign of massive pulmonary embolism. Clin Radiol 1998;53(9):694–698.

86. Ferretti GR, Collomb D, Ravey JN, Vanzetto G, Coulomb M, Bricault I. Severity assessment of acute pulmonary embolism: role of CT angiography. Semin Roentgenol 2005;40(1):25–32.

87. Miller GA, Sutton GC, Kerr IH, Gibson RV, Honey M. Comparison of streptokinase and heparin in treatment of isolated acute massive pulmonary embolism. Br Heart J 1971;33(4):616.

88. Qanadli SD, El Hajjam M, Vieillard-Baron A, et al. New CT index to quantify arterial obstruction in pulmonary embolism: comparison with angiographic index and echocardiography. AJR Am J Roentgenol 2001;176(6):1415–1420.

89. Wu AS, Pezzullo JA, Cronan JJ, Hou DD, Mayo-Smith WW. CT pulmonary angiography: quantification of pulmonary embolus as a predictor of patient outcome—initial experience. Radiology 2004; 230(3):831–835. Epub 2004 Jan 22.

90. Araoz PA, Gotway MB, Trowbridge RL, et al. Helical CT pulmonary angiography predictors of in-hospital morbidity and mortality in patients with acute pulmonary embolism. J Thorac Imaging 2003; 18(4):207–216.

91. Wiest PW, Locken JA, Heintz PH, Mettler FA Jr. CT scanning: a major source of radiation exposure. Semin Ultrasound CT MR 2002;23(5):402–410.

92. Winer-Muram HT, Boone JM, Brown HL, Jennings SG, Mabie WC, Lombardo GT. Pulmonary embolism in pregnant patients: fetal radiation dose with helical CT. Radiology 2002;224(2):487–492.

93. Huda W. When a pregnant patient has a suspected pulmonary embolism, what are the typical embryo doses from a chest CT and a ventilation/perfusion study? Pediatr Radiol 2005;25:25.

94. Kalra MK, Maher MM, Toth TL, et al. Strategies for CT radiation dose optimization. Radiology 2004; 230(3):619–628. Epub 2004 Jan 22.

95. van Erkel AR, van Rossum AB, Bloem JL, Kievit J, Pattynama PM. Spiral CT angiography for suspected pulmonary embolism: a cost-effectiveness analysis. Radiology 1996;201(1):29–36.

96. Perrier A, Nendaz MR, Sarasin FP, Howarth N, Bounameaux H. Cost-effectiveness analysis of diagnostic strategies for suspected pulmonary embolism including helical computed tomography. Am J Respir Crit Care Med 2003;167(1):39–44.

97. Paterson DI, Schwartzman K. Strategies incorporating spiral CT for the diagnosis of acute pulmonary embolism: a cost-effectiveness analysis. Chest 2001;119(6):1791–1800.

98. Quiroz R, Schoepf UJ. CT pulmonary angiography for acute pulmonary embolism: cost-effectiveness analysis and review of the literature. Semin Roentgenol 2005;40(1):20–24.

99. van Erkel AR, van den Hout WB, Pattynama PM. International differences in health care costs in Europe and the United States: Do these affect the cost-effectiveness of diagnostic strategies for pulmonary embolism? Eur Radiol 1999;9(9):1926–1931.

3

The Search for Deep Vein Thrombosis
Evaluation of the Leg Veins

Jan Beyer, MD *and Sebastian M. Schellong,* MD

SUMMARY

Deep vein thrombosis (DVT) and pulmonary embolism (PE) represent two clinical manifestations of the same disease. Therefore, the search for DVT is an integral part of the diagnostic workup of PE. However, out of the wide range of possible tests for diagnosing DVT, only few show acceptable sensitivity and specificity, which also may vary depending on the diagnostic setting in which these tests are performed. This chapter describes the diagnostic procedures for DVT testing, namely clinical examination, pretest probability scores, D-dimers, compression ultrasound, and venography, including computed tomographic and magnetic resonance venography. Advantages and limitations, and the interpretation of test results, are discussed. Because compression ultrasound (CUS) has become the method of choice in suspected DVT, different protocols (2-CUS, E-CUS, and C-CUS) and the validity of their results are described in more detail. Notably, even though the available data suggest that venous ultrasound applied as a single test has low diagnostic sensitivity in suspected PE, it should be an integral part of the diagnostic workup of PE. For example, because lung scans often show indeterminate results, the confirmation of DVT by ultrasound may establish the diagnosis of PE in these patients without further tests. The second domain of venous ultrasound is to reduce the number of direct PE-imaging procedures in patients with high pretest probability and/or positive D-dimer, in whom CUS should be applied first, whenever possible. Venous ultrasound can also be particularly useful if PE is suspected in hemodynamically unstable patients, in whom a fast and reliable diagnosis at the bedside is necessary. The confirmation of DVT by ultrasound establishes the diagnosis of PE in these patients and treatment can be initiated without delay.

Key Words: Deep vein thrombosis; compression ultrasound; algorithms.

From: *Contemporary Cardiology: Management of Acute Pulmonary Embolism*
Edited by: S. Konstantinides © Humana Press Inc., Totowa, NJ

INTRODUCTION

Deep vein thrombosis (DVT) and pulmonary embolism (PE) represent two clinical manifestations of the same disease. Because venous thromboembolism (VTE) is potentially dangerous, an immediate diagnosis is necessary. The approach to the diagnosis or reliable exclusion of DVT is often not standardized and sometimes lacks effectiveness and accuracy owing to the large number of possible diagnostic modalities, the heterogeneity of the tests available in individual institutions, and the differences in experience and expertise among physicians requesting or performing these procedures. This chapter is focused on the diagnostic strategies for DVT, which may vary but principally need to adapt to one of the following typical clinical situations: (1) first episode of suspected DVT in a symptomatic lower extremity; (2) suspicion of recurrent DVT in a symptomatic lower extremity; (3) screening of asymptomatic high-risk patients; and (4) examination of asymptomatic lower extremities in patients with suspected PE.

EVALUATION OF DIAGNOSTIC PROCEDURES FOR DVT

A variety of diagnostic tools are available to confirm or exclude the diagnosis of DVT. The following procedures are those most widely used:

History, Signs, and Symptoms

Although some patients with DVT show typical symptoms, approx 30% of DVT are asymptomatic *(1,2)*. Furthermore, a number of different conditions can present with DVT-like symptoms, which is why the clinical diagnosis of DVT is discarded in approx one-half of the cases after objective testing *(3)*. Therefore, physical examination alone is insufficient and should be followed by more sensitive and specific testing.

Pretest Probability Scores

The easiest way to categorize patients with suspected VTE is to add up basic clinical information on the presence of acquired or inherited risk factors and on clinical symptoms and signs into a semiquantitative assessment of probability for DVT *(see also* Chapter 1). For symptomatic patients, score systems reflecting the combination of these data are useful tools to categorize patients accurately into groups of low, moderate, or high probability for VTE (Table 1, left column) *(4–6)*. Whereas DVT is diagnosed in only 3% of patients considered to have low pretest probability, positive findings in objective testing are much more frequent in the moderate- (17%) and particularly in the high-probability (75%) patient group. In the initial score system published by Wells in 1997, previously documented DVT did not alter the overall score. A slightly modified score was published in 2003 by the same group (Table 1, right column), which included previously documented DVT and divided patients in only two groups, DVT-likely (score > 2) and DVT-unlikely (score < 2) *(7)*. The score accurately reflected the true prevalence of DVT: 54% of the patients were categorized as unlikely to have DVT, and, of these, only 5.5% had DVT diagnosed by objective testing, compared to the 28% frequency of positive findings in patients considered DVT-likely using the Wells score.

D-Dimer Test

D-dimer is a degradation product of cross-linked fibrin, and elevated levels indicate fibrinolysis *(8)*. Because thrombosis is always accompanied by fibrinolysis, increased D-

Table 1
Pretest Probability Scores for Suspected DVT, Evaluated by Wells et al. *(5,7)*

DVT- Pretest probability score (Wells 1997)	Score	*DVT- Pretest probability score (Wells 2003)*	Score
— Active cancer (treatment ongoing or within previous 6 month or palliative)	1	— Active cancer (patient receiving treatment for previous 6 month or currently receiving palliative treatment)	1
— Paralysis, paresis, or recent plaster immobilization of the lower extremities	1	— Paralysis, paresis, or recent plaster immobilization of the lower extremities	1
— Recently bedridden for more than 3 days or major surgery within 4 weeks	1	— Recently bedridden for 3 days or more, or major surgery within the previous 12 weeks requiring general or regional anethesia	1
— Localized tenderness along the distribution of the deep venous system	1	— Localized tenderness along the distribution of the deep venous system	1
— Entire leg swollen	1	— Entire leg swollen	1
— Calf swelling by more than 3 cm when compared with the asymptomatic leg (measured 10 cm below tibial tuberosity)	1	— Calf swelling at least 3 cm larger than on the asymptomatic side (measured 10 cm below tibial tuberosity)	1
— Pitting oedema (greater in the symptomatic leg)	1	— Pitting oedema confined to the symptomatic leg	1
— Collateral superficial vein (nonvaricose)	1	— Collateral superficial vein (nonvaricose)	1
— Alternative diagnosis as likely or greater than that of deep-vein thrombosis	*n.*	— Previously documented deep-vein thrombosis	1
		— Alternative diagnosis at least as likely as deep-vein thrombosis	*n.*

Score 0 or less low probability Score 1 or 2 intermediate probability Score 3 or more high probability	Score less than 2 DVT unlikely Score 2 or more DVT likely

dimers in the circulation are an extremely sensitive marker of thromboembolic events *(9)*. However, because fibrin degradation is also common in nonthromboembolic diseases, false-positive results are common and specifity is low. Thus, the importance of D-dimer testing lies in its negative predictive value. Normal D-dimer levels in combination with low or intermediate pretest probability effectively rule out DVT and PE *(7,10)*.

The value of pretest probability scores combined with D-dimer testing is discussed in more detail in Chapter 1.

Compression Ultrasound (CUS)

Today, real-time venous ultrasound has become the most widely used tool in the diagnostic process of DVT and has replaced continuous-wave Doppler ultrasound. However, the nonstandardized use of various ultrasound modalities such as B-mode, pulsed-wave Doppler, and color Doppler limits the accuracy of this technique. Thus, whereas a high

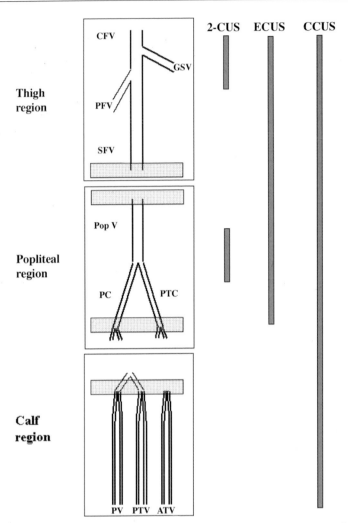

Fig. 1. Comparison of three compression ultrasound protocols *(15)*. 2-CUS, two-point compression ultrasound of the common femoral and popliteal vein; E-CUS, extended compression ultrasound examining the complete thigh veins, popliteal vein and trifurcation; C-CUS, complete compression ultrasound examining the complete deep venous system of thigh and calf. CFV, common femoral vein; GSV, greater saphenous vein; PFV, profound femoral vein; SFV, superficial femoral vein; PopV, popliteal vein; PC, peroneal confluence branch; PTC, posterior tibial confluence branch; PV, peroneal veins; PTV, posterior tibial veins; ATV, anterior tibial veins.

sensitivity and specificity could be shown for diagnosis of proximal DVT (i.e., at the level of the popliteal or femoral vein), a meta-analysis revealed a lack of sensitivity and specificity when examining the calf veins. This was more frequently the case in asymptomatic than in symptomatic patients *(11–14)*.

Because of the limitations of venous ultrasound, simplified or standardized protocols of venous CUS in suspected DVT were developed. These can be categorized into three approaches (Fig. 1): (1) segmental CUS of only two characteristic venous segments, the common femoral vein and the popliteal vein (2-CUS); (2) extended CUS of the complete deep thigh veins and the popliteal vein down to the trifurcation (E-CUS); and (3) com-

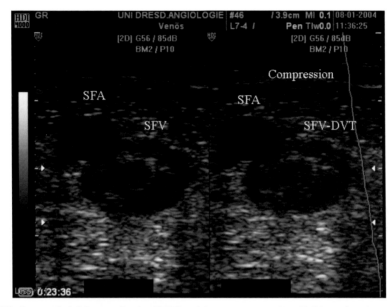

Fig. 2. DVT of superficial femoral vein (SFV), without compression (left), and under compression (right).

plete CUS of all segments of the deep thigh and calf veins (C-CUS) *(15)*. All of these protocols use the noncompressibility of a venous segment as the criterion to diagnose DVT (Fig. 2).

2-CUS

Cogo et al. suggested ultrasound scanning of only the common femoral and popliteal vein (2-point-ultrasound), because most patients with symptomatic DVT present with occlusive proximal thrombosis *(16)*. For this segmental (or rapid) CUS (Fig. 3), Lensing et al. reported a high sensitivity and specifity for proximal symptomatic DVT. On the other hand, diagnosis of distal DVT was shown to be associated with a low sensitivity of only 36% *(17)*.

Using this protocol and a follow-up examination of the groin and popliteal region after 1 week (repeated or serial CUS) has been reported to be a safe strategy in patients with suspected DVT *(18)*. Ascending proximal DVT can be ruled out with the first examination, but this approach will miss segmental proximal thrombi or calf vein thrombosis initially. These thrombi may be found in the follow-up exam should they ascend to the next proximal segment. However, when this protocol is used, all patients with suspected DVT and a normal initial test require a second test, but only about 1–3% of them will ultimately have a positive finding of proximal DVT *(18)*. Because of this, this may not be a cost-effective approach *(19)*.

E-CUS

E-CUS examines all segments of the thigh veins and popliteal vein including the calf vein trifurcation *(20)*. Therefore, segmental thigh thrombi or calf vein thrombosis extending into the trifurcation (or confluence) region are detected, but, again, isolated calf vein thrombosis is missed.

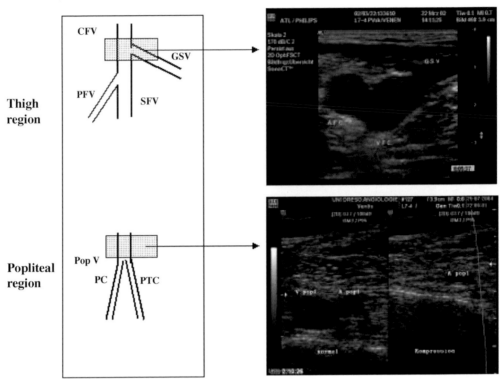

Fig. 3. Compression ultrasound of common femoral and popliteal vein (2-CUS) *(16)*. Abbreviations as in Fig. 1.

C-CUS

The concept of C-CUS uses a standardized protocol *(21)* in which only B-mode ultrasound is applied to cross sections of all venous segments. In exactly defined postures of the patient and venous segments, compression of the entire deep venous system is performed, beginning in the groin and ending at the distal calf veins (Fig. 4). The venous lumen is compressed using the ultrasound probe, following release of compression. Then the transducer is moved further distally for approx 1–2 cm, and again compression is performed. Using this protocol, DVT is diagnosed if a venous segment is not fully compressible (Fig. 2). Thigh veins are examined with the patient in the supine position. For examination of popliteal and calf veins, the patient has to sit up with the legs hanging down. The popliteal vein, all segments of the paired deep calf veins, and the muscle veins are examined sequentially by exerting pressure with the ultrasound probe to every venous segment under investigation. Exclusion of DVT using such a standardized C-CUS protocol was a safe procedure both in retrospective *(22)* and in prospective studies *(21,23,24)*.

We prospectively assessed the safety of a single C-CUS in 1646 consecutive patients with a first episode of suspected DVT. During the 3 months of follow-up, 3 of 1023 patients (0.3%) with negative C-CUS findings experienced a symptomatic VTE event (95% confidence interval [CI], 0.1–0.8%) *(21)*. With comparable study designs, similar results were demonstrated by Elias and Stevens *(23,24)* in 623 and 445 consecutive patients, respectively. In these studies, the incidence of VTE during 3-month follow-up was 0.5% (95% CI, 0.1–1.8%) *(23)* and 0.8% (95% CI, 0.16–2.33%), respectively. The interobserver variability of C-CUS was shown to be low and the duration of the examination as short as

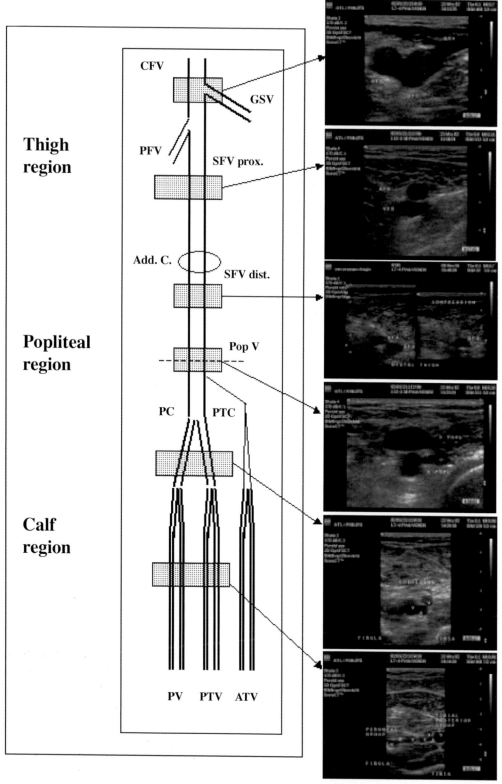

Fig. 4. Complete compression ultrasound *(21)*. Add.C, adductor canal. Other abbreviations as in Fig. 1.

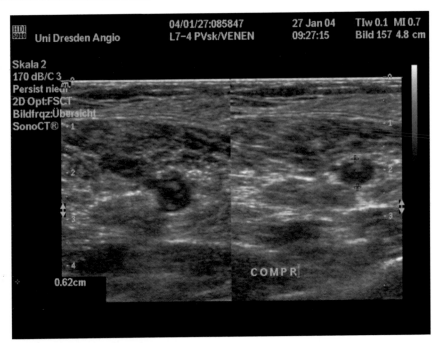

Fig. 5. Acute soleal muscle vein thrombosis (MVT), without compression (left), and under compression (right).

6 minutes per leg *(25)*. Furthermore, with C-CUS, assessment of calf muscle veins is easy, and thrombi in these small veins can be detected even before the deep venous system becomes involved *(26)* (Fig. 5).

Venous Ultrasound in Suspected Recurrent Thrombosis

Reliable diagnosis of recurrent thrombosis is one of the most difficult clinical tasks, because no objective test can safely differentiate between residual and fresh thrombi if no information about the primary DVT episode is available. This is a clinically relevant problem, because residual thrombi can be found in up to 50% of patients 1 year after the first diagnosis of DVT *(27,28)*. Therefore, a systematic approach is even more critical in this setting.

The most reliable differentiation between fresh and residual thrombosis can be made if DVT is detected in previously unaffected venous segments. If the same venous segments are affected, comparison with residual thrombus may still be possible provided that residual thrombus mass was accurately documented in previous sonograms. Therefore, careful assessment and exact documentation of residual thrombus in clearly defined venous segments such as the common femoral vein, the proximal end of the superficial femoral vein, the popliteal vein, and the confluence branches of the popliteal vein is recommended. A compression maneuver of these venous cross-sections is performed and the residual diameter (i.e., residual thrombus thickness under compression) is measured (Fig. 5). An increase of residual thrombus thickness by more than 2 mm at follow-up examination has been proposed to indicate recurrence of DVT *(28)*. If this information is not available, sonographic assessment of recurrence is highly subjective and should therefore also take into account the pretest probability, history, and clinical examination. D-dimer testing could also be a valuable tool, although no data exist on its accuracy in this particular setting.

Because D-dimer concentrations usually return to normal levels within the first 3 months of anticoagulant therapy for thrombembolic disease *(29)*, the recurrence of DVT is less likely in patients with a negative D-dimer test than in D-dimer-positive patients. In case of doubt, we recommend an exact documentation of thrombus mass as described previously and serial testing after 1 week, as suggested by Prandoni et al. *(30)*.

Venography

Venography (or phlebography) is still the gold standard for diagnosis of DVT. Two different methods, the "classic" Rabinov-Paulin venography and the long-leg venography, are used, but it is only for the long-leg venography that a low rate of nondiagnostic results and a high interobserver agreement could be shown *(31)*. DVT is diagnosed when intraluminal filling defects are detectable in more than one projection. However, radiation exposure, nephrotoxic contrast media, and the painful injection into pedal veins are limiting factors leading to primary failure in a significant number of patients *(32)*.

Computed Tomography (CT)

Spiral CT venography has been shown to have similar sensitivity and specificity compared with conventional venography *(33)*, but its high cost and radiation burden preclude routine use *(34,35)*. On the other hand, the possibility of examination of the pulmonary arteries (to confirm or exclude PE) and detection of caval or iliac vein thrombosis in the same session represents a major advantage of CT (*see* Chapter 2).

Magnetic Resonance Venography (MRV)

A high sensitivity and specificity of MRV could be shown in recent studies using different techniques with and without contrast media *(35–37)*, but the high costs and limited availability exclude MRV from routine use. It may prove to be a valuable tool in the diagnosis of recurrent DVT, because the ability to assess the inflammatory reaction in the surrounding tissue may help differentiate between old and fresh thrombi. Furthermore, when caval or iliac vein thrombosis is suspected, MRV may be a safe noninvasive alternative to conventional venography *(38)*.

VALUE OF CUS IN SUSPECTED PE

Although CUS is a safe and reliable method in symptomatic DVT, sensitivity and specificity are low in asymptomatic patients *(11,12,14)*. Because patients with suspicion of PE are usually asymptomatic with regard to the leg veins, the disappointing inaccuracy of CUS seems to apply to this patient group as well. However, the accuracy data on CUS in the examination of asymptomatic legs are derived from screening studies in postoperative patients and do not necessarily reflect the situation of patients with suspected symptomatic PE, in whom the distribution pattern of DVT may be entirely different from "typical" postoperative DVT. For example, although in screening examinations after high-risk surgery most findings are small segmental proximal thrombi, isolated and segmental deep calf-vein thrombi, or muscle vein thrombosis, the source of PE is often proximal ascending DVT. Therefore, the low sensitivity for distal DVT may not necessarily impair the value of CUS in the diagnostic approach to PE. Nevertheless, the available data suggest that 2-CUS and E-CUS have a low diagnostic sensitivity in suspected PE *(39)*. In a prospective multicenter study of 479 patients with suspected PE, a sensitivity of 23% (95% CI, 19–26%) for 2-CUS and 25% (95%, CI 20–28%) for E-CUS could be shown. Thus, including the examination of the trifurcation into the 2-CUS protocol did not improve the sensitivity for PE. To date, no data exist for a standardized C-CUS protocol.

In general, three possible indications exist for CUS in the diagnostic workup of suspected PE: (1) CUS may help in situations of nonconclusive results of PE-imaging procedures such as single-row detector spiral CT or ventilation-perfusion (V/Q) scan; (2) CUS may help reduce the number of patients requiring these tests; and (3) in cases of hemodynamic instability, CUS, used as a bedside test in the intensive care unit, may contribute to rapid diagnosis of PE, thus avoiding patient transport for further imaging techniques.

CUS in Case of Nonconclusive Results of PE-Imaging Studies

If lung scan is the first diagnostic step, a frequent problem is the number of indeterminate test results, i.e., results that do not allow an unequivocal diagnosis. For V/Q scans, the frequency of indeterminate test results may be as high as 50% *(40)*. In these situations, a positive result of venous ultrasound confirms the diagnosis of PE, whereas the interpretation of negative results requires further stratification taking the patient's pretest probability into account. In cases of low or intermediate clinical probability, DVT can safely be ruled out, whereas, in patients with high probability, further diagnostic tests are necessary *(41–43)*. The diagnostic strategy is different when CT is used, especially since the introduction of multi-row detectors. Whereas a study by Van Strijen *(44)* showed a lack of sensitivity of single-row detector in the diagnosis of PE, a meta-analysis including 15 studies with different CT modalities showed a good sensitivity for both single-row and multidetector-row CT *(45)*. Therefore, the need for adjunctive diagnostic procedures to increase CT sensitivity for PE diagnosis is questionable. However, the combination of negative venous ultrasound and a negative spiral CT has been shown to safely rule out PE *(46–48)*. Overall, the combination of D-dimer and venous ultrasound with either V/Q scan or spiral CT has been shown to be a cost-effective strategy for diagnosis of PE *(42,43)* (*see also* Chapter 7).

Use of CUS to Reduce the Number of CT or V/Q Scans

The combination of clinical pretest probability scores, D-dimer-testing, and C-CUS has been shown to result in a significant reduction of CT scans *(49)*. In a prospective study of 965 patients with suspected PE, normal D-dimers ruled out PE in 29%, and positive ultrasound established the diagnosis of PE in 9.5%. Altogether, a CT scan was necessary only in 61% of the patients and showed PE in 12.8%. For patients considered as not having PE, the 3-month thrombembolic risk was 1.5% (95% CI, 0.5–2.1%) *(46)*. Similar results were obtained in another prospective study of 274 patients with suspected PE *(47)*. The combination of pretest probability, D-dimer testing, and venous ultrasound of thigh and calf veins was able to reduce the number of CT scans to 42% of cases. Ultrasound established diagnosis by detection of thigh DVT in 23.7% of patients and of calf DVT in 13.1%. During 3-month follow-up, only one VTE event occurred, yielding an overall incidence of 0.6% (95% CI, 0.1–3.4%). Therefore, if pretest probability scores and D-dimer levels do not rule out PE and imaging techniques are necessary, the diagnostic workup algorithm should include, wherever possible, venous CUS as the first step. Only patients with a negative CUS will require a lung scan or spiral CT.

Reduction of radiation exposure is of particular interest in pregnant women with suspected DVT or PE (*see also* Chapter 17). In pregnancy, diagnosis is complicated because of swelling of the legs unrelated to DVT. Moreover, D-dimer levels may be elevated in pregnancy and are therefore of limited diagnostic value. On the other hand, isolated iliac vein DVT is not uncommon in this setting. Therefore, the ultrasound protocol needs to include pulsed-wave Doppler of the common femoral vein if CUS of the infrainguinal vein is negative. If the flow pattern is normal, isolated iliac vein thrombosis is ruled out. However, owing to increased intraabdominal pressure in pregnancy, venous flow is often impaired and further testing is necessary. An attempt should be made to visualize the iliac veins using color Doppler. If this fails, magnetic resonance imaging (MRI) may be indicated, because data suggest that MRI can safely exclude isolated iliac vein thrombosis in this situation *(50)*.

CUS As a Bedside Test
in Hemodynamically Unstable Patients With Suspected PE

For hemodynamically unstable patients with suspected DVT, a fast and reliable approach at the bedside is necessary (*see also* Chapter 8). Data derived from hemodynamically stable patients showed that clinical signs, D-dimer levels, and the findings of CUS could be used as predictors of large PE *(51)*. This could be particularly true for hemodynamically unstable patients. Therefore, if history and clinical signs are consistent with (massive) PE, the detection of DVT is sufficient to establish the cause of hemodynamical impairment. No further examinations are necessary, because procedure-associated time loss and the need for transportation will only endanger the patient and prevent prompt institution of therapy.

CONCLUSION

CUS is increasingly becoming established as the procedure of choice for diagnosis of DVT. Different protocols exist with a variable quality of results. Serial ultrasound for proximal veins is a safe means for excluding DVT, but a large number of patients need a follow-up examination, and only 1–3% of them will ultimately have a positive finding indicating proximal DVT, making this protocol less cost-effective. For symptomatic patients, C-CUS using a standardized protocol is feasible and has a high sensitivity and specificity. In most cases, one examination will suffice for exact diagnosis.

In suspected PE, venous ultrasound is capable of reducing the number of patients who need spiral CT or V/Q lung scan, leading to a reduction in radiation burden and, in some cases, faster diagnosis of VTE. Furthermore, venous ultrasound is able to confirm or to exclude PE if the lung scan or spiral CT yields inconclusive results.

REFERENCES

1. Haeger K. Problems of acute venous thrombosis: the interpretation of signs and symptoms. Angiology 1969;20:219–223.
2. Kakkar VV, Howe CT, Nicolaides AN, Renney JTG, Clarke MB. Deep vein thrombosis of the leg: is there a "high risk" group? Am J Surg 1970;120:527–530.
3. Kakkar VV, Howe CT, Flanc C, Clarke MB. Natural history of postoperative deep-vein thrombosis. Lancet 1969;2:230–232.
4. Wells PS, Anderson DR, Ginsberg J. Assessment of deep vein thrombosis or pulmonary embolism by the combined use of clinical model and non-invasive tests. Semin Thromb Hemost 2000;26:643–655.
5. Wells PS, Anderson DR, Bormanis J, et al. Value of assessment of pretest probability of deep-vein thrombosis in clinical management. Lancet 1997;350:1795–1798.
6. Perrier A, Desmarais S, Miron MJ, et al. Non-invasive diagnosis of venous thromboembolism in outpatients. Lancet 1999;353:190–195.

 7. Wells PS, Anderson DR, Rodger M, et al. Evaluation of D-dimer in the diagnosis of suspected deep-vein thrombosis. N Engl J Med 2003;349:1227–1235.
 8. Bockenstedt P. D-dimer in venous thrombembolism. N Engl J Med 2003;349:1203–1204.
 9. Kearon C, Julian JA, Newman TE, Ginsberg JS. Noninvasive diagnosis of deep venous thrombosis. Ann Intern Med 1998;128:663–677.
10. Fancher TL, White RH, Kravitz RL. Combined use of rapid D-dimer testing and estimation of clinical probability in the diagnosis of deep vein thrombosis: systematic review. BMJ 2004;329:821.
11. Kassai B, Boissel JP, Cucherat M, Sonie S, Shah NR, Leizorovicz A. A systematic review of the accuracy of ultrasound in the diagnosis of deep venous thrombosis in asymptomatic patients. Thromb Haemost 2004;91:655–666.
12. Kearon C, Ginsberg JS, Hirsh J. The role of venous ultrasonography in the diagnosis of suspected deep venous thrombosis and pulmonary embolism. Ann Intern Med 1998;129:1044–1049.
13. Wells PS, Lensing AW, Davidson BL, Prins MH, Hirsh J. Accuracy of ultrasound for the diagnosis of deep venous thrombosis in asymptomatic patients after orthopedic surgery. A meta-analysis. Ann Intern Med 1995;122(1):47–53.
14. Kearon C, Julian JA, Newman TE, Ginsberg JS. Noninvasive diagnosis of deep venous thrombosis. McMaster Diagnostic Imaging Practice Guidelines Initiative. Ann Intern Med 1998;128(8):663–677.
15. Schellong SM. Complete compression ultrasound for the diagnosis of venous thromboembolism. Curr Opin Pulm Med 2004;10(5):350–355.
16. Cogo A, Lensing AWA, Prandoni P, Hirsh J. Distribution of venous thrombosis in patients with symptomatic deep vein thrombosis. Implications for simplifying the diagnostic process with compression ultrasound. Arch Intern Med 1993;153:2777–2780.
17. Lensing AWA, Prandoni P, Brandjes D, et al. Detection of deep vein thrombosis by real-time B-mode ultrasonography. N Engl J Med 1989;320:342–345.
18. Cogo A, Lensing AWA, Koopman MMW, et al. Compression ultrasonography for diagnostic management of patients with clinically suspected deep vein thrombosis: prospective cohort study. BMJ 1998;316:17–20.
19. Perone N, Bounameaux H, Perrier A. Comparison of four strategies for diagnosing deep vein thrombosis: a cost-effectiveness analysis. AM J Med 2001;110:33–40.
20. Tick LW, Ton E, van Voorthuizen T, Hovens MM, Leeuwenburgh I, Lobatto S. Practical diagnostic management of patients with clinically suspected deep vein thrombosis by clinical probability test, compression ultrasonography, and D-dimer test. Am J Med 2002;113:630–635.
21. Schellong SM, Schwarz T, Halbritter K, et al. Complete compression ultrasonography of the leg as a single test for the diagnosis of deep vein thrombosis. Thromb Haemost 2003;89:228–234.
22. Gottlieb RH, Widjaja J, Tian L, Rubens DJ, Voci SL. Calf sonography for detecting deep venous thrombosis in symptomatic patients: experience and review of the literature. J Clin Ultrasound 1999;27(8):415–420.
23. Elias A, Mallard L, Elias M, et al. A single complete ultrasound investigation of the venous network for the diagnostic management of patients with a clinically suspected first episode of deep venous thrombosis of the lower limbs. Thromb Haemost 2003;89:221–227.
24. Stevens SM, Elliott CG, Chan KJ, Egger MJ, Ahmed KM. Withholding anticoagulation after a negative result on duplex ultrasonography for suspected symptomatic deep venous thrombosis. Ann Intern Med 2004;140(12):985–991.
25. Schwarz T, Schmid BA, Schellong SM. Complete compression ultrasound for clinically suspected deep vein thrombosis: feasibility and inter-observer agreement. Clin. Appl Thromb Hemost 2002;8(1):45–49.
26. Labropoulos N, Webb KM, Kang SS, et al. Patterns and distribution of isolated calf deep vein thrombosis. J Vasc Surg 1999;30:787–791.
27. Hejboer H, Jongbloets LM, Büller HR, Lensing AW, ten Cate JW. Clinical utility of real-time compression ultrasonography for diagnostic management of patients with recurrent venous thrombosis. Acta Radiol 1992;33:297–300.
28. Prandoni P, Cogo A, Bernardi E, et al. A simple ultrasound approach for detection of recurrent proximal vein thrombosis. Circulation 1993;88:1730–1735.
29. Lee AY, Ginsberg JS. The role of D-dimer in the diagnosis of venous thrombembolism. Curr Opin Pul Med 1997;3:275–279.
30. Prandoni P, Lensing AWA, Bernardi E, Villalta S, Bagatella P, Girolami A. The diagnostic value of compression ultrasonography in patients with suspected recurrent deep vein thrombosis. Thromb Haemost 2002;88:402–406.

31. Lensing AWA, Buller HR, Prandoni P, et al. Contrast venography, the gold standard for the diagnosis of deep-vein thrombosis: improvement in observer agreement. Thromb Haemost 1992;67(1):8–12.

32. Heijboer H, Cogo A, Buller HR, Prandoni P, ten Cate JW. Detection of deep vein thrombosis with impedance plethysmography and real-time compression ultrasonography in hospitalized patients. Arch Intern Med 1992;152:1901–1903.

33. Baldt MM, Zontsich T, Stümpflen A, et al. Deep venous thrombosis of the lower extremity: efficiacy of spiral CT venography compared with conventional venography in diagnosis. Radiology 1996;200: 423–428.

34. Begemann PG, Bonacker M, Kemper J, et al. Evaluation of the deep venous system in patients with suspected pulmonary embolism with multi-detector CT: a prospective study in comparison to doppler-sonography. J Comput Assist Tomogr 2003;27:399–409.

35. Kanne JP, Lalani TA. Role of computed tomography and magnetic resonance imaging for deep venous thrombosis and pulmonary embolism. Ciculation 2004;109:I15–I21.

36. Spritzer CE, Norconk JJ Jr, Sostman HD, Coleman RE. Detection of deep venous thrombosis by magnetic resonance imaging. Chest 1993;104:54–60.

37. Evans AJ, Sostman HD, Knelson MH, et al. Am J Radiol 1993;161:131–139.

38. Dupas B, El Kouri D, Curtet C, et al. Angiomagnetic resoonance imaging of iliofemoral venous thrombosis. Lancet 1995;346:17–19.

39. Mac Gillavry MR, Sanson BJ, Buller HR, Brandjes DP; ANTELOPE Study Group. Compression ultrasonography of the leg veins in patients with clinically suspected pulmonary embolism: is a more extensive assessment of compressibility useful? Thromb Haemost 2000;84(6):973–976.

40. Value of the ventilation/perfusion scan in acute pulmonary embolism. Results of the prospective investigation of pulmonary embolism diagnosis (PIOPED). The PIOPED Investigators. JAMA 1990;263(20): 2753–2759.

41. Perrier A, Bounameaux H. Ultrasonography of leg veins in patients suspected of having pulmonary embolism. Ann Intern Med 1998;128(3):243–251.

42. Perrier A, Buswell L, Bounameaux H, et al. Cost-effectiveness of noninvasive diagnostic aids in suspected pulmonary embolism. Arch Intern Med 1997;157(20):2309–2316.

43. Perrier A, Nendaz MR, Sarasin FP, Howarth N, Bounameaux H. Cost-effectiveness analysis of diagnostic strategies for suspected pulmonary embolism including helical computed tomography. Am J Respir Crit Care Med 2003;167(1):39–44.

44. Van Strijen MJ, De Monye W, Kieft GJ, Pattynama PM, Prins MH, Huisman MV. Accuracy of single-detector spiral CT in the diagnosis of pulmonary embolism: a prospective multicenter cohort study of consecutive patients with abnormal perfusion scintigraphy. J Thromb Haemost 2005;3(1):17–25.

45. Quiroz R, Kucher N, Zou KH, et al. Clinical validity of a negative computed tomography scan in patients with suspected pulmonary embolism: a systematic review. JAMA 2005;293(16):2012–2017.

46. Perrier A, Roy PM, Aujesky D, et al. Diagnosing pulmonary embolism in outpatients with clinical assessment, D-dimer measurement, venous ultrasound, and helical computed tomography: a multicenter management study. Am J Med 2004;116(5):291–299.

47. Elias A, Cazanave A, Elias M, et al. Diagnostic management of pulmonary embolism using clinical assessment, plasma D-dimer assay, complete lower limb venous ultrasound and helical computed tomography of pulmonary arteries. A multicentre clinical outcome study. Thromb Haemost 2005;93(5):982–988.

48. Musset D, Parent F, Meyer G, et al.; Evaluation du Scanner Spirale dans l'Embolie Pulmonaire Study Group. Diagnostic strategy for patients with suspected pulmonary embolism: a prospective multicentre outcome study. Lancet 2002;360(9349):1914–1920.

49. Michiels JJ, Gadisseur A, Van Der Planken M, et al. A critical appraisal of non-invasive diagnosis and exclusion of deep vein thrombosis and pulmonary embolism in outpatients with suspected deep vein thrombosis or pulmonary embolism: how many tests do we need? Int Angiol 2005;24(1):27–39.

50. Spritzer CE, Evans AC, Kay HH. Magnetic resonance imaging of deep venous thrombosis in pregnant women with lower extremity edema. Obstet Gynecol 1995;85:603–607.

51. Galle C, Papazyan JP, Miron MJ, Slosman D, Bounameaux H, Perrier A. Prediction of pulmonary embolism extent by clinical findings, D-dimer level and deep vein thrombosis shown by ultrasound. Thromb Haemost 2001;86(5):1156–1160.

4 Risk Stratification of Pulmonary Embolism

Detection and Prognostic Impact of Right Ventricular Dysfunction

Stavros V. Konstantinides, MD

CONTENTS

SUMMARY

The appropriate management of patients with acute pulmonary embolism (PE) who present with right ventricular (RV) dysfunction but normal arterial blood pressure (i.e., those with submassive PE) continues to be highly controversial. Recently, a number of studies have improved our understanding of subclinical RV dysfunction in PE. Despite the limitations of echocardiographic criteria for diagnosing the enlargement and/or dysfunction of the right ventricle, ample evidence supports the notion that RV dysfunction diagnosed by echocardiography (echo) is an independent predictor of early mortality and complications in normotensive patients with PE. Retrospective studies showed that similar prognostic data can be obtained using multidetector-row chest computed tomography (CT). Moreover, very recent reports indicate that biomarker, particularly troponin, testing followed by echocardiographic or CT imaging of the right ventricle may be an efficient and reliable strategy both for excluding (ruling out) and for predicting (ruling in) a poor outcome in patients with PE. Thus, novel risk stratification algorithms help identify possible candidates for early thrombolytic treatment in PE and thus provide the background for a large controlled trial that will hopefully resolve the 30-year-old debate on the benefits of thrombolysis in normotensive patients with PE and RV dysfunction.

From: *Contemporary Cardiology: Management of Acute Pulmonary Embolism*
Edited by: S. Konstantinides © Humana Press Inc., Totowa, NJ

Key Words: Right ventricle; prognosis; biomarkers; echocardiography; computed tomography.

INTRODUCTION

As early as 35 yr ago, McIntyre and Sasahara demonstrated that right ventricular (RV) pressure overload and dysfunction are critical events in the pathophysiology of pulmonary embolism (PE), and that they may be important determinants of the patients' outcome in the acute phase *(1,2)*. At present, it is widely acknowledged that RV dilation and hypokinesis resulting from acute pressure overload is capable of initiating a vicious cycle of increased myocardial oxygen demand, myocardial ischemia (or infarction), left ventricular preload reduction, and, ultimately, inability to maintain the cardiac index and arterial pressure *(3)*. If left untreated, this sequence of events will lead to cardiogenic shock, and, in fact, most PE-related deaths are due to refractory cardiac (rather than respiratory) failure.

Overt RV failure with hemodynamic instability and shock due to massive, fulminant PE does not pose diagnostic problems, and its detection certainly does not require sophisticated imaging procedures or biochemical tests (*see* Chapter 8). This condition is associated with a very poor prognosis and mortality rates of up to 65% in the acute phase *(4)*. As a result, there is consensus *(5–7)*, even in the absence of large randomized trials *(8)*, that hemodynamically unstable patients with PE should undergo emergency pulmonary artery recanalization using thrombolytic agents (*see* Chapters 10 and 11), or by means of surgical (*see* Chapter 12) or interventional (*see* Chapter 13) procedures. On the other hand, it remains highly controversial whether the diagnosis of RV dysfunction in *normotensive* patients with acute PE (so-called *submassive* PE) should also alert clinicians and prompt them to administer thrombolytic treatment in order to prevent (rather than treat) cardiogenic shock *(9–12)*. In fact, the results of meta-analyses of the randomized trials that tested thrombolysis in PE appear to contradict its (presumed) clinical benefits in this setting *(13,14)*.

This and the following chapter will focus on recent studies that improved our understanding of subclinical RV dysfunction in PE. The data obtained in these trials provide the background for emerging risk stratification algorithms, which will hopefully succeed in identifying high-risk normotensive patients and thus help resolve the ongoing debate on the possible indications for thrombolysis in submassive PE.

CAN THE ELECTROCARDIOGRAM SUGGEST RV DYSFUNCTION?

Although the electrocardiogram (ECG) on admission can, by itself, neither confirm nor exclude the diagnosis of acute PE in a given patient, a number of earlier reports suggested that specific ECG changes may correlate with the severity of PE *(15–17)*. More recently, Geibel et al. provided data to support the notion that simple ECG parameters could serve as a noncostly, ubiquitously available tool for initial triage of patients with PE, i.e., for raising the suspicion of RV dysfunction and for prompting further risk stratification of PE *(18)*. The authors performed multivariate analysis in 508 patients with acute massive or submassive PE derived from the 1001-patient Management Strategies and Prognosis in Pulmonary Embolism (MAPPET) registry *(19)*. The presence of at least one of prespecified ECG abnormalities (atrial arrhythmias, complete right bundle branch block, peripheral low voltage, pseudoinfarction pattern in leads III and aVF, or ST segment changes over the left precordial leads) on admission was associated with an elevated in-hospital death risk (odds ratio [OR], 2.56; 95% confidence interval [CI], 1.49–4.57; $p < 0.001$) after adjustment for clinical baseline parameters. These results appear encouraging, and it has indeed been a long-standing hypothesis that the ECG changes frequently observed in acute PE may reflect acute myocardial ischemia and/or RV wall stress. However, studies using scintigraphic and enzymatic assessment were unable to consistently confirm the presence of ischemia in patients with T-wave changes over the anterior precordial leads (20). Moreover, not all investigators agree that ECG abnormalities can reliably predict severe PE (21), and it is often impossible for the clinician in the emergency room or intensive care unit to find out whether the ECG changes present on admission are preexisting or of new onset. Thus, although the ECG findings can be used in combination with other parameters to assess the clinical pretest probability of PE (see Chapter 1), the available evidence is not sufficient to support a clinically relevant role for the ECG as an independent baseline risk stratification test.

THE VALUE OF ECHOCARDIOGRAPHY: STRENGTHS AND LIMITATIONS

As early as two decades ago, it was reported that echocardiography (echo) is capable of visualizing the enlargement of the right ventricle that results from acute submassive and massive PE, and that it may even detect thrombi of venous origin appearing in the right heart cavities in transit to the pulmonary circulation (22–24). Since that time, a number of echocardiographic findings, including RV enlargement and/or hypokinesis of the free wall (Fig. 1A), leftward septal shift (Fig. 1A and B), and evidence of pulmonary hypertension, have been proposed for noninvasive diagnosis of RV dysfunction at the bedside. These criteria were recently reviewed by Goldhaber (25,26). Currently, echo is established in many (particularly European) institutions as the method of choice for identifying high-risk patients with acute PE, because a number of studies could demonstrate an association between abnormal echocardiographic findings and an adverse in-hospital outcome in terms of PE-related death and complications (27–30). Notwithstanding, the prognostic value of cardiac ultrasound in *normotensive* patients with confirmed PE has not been unequivocally demonstrated and is therefore not universally accepted. For example, in a recent systematic review of the literature (31), ten Wolde et al. found seven studies that assessed the impact of RV dysfunction diagnosed by ultrasound on the outcome of patients with PE. They pointed out some important methodological limitations of these studies, including lack of confirmation of PE in some of the cases, the inclusion of both hemodynamically stable and unstable patients (i.e., a mixed population of submassive and massive PE), and the possible confounding effects of early (thrombolytic) treatment. Overall, a twofold elevation in the risk of PE-related mortality (4–18% increase in absolute terms) was found in patients with RV dysfunction, the prevalence of which ranged from 40–70%. However, focusing on those studies that excluded patients with overt hemodynamic instability at presentation revealed a much less pronounced difference, which did not exceed 4–5% in absolute terms. These findings led ten Wolde et al. to question the value of echo for risk stratification of PE and its therapeutic implications in the absence of cardiogenic shock (31). Similarly, a retrospective cohort study suggested that echocardiographic detection of RV dysfunction does not suffice to set the indication for thrombolysis in hemodynamically stable patients with PE (32), although an earlier analysis of the MAPPET registry had found that the relative risk of in-hospital death might be reduced by as much as 70% in this patient group (33).

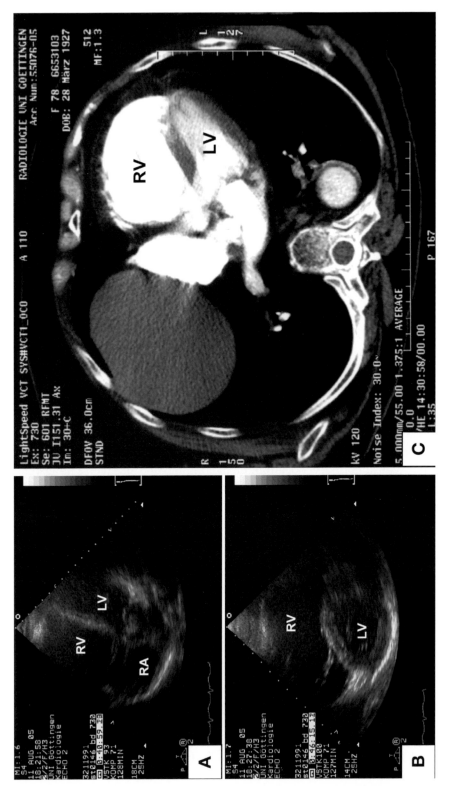

Fig. 1. RV dysfunction in 78-yr-old patient with acute submassive PE. **A,B:** echocardiographic imaging using the apical four-chamber view (**A**) and the parasternal short-axis view (**B**) revealed pronounced RV enlargement compared to the size of the left ventricle (**A,B**), which was accompanied by leftward displacement (flattening) of the interventricular septum (**B**). A four-chamber view of the heart on multidetector-row chest CT yielded very similar findings, further supporting the diagnosis of RV dysfunction (**C**).

How should these controversial data be interpreted? Should echo still be used in the differential diagnosis of cardiogenic shock in order to confirm (or exclude) massive PE (*see* Chapter 8) but otherwise be omitted in patients who are normotensive at presentation? Although no definite answer can be given to this question at present, a very recent report provided further evidence to support the prognostic importance of echo (even) in apparently stable patients with PE *(34)*. The authors evaluated 1035 patients included in the International Cooperative Pulmonary Embolism Registry (ICOPER) *(35)*. The patients analyzed were those who presented with systemic blood pressure of 90 mmHg or higher and underwent echo within 24 h of diagnosis. The prevalence of RV dysfunction was 39%, and, on multivariate analysis, RV hypokinesis remained an independent predictor of 30-d mortality (hazard ratio, 1.94; 95% CI, 1.23–3.06) after adjusting for a number of clinical baseline parameters and the administration of thrombolytic agents.

Personally, I am convinced that transthoracic echo is a valuable nonexpensive bedside test that often yields prognostically relevant findings and may guide therapeutic decisions in many patients with acute PE, particularly in those who are not (yet) in cardiogenic shock at presentation. In fact, a recent randomized trial showed that early thrombolytic treatment of patients with submassive PE may prevent hemodynamic deterioration and obviate the need for emergency esacalation of treatment during the in-hospital period *(36)*. On the other hand, it is indeed appropriate and necessary to point out the limitations of this technique and the studies that were performed to validate it. These limitations include: (1) the diversity and lack of standardization of echocardiographic criteria (not only among various institutions, but also among examiners in the same hospital) for assessing the function of the right ventricle; (2) the need for an experienced echocardiographer on a round-the-clock basis; (3) the poor quality of transthoracic imaging in certain individuals, inconclusive findings in some individuals, particularly in those who are obese, on mechanical ventilation, or have severe pulmonary emphysema; and (4) the fact that transesophageal echo, which offers superior image resolution and the potential to visualize proximally located pulmonary artery thrombi, is poorly tolerated by most patients with acute PE. Finally, differential diagnosis between acute PE and chronic thromboembolic pulmonary hypertension may be particularly difficult, although some echocardiographic criteria have been proposed to distinguish between acute and chronic cor pulmonale *(37)*. Therefore, risk stratification strategies need to assess the value of further imaging and nonimaging procedures, which can either be used as an alternative to echo or in combination with ultrasound imaging to reliably confirm (or exclude) dysfunction of and/or injury to the right ventricle in submassive PE.

THE EMERGING ROLE OF CHEST COMPUTED TOMOGRAPHY (CT) AS AN ALTERNATIVE TO ECHOCARDIOGRAPHY

Four-chamber views of the heart on chest CT may, according to recent preliminary data, reliably detect right ventricular enlargement due to PE (Fig. 1C) and predict early death (*see also* Chapter 2). In a large retrospective series of 431 patients, Schoepf et al. found that 30-d mortality was 15.6% in patients with RV enlargement (reconstructed four-chamber views), defined as right/left ventricular dimension ratio greater than 0.9 (calculated by receiver operating characteristic analysis), on multidetector-row chest CT, compared to 7.7% in those without this finding *(38)*. Multivariate analysis revealed that RV enlargement independently predicted 30-d mortality (hazard ratio, 5.17; 95% CI, 1.63–16.35; $p = 0.005$). Thus, by analyzing a sufficiently large patient population, this study confirmed and extended the results of a previous retrospective analysis by the same group *(39)*. Another retrospective study on 120 patients evaluated the prognostic value of a predefined right/left ventricular short-axis diameter ratio of 1.0 during 3-mo follow-up *(40)*. The negative predictive value of a small right ventricle on helical CT was excellent, reaching 100%, whereas the positive predictive value of a right/left ventricular ratio greater than 1.0 for PE-related mortality was rather low (10.1%) and appeared to be inferior to a pulmonary artery obstruction index of 40% or higher. Of course, some important limitations of CT also need to be kept in mind. They include, besides the exposure to radiation and contrast medium, the inability to assess RV function in real time and thus the need to use RV enlargement as a surrogate parameter. Nevertheless, if these encouraging data are confirmed by further, prospective studies, multidetector-row chest CT may become a reasonable alternative to echo for diagnosing RV dysfunction in many institutions. This is particularly important, because this imaging technique does not share the limitations and uncertainties of echo (mentioned in the previous section) and is currently evolving into the gold standard in the diagnostic workup of patients with suspected PE *(41)* (*see* Chapter 7). Therefore, CT has the potential to become the link between diagnostic and risk stratification strategies in this setting.

BEYOND RV IMAGING: CARDIAC BIOMARKERS
Cardiac Troponins I and T

A number of studies published between 2000 and 2003 *(42–45)* and comprehensively summarized by Kucher and Goldhaber *(46)* demonstrated that elevated cardiac troponin I (TnI) or T (TnT) levels, which are sensitive indicators of myocardial cell damage and microscopic myocardial necrosis, are found in 11 to 50% of patients with acute PE. Cardiac troponin elevation correlated with the presence of RV dysfunction on echo and exhibited a very high (97–100%) negative predictive value with regard to death or complication risk in the acute phase. This implies that normal troponin levels on admission may suffice to *rule out* an adverse outcome in patients with PE *(46)*. Subsequent studies *(47–49)* added further evidence to support the prognostic importance of cardiac troponins in PE.

Because the critical (and controversial) issue is, as previously emphasized, early risk stratification of normotensive patients and thus prevention (rather than treatment) of cardiogenic shock, a recent study by Douketis et al. focused on the subpopulation of hemodynamically stable patients with nonmassive PE *(50)*. The study population (458 patients) was derived from a large randomized trial that investigated the benefits of fondaparinux treatment in patients with acute symptomatic PE *(51)*. The authors found that 14% of the study patients without clinical evidence of RV dysfunction had TnI levels greater than 0.5 ng/mL within 24 h of presentation. Importantly, this elevation was associated with an increased risk of all-cause death during the 3-mo follow-up period (OR, 3.5; 5% CI, 1.0–11.9), although it did not appear to affect the risk of recurrent venous thromboembolism. Thus, in view of the available data, there can be little doubt that cardiac troponin levels are a useful laboratory parameter and should be integrated into a risk stratification algorithm for patients presenting with acute PE.

The limitations of troponin testing also need to be kept in mind. For example, despite some reports presenting cardiac troponins as independent predictors of mortality *(48)*, the overall positive predictive value of these biomarkers is low, ranging between 12 and 44% *(46)*. Therefore, troponin elevation alone may not be sufficient to predict *(rule in)* early death or major complications in patients with acute PE, and it cannot, by itself, identify hemodynamically stable patients who may benefit from thrombolytic treatment. Moreover, and importantly, it has been shown both in patients with acute coronary syndromes *(52)* and in those with acute PE *(53,54)* that cardiac troponin elevation may not occur until 6–12 h after the onset of symptoms. Consequently, the troponin levels measured on admission may not suffice for assessment of prognosis and guidance of early therapeutic decisions. Instead, repeated troponin measurements over the first 24 h of hospitalization may be necessary for reliable risk assessment *(44,53)*.

Natriuretic Peptides

Natriuretic peptides are released as a result of cardiomyocyte stretch and are very sensitive indicators of neurohormonal activation due to ventricular dysfunction (*see* Chapter 5). Both the biologically active C-terminal peptide 77-108 (BNP) and the inactive N-terminal fragment 1-76 (NT-proBNP) are detectable in human plasma, and their levels have been determined and evaluated in patients presenting with acute PE *(55–58)*. NT-proBNP exhibits more pronounced increments and a wider spectrum of plasma concentrations compared to BNP, thus offering the theoretical advantage of more precise assessment of the severity of heart failure *(59)*. However, the clinical relevance of this difference is probably negligible. In general, both BNP and NT-proBNP are characterized by extreme prognostic sensitivity and a negative prognostic value that is probably even higher than that of the cardiac troponins and approaches or equals 100% *(46)*. This fact makes natriuretic petides, at least theoretically, a valuable tool for the initial triage of hemodynamically stable patients with acute PE, and particularly for ruling out a high death or complication risk during the in-hospital phase. On the other hand, their high sensitivity goes at the cost of a very low specificity and a disappointingly low positive prognostic value in the range of 12 to 25%. In fact, two recent trials reported that BNP elevation alone does not independently predict (rule in) mortality or in-hospital complications in PE *(53,60)*. Furthermore, the appropriate cut-off levels for distinguishing between a "positive" and a "negative" BNP or NT-proBNP test remain rather arbitrary, as they have not yet been prospectively validated *(61)*.

Other Biomarkers

Fatty acid-binding proteins (FABPs) are relatively small cytoplasmic proteins (12–15 kDa) that are abundant in tissues with active fatty acid metabolism, including the heart *(62)*. In fact, heart-type FABP (H-FABP) is particularly important for myocardial homeostasis, because 50–80% of the heart's energy is provided by lipid oxidation, and H-FABP ensures intracellular transport of insoluble fatty acids *(63)*. Following myocardial cell damage, this small protein diffuses much more rapidly than troponins through the interstitial space and appears in the circulation as early as 90 min after symptom onset, reaching its peak within 6 h *(63)*. These features make H-FABP an excellent candidate marker of myocardial injury *(64)*, and very recent data suggested that it may indeed provide prognostic information superior to that of cardiac troponins in the early hours of acute coronary syndromes *(65,66)*. In 107 consecutive patients with proven PE, we compared the prognostic value of H-FABP to that of cardiac TnT and NT-proBNP (Puls et al., unpublished data). The end points were major PE-related complications and overall in-hospital mortality. Overall, 29 patients (27%) had abnormal (>6 ng/mL) H-FABP levels at presentation. Of those, 12 (41%) had a complicated course, whereas none of the patients with normal baseline H-FABP experienced PE-related complications (mean OR, 71.45; $p <$ 0.0001). On multivariate analysis, H-FABP (OR, 36.74; $p < 0.0001$) but not cTnT ($p = 0.13$)

or NT-proBNP ($p = 0.36$) remained an independent predictor of overall mortality or PE-related complications. Thus, H-FABP is a promising and, importantly, a very early indicator of RV injury and dysfunction in acute PE.

EMERGING ALGORITHMS
FOR IMPROVING THE DIAGNOSIS OF RV DYSFUNCTION
Cardiac Biomarkers Followed by Imaging Procedures

In a recently published study *(53)*, our group hypothesized that combination of biomarker testing with ECG might improve the prognostic specificity of either method alone and help identify not only the low-risk but also the high-risk patients with PE. In this study of 124 patients, it was confirmed that a negative TnT test or "low" (<1,000 pg/mL) NT-proBNP levels over the first 24 h after admission virtually excluded an adverse outcome. Importantly, the risk of an adverse outcome increased 10-fold in patients with both an elevation of TnT levels and RV dysfunction on echo (15% of the total study population; $p = 0.004$). Similarly, patients with both an elevation of circulating NT-proBNP and an abnormal echocardiogram had a more than 12-fold increase of in-hospital death or complication risk ($p = 0.002$). These results are in agreement with those reported by Scridon et al. in a retrospective study that examined the prognostic significance of combined TnI testing and echo in 141 patients *(67)*. In this latter report, the combination of elevated troponin and RV enlargement predicted a high mortality risk in *normotensive* patients with PE (hazard ratio in this group, 5.6; 95% CI, 1.2–25.9).

Beyond the established biomarkers, i.e., the cardiac troponins and natriuretic peptides discussed in detail previously, our recent data (Puls et al. 2006; submitted) suggest that heart-type fatty acid-binding protein may be particularly suitable for combination with ECG as part of a risk stratification algorithm. In this study, cardiac ultrasound offered no additional prognostic information and was thus "unnecessary" in the presence of a negative H-FABP test, because all of these patients had an excellent short-term outcome. On the other hand, in patients with high H-FABP levels (>6 ng/mL) on admission (27% of the entire study population), complication rates doubled and the relative risk of an adverse outcome was four times higher in the presence of RV dysfunction on echo.

CONCLUSIONS

Despite the accumulating evidence that RV dysfunction may identify a high-risk group among hemodynamically stable, i.e., normotensive patients with PE, the therapeutic implications of this finding remain uncertain *(11,12)*. To date, only one prospective randomized trial tested the hypothesis that early thrombolytic treatment could improve the in-hospital outcome of patients with RV dysfunction *(36)*. In that study, the incidence of in-hospital mortality or need for escalation of treatment was significantly lower in patients treated with heparin plus alteplase compared to those who received heparin plus placebo. However, mortality was low in both treatment groups, and the reduction in the need for treatment escalation (mostly secondary thrombolysis) has not been widely accepted as definitive evidence favoring early thrombolytic treatment in this setting. The recent data summarized in this chapter indicate that we now have much more accurate and reliable parameters for detecting and assessing RV dysfunction in acute PE. In particular, a new concept is emerging that supports combination of biomarker testing with RV imaging procedures as a part of risk stratification algorithms *(46)* (Fig. 2). Thus, it appears that the time has come for a

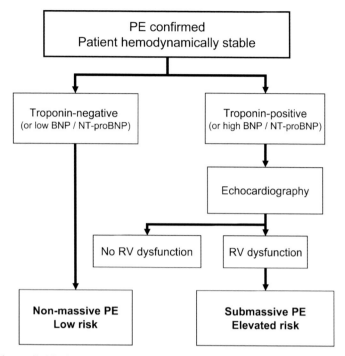

Fig. 2. Currently available data support a risk stratification algorithm for hemodynamically stable patients with proved pulmonary embolism (PE). Natriuretic peptide (BNP or NT-proBNP) or, preferably, troponin I or T testing should be followed by echocardiography only if the cardiac biomarker is abnormally elevated. Patients with a negative biomarker test can be classified as having a low risk of PE-related in-hospital complications and mortality, and they can safely be treated with anticoagulation alone. On the other hand, it remains unclear whether higher-risk patients with an abnormal biomarker test and a positive echocardiogram (submassive PE) necessitate thrombolytic treatment. (Modified from ref. *43*).

large international multicenter study that will use a contemporary inclusion algorithm and assess prognostically relevant end points (e.g., death or hemodynamic collapse) in order to resolve the long-standing debate on the (possible) benefits of thrombolysis in normotensive patients with PE and RV dysfunction (*see* Chapter 10). This trial is planned to begin in 2006 and is expected to enroll up to 1000 patients in North America and Europe.

REFERENCES

1. McIntyre KM, Sasahara AA. Determinants of right ventricular function and hemodynamics after pulmonary embolism. Chest 1974;65:534–543.
2. McIntyre KM, Sasahara AA. The hemodynamic response to pulmonary embolism in patients without prior cardiopulmonary disease. Am J Cardiol 1971;28:288–294.
3. Lualdi JC, Goldhaber SZ. Right ventricular dysfunction after acute pulmonary embolism: pathophysiologic factors, detection, and therapeutic implications. Am Heart J 1995;130:1276–1282.
4. Kasper W, Konstantinides S, Geibel A, et al. Management strategies and determinants of outcome in acute major pulmonary embolism: results of a multicenter registry [see comments]. J Am Coll Cardiol 1997;30:1165–1171.
5. European Society of Cardiology TFoPE. Guidelines on diagnosis and management of acute pulmonary embolism. Eur Heart J 2000;21:1301–336.
6. British Thoracic Society. Guidelines for the management of suspected acute pulmonary embolism. Thorax 2003;58:470–483.

7. Kucher N, Goldhaber SZ. Management of massive pulmonary embolism. Circulation 2005;112:e28–e32.

8. Jerjes-Sanchez C, Ramírez-Rivera A, de Lourdes G, et al. Streptokinase and heparin versus heparin alone in massive pulmonary embolism: a randomized controlled trial. J Thromb Thrombolysis 1995; 2:227–229.

9. Dalen JE. Thrombolysis in submassive pulmonary embolism? No. J Thromb Haemost 2003;1:1130–1132.

10. Konstantinides S. Thrombolysis in submassive pulmonary embolism? Yes. J Thromb Haemost 2003;1: 1127–1129.

11. Goldhaber SZ. Thrombolytic therapy for patients with pulmonary embolism who are hemodynamically stable but have right ventricular dysfunction: Pro. Arch Intern Med 2005;165:2197–2199.

12. Thabut G, Logeart D. Thrombolysis for pulmonary embolism in patients with right ventricular dysfunction: Con. Arch Intern Med 2005;165:2200–2203.

13. Thabut G, Thabut D, Myers RP, et al. Thrombolytic therapy of pulmonary embolism: a meta-analysis. J Am Coll Cardiol 2002;40:1660–1667.

14. Wan S, Quinlan DJ, Agnelli G, Eikelboom JW. Thrombolysis compared with heparin for the initial treatment of pulmonary embolism: a meta-analysis of the randomized controlled trials. Circulation 2004; 110:744–749.

15. Daniel KR, Courtney DM, Kline JA. Assessment of cardiac stress from massive pulmonary embolism with 12-lead ECG. Chest 2001;120:474–481.

16. Ferrari E, Imbert A, Chevalier T, Mihoubi A, Morand P, Baudouy M. The ECG in pulmonary embolism. Predictive value of negative T waves in precordial leads—80 case reports [see comments]. Chest 1997; 111:537–543.

17. Stein PD, Dalen JE, McIntyre KM, Sasahara AA, Wenger NK, Willis PW III. The electrocardiogram in acute pulmonary embolism. Prog Cardiovasc Dis 1975;17:247–257.

18. Geibel A, Zehender M, Kasper W, Olschewski M, Klima C, Konstantinides SV. Prognostic value of the ECG on admission in patients with acute major pulmonary embolism. Eur Respir J 2005;25:843–848.

19. Kasper W, Konstantinides S, Geibel A, et al. Management strategies and determinants of outcome in acute major pulmonary embolism: results of a multicenter registry [see comments]. J Am Coll Cardiol 1997;30:1165–1171.

20. Wood KE. Major pulmonary embolism: review of a pathophysiologic approach to the golden hour of hemodynamically significant pulmonary embolism. Chest 2002;121:877–905.

21. Sreeram N, Cheriex EC, Smeets JL, Gorgels AP, Wellens HJ. Value of the 12-lead electrocardiogram at hospital admission in the diagnosis of pulmonary embolism. Am J Cardiol 1994;73:298–303.

22. Kasper W, Meinertz T, Henkel B, et al. Echocardiographic findings in patients with proved pulmonary embolism. Am Heart J 1986;112:1284–1290.

23. Come PC, Kim D, Parker JA, Goldhaber SZ, Braunwald E, Markis JE. Early reversal of right ventricular dysfunction in patients with acute pulmonary embolism after treatment with intravenous tissue plasminogen activator. J Am Coll Cardiol 1987;10:971–978.

24. Jardin F, Dubourg O, Gueret P, Delorme G, Bourdarias JP. Quantitative two-dimensional echocardiography in massive pulmonary embolism: emphasis on ventricular interdependence and leftward septal displacement. J Am Coll Cardiol 1987;10:1201–1206.

25. Goldhaber SZ. Echocardiography in the management of pulmonary embolism. Ann Intern Med 2002; 136:691–700.

26. Goldhaber SZ. Pulmonary embolism. Lancet 2004;363:1295–1305.

27. Vieillard-Baron A, Page B, Augarde R, et al. Acute cor pulmonale in massive pulmonary embolism: incidence, echocardiographic pattern, clinical implications and recovery rate. Intensive Care Med 2001; 27:1481–1486.

28. Grifoni S, Olivotto I, Cecchini P, et al. Short-term clinical outcome of patients with acute pulmonary embolism, normal blood pressure, and echocardiographic right ventricular dysfunction. Circulation 2000; 101:2817–2822.

29. Ribeiro A, Lindmarker P, Johnsson H, Juhlin-Dannfelt A, Jorfeldt L. Pulmonary embolism: one-year follow-up with echocardiography doppler and five-year survival analysis [see comments]. Circulation 1999;99:1325–1330.

30. Kasper W, Konstantinides S, Geibel A, Tiede N, Krause T, Just H. Prognostic significance of right ventricular afterload stress detected by echocardiography in patients with clinically suspected pulmonary embolism. Heart 1997;77:346–349.

31. ten Wolde M, Sohne M, Quak E, Mac Gillavry MR, Buller HR. Prognostic value of echocardiographically assessed right ventricular dysfunction in patients with pulmonary embolism. Arch Intern Med 2004; 164:1685–1689.

32. Hamel E, Pacouret G, Vincentelli D, et al. Thrombolysis or heparin therapy in massive pulmonary embolism with right ventricular dilation: results from a 128-patient monocenter registry. Chest 2001;120: 120–125.
33. Konstantinides S, Geibel A, Olschewski M, et al. Association between thrombolytic treatment and the prognosis of hemodynamically stable patients with major pulmonary embolism: results of a multicenter registry. Circulation 1997;96:882–888.
34. Kucher N, Rossi E, De Rosa M, Goldhaber SZ. Prognostic role of echocardiography among patients with acute pulmonary embolism and a systolic arterial pressure of 90 mm Hg or higher. Arch Intern Med 2005;165:1777–1781.
35. Goldhaber SZ, Visani L, De Rosa M. Acute pulmonary embolism: clinical outcomes in the International Cooperative Pulmonary Embolism Registry (ICOPER). Lancet 1999;353:1386–1389.
36. Konstantinides S, Geibel A, Heusel G, Heinrich F, Kasper W. Heparin plus alteplase compared with heparin alone in patients with submassive pulmonary embolism. N Engl J Med 2002;347:1143–1150.
37. Kasper W, Geibel A, Tiede N, et al. Distinguishing between acute and subacute massive pulmonary embolism by conventional and Doppler echocardiography. Br Heart J 1993;70:352–356.
38. Schoepf UJ, Kucher N, Kipfmueller F, Quiroz R, Costello P, Goldhaber SZ. Right ventricular enlargement on chest computed tomography: a predictor of early death in acute pulmonary embolism. Circulation 2004;110:3276–3280.
39. Quiroz R, Kucher N, Schoepf UJ, et al. Right ventricular enlargement on chest computed tomography: prognostic role in acute pulmonary embolism. Circulation 2004;109:2401–2404.
40. van der Meer RW, Pattynama PM, van Strijen MJ, et al. Right ventricular dysfunction and pulmonary obstruction index at helical CT: prediction of clinical outcome during 3-month follow-up in patients with acute pulmonary embolism. Radiology 2005;235:798–803.
41. Perrier A, Roy PM, Sanchez O, et al. Multidetector-row computed tomography in suspected pulmonary embolism. N Engl J Med 2005;352:1760–1768.
42. Janata K, Holzer M, Laggner AN, Mullner M. Cardiac troponin T in the severity assessment of patients with pulmonary embolism: cohort study. BMJ 2003;326:312–313.
43. Pruszczyk P, Bochowicz A, Torbicki A, et al. Cardiac troponin T monitoring identifies high-risk group of normotensive patients with acute pulmonary embolism. Chest 2003;123:1947–1952.
44. Konstantinides S, Geibel A, Olschewski M, et al. Importance of cardiac troponins I and T in risk stratification of patients with acute pulmonary embolism. Circulation 2002;106:1263–1268.
45. Giannitsis E, Muller-Bardorff M, Kurowski V, et al. Independent prognostic value of cardiac troponin T in patients with confirmed pulmonary embolism. Circulation 2000;102:211–217.
46. Kucher N, Goldhaber SZ. Cardiac biomarkers for risk stratification of patients with acute pulmonary embolism. Circulation 2003;108:2191–2194.
47. Bova C, Crocco F, Ricchio R, Serafini O, Greco F, Noto A. Importance of troponin T for the risk stratification of normotensive patients with pulmonary embolism. A prospective, cohort study with a three-month follow-up. Haematologica 2005;90:423–424.
48. La Vecchia L, Ottani F, Favero L, et al. Increased cardiac troponin I on admission predicts in-hospital mortality in acute pulmonary embolism. Heart 2004;90:633–637.
49. Yalamanchili K, Sukhija R, Aronow WS, Sinha N, Fleisher AG, Lehrman SG. Prevalence of increased cardiac troponin I levels in patients with and without acute pulmonary embolism and relation of increased cardiac troponin I levels with in-hospital mortality in patients with acute pulmonary embolism. Am J Cardiol 2004;93:263–264.
50. Douketis JD, Leeuwenkamp O, Grobara P, et al. The incidence and prognostic significance of elevated cardiac troponins in patients with submassive pulmonary embolism. J Thromb Haemost 2005;3:508–513.
51. Buller HR, Davidson BL, Decousus H, et al. Subcutaneous fondaparinux versus intravenous unfractionated heparin in the initial treatment of pulmonary embolism. N Engl J Med 2003;349:1695–1702.
52. Gibler WB, Cannon CP, Blomkalns AL, et al. Practical implementation of the Guidelines for Unstable Angina/Non-ST-Segment Elevation Myocardial Infarction in the emergency department. Ann Emerg Med 2005;46:185–197.
53. Binder L, Pieske B, Olschewski M, et al. N-terminal pro-brain natriuretic peptide or troponin testing followed by echocardiography for risk stratification of acute pulmonary embolism. Circulation 2005; 112:1573–1579.
54. Muller-Bardorff M, Weidtmann B, Giannitsis E, Kurowski V, Katus HA. Release kinetics of cardiac troponin T in survivors of confirmed severe pulmonary embolism. Clin Chem 2002;48:673–675.

55. Kucher N, Printzen G, Doernhoefer T, Windecker S, Meier B, Hess OM. Low pro-brain natriuretic peptide levels predict benign clinical outcome in acute pulmonary embolism. Circulation 2003;107: 1576–1578.

56. Kucher N, Printzen G, Goldhaber SZ. Prognostic role of brain natriuretic peptide in acute pulmonary embolism. Circulation 2003;107(20):2545–2547.

57. Pruszczyk P, Kostrubiec M, Bochowicz A, et al. N-terminal pro-brain natriuretic peptide in patients with acute pulmonary embolism. Eur Respir J 2003;22:649–653.

58. ten Wolde M, Tulevski II, Mulder JW, et al. Brain natriuretic peptide as a predictor of adverse outcome in patients with pulmonary embolism. Circulation 2003;107:2082–2084.

59. Richards AM, Nicholls MG, Yandle TG, et al. Plasma N-terminal pro-brain natriuretic peptide and adreno-medullin: new neurohormonal predictors of left ventricular function and prognosis after myocardial infarction. Circulation 1998;97:1921–1929.

60. Krüger S, Graf J, Merx MW, et al. Brain natriuretic peptide predicts right heart failure in patients with acute pulmonary embolism. Am Heart J 2004;147:60–65.

61. Giannitsis E, Katus HA. Risk stratification in pulmonary embolism based on biomarkers and echocardiography. Circulation 2005;112:1520–1521.

62. Storch J, Thumser AE. The fatty acid transport function of fatty acid-binding proteins. Biochim Biophys Acta 2000;1486:28–44.

63. Alhadi HA, Fox KA. Do we need additional markers of myocyte necrosis: the potential value of heart fatty-acid-binding protein. QJM 2004;97:187–198.

64. Pelsers MM, Hermens WT, Glatz JF. Fatty acid-binding proteins as plasma markers of tissue injury. Clin Chim Acta 2005;352:15–35.

65. Ishii J, Ozaki Y, Lu J, et al. Prognostic value of serum concentration of heart-type fatty acid-binding protein relative to cardiac troponin T on admission in the early hours of acute coronary syndrome. Clin Chem 2005;51:1397–1404.

66. Kilcullen N, Das R, Morrell C, Barth JH, Hall AS. Heart-type fatty acid-binding protein predicts long-term mortality in troponin-negative patients with acute coronary syndrome [abstr]. Circulation 2005;112 (Suppl II):II–388.

67. Scridon T, Scridon C, Skali H, Alvarez A, Goldhaber SZ, Solomon SD. Prognostic significance of troponin elevation and right ventricular enlargement in acute pulmonary embolism. Am J Cardiol 2005; 96:303–305.

5

Cardiac Biomarkers in the Diagnostic Workup of Pulmonary Embolism

Evangelos Giannitsis, MD
and Hugo A. Katus, MD

CONTENTS

SUMMARY

Confirmation of pulmonary embolism (PE) must be followed by risk stratification in order to obtain information on short-term prognosis and determine the need for more aggressive therapy such as thrombolysis or surgical/interventional embolectomy. The cardiospecific troponins, I and T, and the brain-type natriuretic peptide (BNP) or its biologically inactive N-terminal fragment, NT-pro BNP, are frequently elevated in PE. Although the exact mechanisms are still unknown, there is a link between the presence of cardiac troponins, BNP, or NT-pro BNP in blood and the presence and severity of right ventricular dysfunction resulting from PE. Thus, absence of cardiac troponin or natriuretic peptide elevation is associated with a benign clinical course that justifies conservative treatment, i.e., heparin anticoagulation followed by oral vitamin K antagonists. On the other hand, the presence of elevated cardiac troponins, BNP, or NT-pro BNP does not necessarily predict an adverse outcome when biomarker tests are used alone for risk stratification of PE. The following chapter presents an overview of the pathophysiology and prevalence of elevated biomarkers in PE and summarizes the evidence supporting a novel risk stratification algorithm based on biomarker testing and echocardiography or other imaging modalities.

Key Words: Cardiac troponins; natriuretic peptides; right ventricular dysfunction; prognosis.

From: *Contemporary Cardiology: Management of Acute Pulmonary Embolism*
Edited by: S. Konstantinides © Humana Press Inc., Totowa, NJ

INTRODUCTION

Traditionally, cardiac biomarkers have been used for classification and risk stratification of suspected acute coronary syndromes, and for retrospective confirmation of acute myocardial infarction. More recently however, cardiac troponins and the natriuretic peptides BNP and NT-pro BNP were also shown to be useful for risk stratification of patients with confirmed pulmonary embolism (PE). The following chapter will summarize the results of contemporary clinical trials on cardiac troponins and natriuretic peptides with regard to risk assessment in the setting of acute PE, and discuss how these biomarker results might be integrated into the management strategy of patients with PE.

PATHOMECHANISM OF BIOMARKER RELEASE IN ACUTE PE

Cardiac Troponins

As explained in the previous chapter, embolization of thrombotic material into the pulmonary artery leads to an acute increase of pulmonary vascular resistance, which, in turn, increases right-ventricular afterload and causes right-ventricular dysfunction. Reduced right-ventricular output and shift of the interventricular septum may impair left-ventricular performance, resulting in systemic hypotension. Impaired coronary perfusion and reduced oxygen supply ultimately cause myocardial ischemia, which is amplified in a vicious cycle *(1)*. As a consequence of myocardial damage, the cardiac troponins T (cTnT) and I (cTnI) are released into the circulation.

Whether troponin release is due to irreversible myocardial damage or, rather, to membrane leakage following severe but reversible myocardial ischemia remains speculative at present. In principle, cTnT and cTnI are structurally bound to the myofilaments. Only a small cytosolic fraction of approx 6 and 3%, respectively, is unbound, and it is released prior to the degradation of the structurally bound troponin after ischemic injury *(2)*. Thus, in patients with large acute myocardial infarction, cTnT and cTnI appear in the blood as soon as 2 h after the onset of ischemia and persist for at least 10 d *(2,3)*. In PE, however, the release pattern of troponins is distinct from that seen in patients with large non-ST segment elevation (NSTEMI) or ST-segment elevation myocardial infarction (STEMI). For example, in an observational study, cTnT levels were measured consecutively in nine patients who survived confirmed moderate or severe PE. In these patients, cTnT was detectable only for 1 to 3 d after the index event *(4)*. The peak concentrations were quantitatively lower than typically observed in STEMI (Fig. 1). These findings have generated the hypothesis that only the structurally unbound troponin pool is being released in PE unless true right-ventricular infarction complicates the thromboembolic event *(5)*. Regardless of the exact pathomechanism of troponin release, the narrow diagnostic window must be kept in mind when using this biomarker for risk stratification of patients with suspected or confirmed PE *(4,6,7)*. Finally, although the prognostic value of cTnI is superior to that of cTnT in particular settings such as chronic renal failure *(8)*, there appear to be no appreciable clinical differences between cTnT and cTnI with regard to evaluation of the severity of PE *(6)*.

Natriuretic Peptides

The principal stimulus for brain natriuretic peptide (BNP) synthesis and secretion is cardiomyocyte stress *(9)*. After *de novo* synthesis, the prohormone is cleaved within the

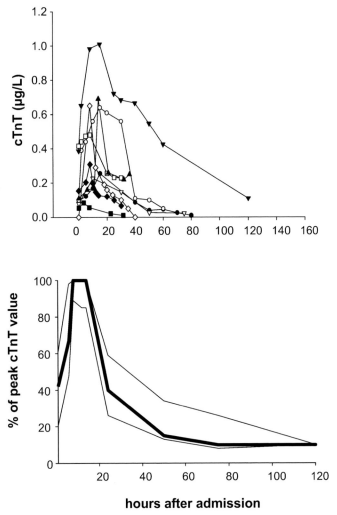

Fig. 1. Upper panel displays the release of cTnT over time in nine patients surviving acute PE. The lower panel displays the time release of cTnT relative to peak levels over time (values are given as percentage of peak).

cardiomyocyte, and equal amounts of the biologically active neuropeptide, BNP, and the inactive signal peptide, N-terminal (NT)-pro BNP, are secreted into the blood. Abnormal natriuretic peptide levels are not specific for acute PE and are also increased in other conditions associated with right ventricular pressure overload including primary pulmonary hypertension, chronic thromboembolic pulmonary hypertension, and chronic lung disease *(10–12)*.

There are considerable differences between NT-pro BNP and BNP with respect to biological activity, plasma clearance and half-life times, as well as preanalytical and analytical properties *(13)*. Nevertheless, head-to-head comparison of BNP and NT-pro BNP demonstrates that both peptides are principally suitable for evaluation of the severity of PE without appreciable differences in clinical practice *(14,15)*.

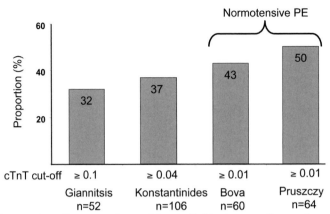

Fig. 2. Prevalence of cardiac troponin-positive individuals according to the cut-off applied.

FREQUENCY OF DETECTABLE BIOMARKER LEVELS IN PE AND CORRELATION WITH RIGHT VENTRICULAR FUNCTION

Cardiac Troponins

The proportion of patients with PE who have increased cardiac troponin levels is strongly related to the diagnostic cutoff levels chosen. In a series by our own group, 16 of 56 patients (32%) were classified as cTnT-positive using a diagnostic cut-off of 0.1 μg/L *(16)*. Subsequently, the use of more sensitive assays allowed application of lower diagnostic cut-off levels. Accordingly, the prevalence of troponin-positive individuals increased to values between 37 and 50%, even among normotensive patients *(6,16–18)* (Fig. 2).

cTnT or cTnI offers several advantages compared to creatine kinase (CK) or CK-MB, including cardiospecificity (increases exclusively resulting from myocardial damage) and superior diagnostic sensitivity. Accordingly, less than half of the patients with detectable cardiac troponin levels have CK or CK-MB levels greater than the upper reference limit *(6,16,17)*.

As proof of concept, several studies established that increased cardiac troponin levels were closely associated with the presence of right ventricular dysfunction in PE *(6,16,19, 20)*. We examined 56 consecutive patients with PE and found that all patients with elevated cTnT had echocardiographic (echo) evidence for right ventricular dysfunction, whereas only 66% of the patients without cTnT elevation had right ventricular dysfunction on transthoracic echo *(16)*. Moreover, right ventricular dimensions were larger (36 vs 33 mm, $p = 0.05$) in patients with troponin elevation than in those without detectable biomarker in the circulation (Fig. 3). In agreement with these findings, Meyer et al. studied 36 patients with acute PE and reported that 63% of those with right ventricular dilation had increased cTnI levels. From a different perspective, only 29% of cTnI-positive patients had normal right ventricular dimensions *(19)*. Moreover, patients with positive cTnI tests had a significantly larger number of segmental defects on ventilation/ perfusion scan than patients with normal serum troponin I. In another study, Konstantinides et al. enrolled 106 consecutive patients with acute PE and confirmed that cTnT or cTnI were closely associated with right ventricular dysfunction on echo *(6)*. Thus, a substantial body of evidence has established beyond doubt that elevation of cTnT or cTnI is fre-

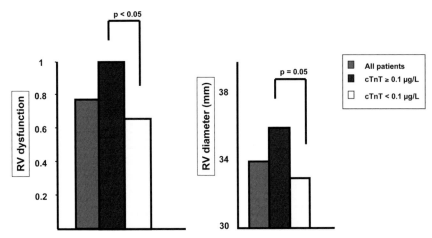

Fig. 3. Association between right ventricular dysfunction and right ventricular dimensions with cTnT.

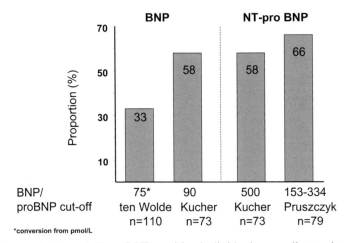

Fig. 4. Prevalence of BNP or NT-proBNP-positive individuals according to the cut-off applied.

quently present in *submassive* PE and may be regarded as a surrogate for right ventricular dysfunction or right ventricular enlargement.

BNP/NT-pro BNP

As with cardiac troponins, the proportion of patients with abnormal NT-pro BNP levels is inversely related to the diagnostic cut-off levels used. Hence, the frequency of a positive BNP or NT-pro BNP test result varies between 33 and 66% in patients with PE (Fig. 4). BNP concentrations indicating right ventricular strain are seemingly lower than cut-off levels used in the setting of congestive left heart failure. Applying a BNP concentration threshold of 50 or 90 ng/mL allows identification of right ventricular dysfunction (64 vs 6%) or enlargement with high sensitivity *(15,21)*. Likewise, a receiver operating curve (ROC)-determined NT-pro BNP level greater than 500 pg/mL was associated with higher rates of right ventricular dysfunction (76 vs 3%, $p < 0.001$) and greater dimensions (45 vs 38 mm, $p < 0.001$) of the right ventricle *(14)*. Thus, like cardiac troponins, elevated levels of BNP or NT-pro BNP can serve as surrogates of right ventricular dysfunction.

Table 1
Overview of Cardiac Troponin Studies in PE

Reference	Marker	n	Cut-off	Tested +	NPV	PPV
Giannitsis	cTnT	56	0.1	32	97	44
Konstantinides	cTnT	106	0.04	37	97	12
Janata	cTnT	106	0.09	11	99	34
Pruszczyk	cTnT	64	0.01	50	100	25
Konstantinides	cTnT	106	0.07	41	98	14

The table displays numbers of patients, cut-off levels, prevalence, and positive and negative predictive values. NPV, negative predictive value; PPV, positive predictive value.

PROGNOSTIC IMPLICATIONS

Cardiac Troponins

Numerous studies and registries have shown that the presence of right ventricular dysfunction is associated with an adverse prognosis, even in initially normotensive patients with PE (22–25). Despite the fact that, as mentioned previously, a strong correlation exists between the presence of right ventricular dysfunction (as confirmed by echo) and the release of cardiac troponins in the circulation, several studies have suggested that elevation of cTnT or cTnI may confer additive and independent prognostic information with respect to in-hospital complications and death (6,16). Detectable troponin levels were associated with higher rates of in-hospital death and complications, and the risk of an adverse outcome increased in proportion to the magnitude of troponin release (6). However, the overall specificity is rather low, and the positive predictive value of cardiac troponins for identification of a high-risk patient is only 12 to 44% (6,16,17,20) (Table 1). Notably, recent data suggest that combining the troponin test with echo imaging of the right ventricle may increase the positive predictive value of the biomarker (26). Scridon et al. examined 141 patients with PE and found that patients with both elevated troponin and right ventricular dysfunction were at higher risk of death at 30-d follow-up compared to those with only one or none of these findings (27). More recently, Binder et al. found that right ventricular dysfunction combined with a positive biomarker test was associated with a 10-fold higher risk of suffering in-hospital complications related to PE (28). In contrast, neither the presence of right ventricular dysfunction on echo nor elevation of cTnT alone showed a significant excess risk. Thus, such a combined approach may prove useful for choosing the appropriate candidates for thrombolytic therapy.

In contrast to the difficulties arising from low specificity, a large body of evidence indicates that troponin testing is particularly helpful for identification of low-risk patients with PE, because absence of cardiac troponin elevation predicts a favorable in-hospital outcome with high sensitivity. The negative predictive values for ruling out life-threatening PE range between 97 and 100% (6,16,17,20) (Table 1).

The timing of blood collection for troponin testing appears crucial for proper risk stratification. Müller-Bardorff et al. reported on time-release curves of cTnT in nine patients surviving submassive PE and could show that cTnT was detectable only for a median duration of 30 h (4). Although there is currently no recommendation for the exact timing of blood collection, repeated blood sampling for cardiac troponin testing appears necessary

Table 2
Overview of BNP/NT-pro BNP Studies in PE

Reference	Marker	n	Cut-off	Tested +	NPV	PPV
Kucher	NT-pro BNP	73	500	58	100	12
Kucher	BNP	73	50	58	100	12
ten Wolde	BNP	110	21.7*	33	99	17
Pruszczyk	NT-pro BNP	79	153-334	66	100	23

The table displays number of patients, cut-off levels, prevalence, positive and negative predictive values. NPV, negative predictive value; PPV, positive predictive value.

All values given as pg/mL, except for [a]pmol/L.

during the early hospital course to avoid underestimation of risk from too early sampling. In addition, some underestimation may be expected in patients presenting late after the onset of symptoms.

BNP/NT-pro BNP

Acute right ventricular strain stimulates the secretion of BNP or NT-pro BNP. Several studies support the notion that "abnormal" increase of natriuretic peptide levels is associated with poor prognosis and higher in-hospital complication rates (14,15,29,30). For example, Kucher et al. measured NT-pro BNP in 73 patients with acute PE (14). Patients with an adverse outcome had higher NT-pro BNP levels than patients with an uneventful clinical course (4250 vs 121 pg/mL; $p < 0.0001$). A ROC-optimized cut-off level of 500 pg/mL remained independently predictive for adverse outcome after adjustment for cardiac troponin concentrations. However, the positive predictive value was only 45%. Likewise, increased BNP levels were higher in patients with adverse events compared to those with a favorable clinical course. The positive predictive value of BNP greater than 50 pg/mL was 57% (15). In another study, ten Wolde et al. reported on the role of BNP in 110 consecutive patients with PE (29). Rates of PE-related death increased with BNP concentrations; mortality rates were 16.7% in the highest BNP tertile (>21.7 pmol/L) and 2.7% in the intermediate tertile (2.5 to 21.7 pmol/L), whereas no deaths occurred in the lowest tertile (<2.5 pmol/L). Again, the positive predictive value of BNP was low (17%). Along with increased in-hospital mortality, abnormally high NT-pro BNP and BNP levels predict a more frequent need for inotropic drug support, mechanical ventilation, rescue thrombolytic therapy, or cardiopulmonary resuscitation (14,15,29).

Although (and as with troponin testing) the positive predictive value of abnormal natriuretic peptide levels alone appears to be disappointingly low (Table 2), it is tempting to speculate that the combination with transthoracic or transesophageal echo will improve the predictive power of BNP testing substantially (31). Very recent data from Binder et al. have nicely supported this hypothesis (28). Among 124 patients with proven PE, those with a combination of right ventricular dysfunction on echo and an elevation of NT-pro BNP greater than 1000 pg/mL had a more than 12-fold higher risk for a complicated in-hospital course. On the other hand, several recent studies have consistently shown that the negative predictive values of NT-pro BNP and BNP approach 100% (Table 2). Thus, the absence of natriuretic peptide elevation has appeared particularly helpful for ruling out life-threatening PE, and may be helpful for the identification of low-risk patients in whom conservative therapy is warranted.

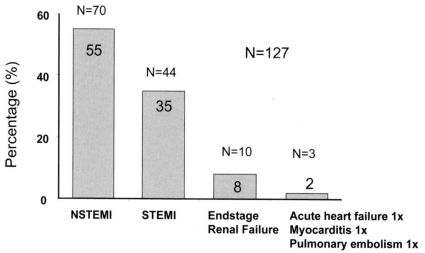

Fig. 5. Causes of cTnT elevation in patients with acute chest pain triaged in the emergency room (*n* = 127). Data from ref. *35*.

CAN BIOMARKER TESTING BE USED TO *DIAGNOSE* PE?

Elevation of cardiac troponins or natriuretic peptide levels is not restricted to patients with PE *(8)*. Although troponins are highly specific markers for cardiomyocyte damage, multiple clinical conditions, including, of course, acute coronary syndromes, are associated with elevation of their concentrations in blood. The diagnosis of acute myocardial infarction requires the presence of ischemic signs or symptoms in addition to a cardiac troponin concentration exceeding the 99th percentile of a healthy reference population *(32)*. In patients in whom an acute coronary syndrome can be ruled out, other causes of an abnormal troponin result should be considered.

The clinical presentation of acute PE is highly variable and sometimes oligosymptomatic. Therefore, the diagnosis of mild to moderate PE may be missed unless the diagnosis is actively persued. For this purpose, the use of clinical scoring systems like the Wells score or the Geneva score are considered helpful *(33,34)*. The number of patients with retrospectively confirmed PE that will be identified by chance from an abnormal troponin result has not been assessed systematically. According to the Bayes theorem, screening with cardiac troponins for PE is not very useful in patients admitted to an emergency department or chest pain unit with suspected acute coronary syndrome (Fig. 5). In contrast, screening for PE with cardiac troponins after, for instance, orthopedic surgery, may be useful given the high prevalence of venous thrombembolism in this setting. However, whether troponin testing might be helpful as part of a screening strategy in the postoperative setting has not been addressed by prospective studies. The possible role of natriuretic peptides for diagnosis of acute PE is even less clear than that of cardiac troponins, because BNP and NT-pro BNP lack cardiospecificity.

CONCLUSION

Cardiac troponins and the natriuretic peptides BNP and NT-pro BNP were consistently shown to be useful for risk stratification in acute PE. Both biomarkers allow identification of patients at higher risk for in-hospital death or a complicated clinical course. However, the low positive predictive value precludes the active selection of these patients for thrombolytic therapy. Combination of biomarker testing with ECG findings could be more useful for guiding therapeutic decisions, and this important issue will be addressed by a forthcoming international multicenter trial. On the other hand, both biomarkers, particularly BNP or NT-pro BNP, are characterized by a very high negative predictive value in the range of 97 to 100%. Thus, a negative result can be used to identify patients who are at low risk for death or clinical deterioration and should be treated conservatively. Finally, the usefulness of cardiac biomarker testing as part of a screening panel for diagnosis of PE is still unsettled. Theoretically, the measurement of cardiac troponin could be helpful in a clinical setting with a high prevalence of PE as, for example, after hip or knee surgery.

REFERENCES

1. Lualdi JC, Goldhaber SZ. Right ventricular dysfunction after acute pulmonary embolism: pathophysiologic factors, detection, and therapeutic implications. Am Heart J 1995;130:1276–1282.
2. Katus HA, Remppis A, Scheffold T, Diederich KW, Kuebler W. Intracellular compartmentation of cardiac troponin T and its release kinetics in patients with reperfused and nonreperfused myocardial infarction. Am J Cardiol 1991;67:1360–1367.
3. Giannitsis E, Katus HA. Comparison of cardiac troponin T and troponin I assays—implications of analytical and biochemical differences on clinical performance. Clin Lab 2004;50:521–528.
4. Muller-Bardorff M, Weidtmann B, Giannitsis E, et al. Release kinetics of cardiac troponin T in survivors of confirmed severe pulmonary embolism. Clin Chem 2002;48:673–675.
5. Coma-Canella I, Gamallo C, Martinez Onsurbe P, et al. Acute right ventricular infarction secondary to massive pulmonary embolism. Eur Heart J 1988;9:534–540.
6. Konstantinides S, Geibel A, Olschewski M, et al. Importance of cardiac troponins I and T in risk stratification of patients with acute pulmonary embolism. Circulation 2002;106:1263–1268.
7. Punukollu G, Khan IA, Gowda RM, Lakhanpal G, Vasavada BC, Sacchi TJ. Cardiac troponin I release in acute pulmonary embolism in relation to the duration of symptoms. Int J Cardiol 2005;99:207–211.
8. Hamm CW, Giannitsis E, Katus HA. Cardiac troponin elevations in patients without acute coronary syndrome. Circulation 2002;106:2871–2872.
9. Yasue H, Yoshimura M, Sumida H, et al. Localization and mechanism of secretion of B-type natriuretic peptide in comparison with those of A-type natriuretic peptide in normal subjects and patients with heart failure. Circulation 1994;90:195–203.
10. Nagaya N, Nishikimi T, Okano Y, et al. Plasma brain natriuretic peptide levels increase in proportion to the extent of right ventricular dysfunction in pulmonary hypertension. J Am Coll Cardiol 1998;31:202–208.
11. Bando M, Ishii Y, Sugiyama Y, Kitamura S. Elevated plasma brain natriuretic peptide levels in chronic respiratory failure with cor pulmonale. Respir Med 1999;93:507–514.
12. Nagaya N, Nishikimi T, Uematsu M, et al. Plasma brain natriuretic peptide as a prognostic indicator in patients with primary pulmonary hypertension. Circulation 2000;102:865–870.
13. Pfister R, Schneider CA. Natriuretic peptides BNP and NT-pro-BNP: established laboratory markers in clinical practice or just perspectives? Clin Chim Acta 2004;349:25–38.
14. Kucher N, Printzen G, Doernhoefer T, Windecker S, Meier B, Hess OM. Low pro-brain natriuretic peptide levels predict benign clinical outcome in acute pulmonary embolism. Circulation 2003;107:1576–1578.
15. Kucher N, Printzen G, Goldhaber SZ. Prognostic role of brain natriuretic peptide in acute pulmonary embolism. Circulation 2003;107:2545–2547.
16. Giannitsis E, Muller-Bardorff M, Lehrke S, et al. Independent prognostic value of cardiac troponin T in patients with confirmed pulmonary embolism. Circulation 2000;102:211–217.
17. Pruszczyk P, Bochowicz A, Torbicki A, et al. Cardiac troponin T monitoring identifies high-risk group of normotensive patients with acute pulmonary embolism. Chest 2003;123:1947–1952.
18. Bova C, Crocco F, Ricchio R, Serafini O, Greco F, Noto A. Importance of troponin T for the risk stratification of normotensive patients with pulmonary embolism. A prospective, cohort study with a three-month follow-up. Haematologica 2005;90:423–424.
19. Meyer T, Binder L, Hruska N, Luthe H, Buchwald AB. Cardiac troponin I elevation in acute pulmonary embolism is associated with right ventricular dysfunction. J Am Coll Cardiol 2000;36:1632–1636.

20. Janata K, Holzer A, Laggner AN, et al. Cardiac troponin T in the severity assessment of patients with pulmonary embolism: cohort study. BMJ 2003;326:312–313.
21. Kruger S, Graf J, Merx MW, et al. Brain natriuretic peptide predicts right heart failure in patients with acute pulmonary embolism. Am Heart J 2004;147:60–65.
22. Goldhaber SZ, Visani L, De Rosa M. Acute pulmonary embolism: clinical outcomes in the International Cooperative Pulmonary Embolism Registry (ICOPER). Lancet 1999;353:1386–1389.
23. Kasper W, Konstantinides S, Geibel A, Tiede N, Krause T, Just H. Prognostic significance of right ventricular afterload stress detected by echocardiography in patients with clinically suspected pulmonary embolism. Heart 1997;77:346–349.
24. Grifoni S, Olivotto I, Cecchini P, et al. Short-term clinical outcome of patients with acute pulmonary embolism, normal blood pressure, and echocardiographic right ventricular dysfunction. Circulation 2000;101:2817–2822.
25. Ribeiro A, Lindmarker P, Juhlin-Dannfelt A, et al. Echocardiography Doppler in pulmonary embolism: right ventricular dysfunction as a predictor of mortality rate. Am Heart J 1997;134:479–487.
26. Kucher N, Wallmann D, Carone A, et al. Incremental prognostic value of troponin I and echocardiography in patients with acute pulmonary embolism. Eur Heart J 2003;24:1651–1656.
27. Scridon T, Scridon C, Skali H, Alvarez A, Goldhaber SZ, Solomon SD. Prognostic significance of troponin elevation and right ventricular enlargement in acute pulmonary embolism. Am J Cardiol 2005;96: 303–305.
28. Binder L, Pieske B, Olschewski M, et al. N-terminal pro-brain natriuretic peptide or troponin testing followed by echocardiography for risk stratification of acute pulmonary embolism. Circulation 2005; 112:1573–1579.
29. ten Wolde M, Tulevski II, Mulder JW, et al. Brain natriuretic peptide as a predictor of adverse outcome in patients with pulmonary embolism. Circulation 2003;107:2082–2084.
30. Pruszczyk P, Kostrubiec M, Bochowicz A, et al. N-terminal pro-brain natriuretic peptide in patients with acute pulmonary embolism. Eur Respir J 2003;22:649–653.
31. Kucher N, Goldhaber SZ. Cardiac biomarkers for risk stratification of patients with acute pulmonary embolism. Circulation 2003;108:2191–2194.
32. Alpert JS, Thygesen K, Antman E, Bassand JP. Myocardial infarction redefined—a consensus document of The Joint European Society of Cardiology/American College of Cardiology Committee for the redefinition of myocardial infarction. J Am Coll Cardiol 2000;36:959–969.
33. Wells PS, Anderson DR, Rodger M, et al. Derivation of a simple model to categorize patients probability of pulmonary embolism: increasing the model's utility with the SimpliRED D-dimer. Thromb Haemost 2000;83:416–420.
34. Wicki J, Perneger TV, Junod AF, Bounameaux H, Perrier A. Assessing clinical probability of pulmonary embolism in the emergency ward: a simple score. Arch Intern Med 2001;161:92–97.
35. Hamm CW, Goldmann BU, Heeschen C, Kreymann G, Berger J, Meinertz T. Emergency room triage of patients with acute chest pain by means of rapid testing for cardiac troponin T or troponin I. N Engl J Med 1997;337:1648–1653.

6

Importance of a Patent Foramen Ovale

Annette Geibel, MD, Manfred Zehender, MD, and Wolfgang Kasper, MD

SUMMARY

Patent foramen ovale (PFO) is a relatively frequent remnant of the fetal circulation, causing transient right-to-left shunt. Its potential consequences include arterial hypoxemia and paradoxical embolism. Echocardiographic contrast imaging techniques make the detection of PFO possible during life. Over the past 20 yr, clinical research focused on the association between PFO and cryptogenic stroke, peripheral embolism, decompression sickness, platypnea-orthodeoxia, and fat embolism. However, although right-to-left shunt through a PFO can occur in the presence of normal right-side hemodynamics, patients with pulmonary embolism (PE) and elevated pressures in the right ventricle and atrium may be at particularly high risk to suffer hypoxemia and paradoxical embolism. In a study performed by our group, PFO was diagnosed in 35% of the patients with PE. These patients had an in-hospital death rate of 33% as opposed to 14% in patients without a PFO. Logistic regression analysis demonstrated that the only independent predictors of mortality were a PFO and arterial hypotension at presentation. Patients with a PFO also had a higher incidence of ischemic stroke and peripheral embolism. Moreover, significant differences were observed in arterial oxygen tension depending on the presence or absence of a PFO. Overall, the risk of a complicated in-hospital course was 5.2 times higher in patients with a PFO. Thus, in patients with PE and right ventricular dysfunction, PFO indicates a particularly high risk of death and arterial thromboembolic complications, and it is, in fact, one of the independent predictors of an adverse clinical outcome.

Key Words: Patent foramen ovale; echocardiography; paradoxical embolism; prognosis.

From: *Contemporary Cardiology: Management of Acute Pulmonary Embolism*
Edited by: S. Konstantinides © Humana Press Inc., Totowa, NJ

INTRODUCTION

The clinical relevance of patent foramen ovale (PFO), a relatively frequent remnant of fetal circulation *(1)*, has remained obscure for many decades. In fact, before the development of echocardiographic (echo) imaging techniques, detection of a PFO during life and clinical diagnosis of paradoxical embolism were rarely possible *(2,3)*. This was due to the fact that, since the first description of paradoxical embolism by Cohnheim in 1877 *(4)*, confirmation of the diagnosis essentially required the detection of a right atrial thrombus crossing the foramen ovale *(5)*. In fact, even with recent advances in noninvasive visualization of the cardiac cavities, direct observation of this phenomenon during life remains confined to isolated echo reports *(6,7)*. Thus, in clinical practice, the diagnosis of paradoxical embolism is almost always presumptive and relies on indirect signs such as the presence of a PFO and the diagnosis of arterial embolism *(5,8,9)*. During the past 20 yr, initial studies reporting noninvasive detection of right-to-left-shunt by contrast echo *(10,11)* were followed by extensive clinical research on the association between PFO and several pathological processes including cryptogenic stroke *(12–15)*, peripheral embolism *(14, 16)*, brain abscesses *(17)*, decompression sickness *(18–20)*, platypnea-orthodeoxia *(21)*, and fat embolism syndrome *(22)*. In these studies, PFO was suggested as a source of paradoxical embolism caused by air, thromboemboli, and fat emboli.

Transient right-to-left shunt through a PFO can occur in the presence of normal right-side hemodynamics *(10,23,24)*. However, patients with submassive and massive pulmonary embolism (PE), i.e., those with pulmonary hypertension and right-ventricular dysfunction, may be at particularly high risk of paradoxical embolism if they happen to have a PFO, with a substantial impact on their in-hospital morbiditiy and mortality *(25,16)*. In fact, our own group could demonstrate in a large series of patients with submassive and massive PE that PFO was an important independent predictor of an adverse clinical outcome *(26)*.

EMBRYOLOGY AND INCIDENCE

PFO is a remnant of fetal circulation. Oxygenated placental blood enters the right atrium via the inferior vena cava and crosses the foramen ovale to enter the systemic arterial system. At birth, pulmonary vascular resistance and right-sided cardiac pressures drop with a reversal of the right-to-left atrial pressure gradient. The flap of the foramen ovale closes against the atrial septum with fusion usually occurring within the first 2 yr of life. This anatomic configuration determines the properties of a PFO as a potential one-way passage for blood from the right to the left atrial cavity (Fig. 1). The extent of the shunt is determined by the size of the PFO and the pressure differences between the right and the left atrium. A right-to-left shunt through a PFO may occur under certain physiological circumstances such as coughing and the Valsalva maneuver *(10,23,24)*.

The prevalence of a PFO in adults ranged from 25 to 35% in autopsy series *(1,27)*, and from 5 to 31% in healthy volunteers *(11–13,15)*. In a series of 965 autopsy specimens from the Mayo Clinic, the size of the foramen ovale in normal hearts varied between 1 and 19 mm with a mean of 4.9 mm *(1)*. Neither the prevalence of PFO nor its size differed significantly between the two genders, but there was a correlation with age. Thus, the overall frequency was 27.3%, declining from 34.3% in the first three decades of life to 25% in the fourth to the eighth decades. In patients older than 80 yr, it decreased to 20.2%. The reasons for these differences remain speculative and include age-dependent closure of the PFO

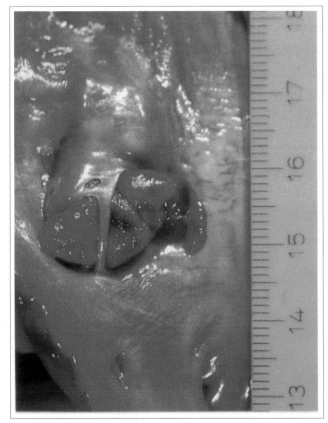

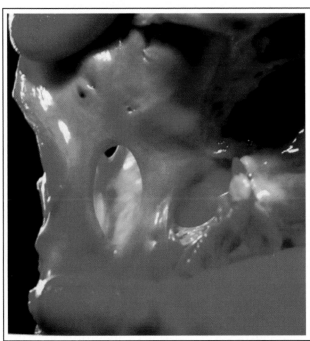

Fig. 1. Anatomic view of a PFO (left panel) and of a thrombus crossing the PFO (right panel).

81

Table 1
Ultrasound Techniques for PFO Diagnosis: Diagnostic Accuracy
in Comparison to Transesophageal Contrast Echocardiography

	Sensitivity	Specificity	PPV	NPV
Contrast TTE	37–54%	92–100%	68–82%	72–84%
Color flow TEE	79%	75%	78%	76%
Color flow TTE	7%	85–100%	50%	65%
TDC	68–100%	92–100%	91–100%	87–100%

NPV, negative predictive value; PPV, positive predictive value; TDC, transcranial
Doppler; TEE, transesophageal echocardiography; TTE, transthoracic echocardiography.

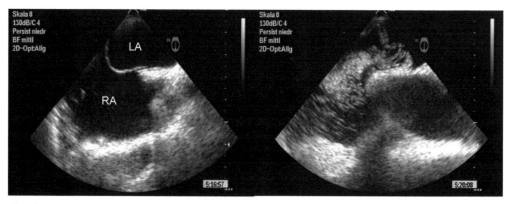

Fig. 2. Echo examination without (left panel) and with echo contrast injection (right panel) in a patient with a PFO.

as well as possible selection bias, if adults with a PFO were, in fact, more likely to die earlier.

DIAGNOSIS OF PFO

The presence of a PFO generally does not affect the patient's history, clinical findings, ECG, or chest radiograph. Either invasive or noninvasive methods can be used for detection of an intracardiac shunt. Routine right- and left-side cardiac catheterization is generally inadequate for definite diagnosis of a PFO, and specialized techniques are required for shunt diagnosis (3).

Ultrasound techniques have emerged as the principal method for diagnosis and assessment of PFO in clinical practice. Transthoracic and transesophageal echocardiography, color flow Doppler and transcranial Doppler are commonly used (Table 1) (15,28–32). During visualization of the interatrial septum from the transthoracic apical four-chamber view, or from a transesophageal window, echo-contrast opacification of the right atrium can be achieved by rapidly injecting, for example, 10 mL of agitated 5.5% oxypolygelatine solution or 10 mL of agitated saline through an antecubital vein (11–14,16,33). The detection of five or more microbubbles in the left heart cavities within three cardiac cycles after their appearance in the right atrium is considered an indication of a PFO (23) (Fig. 2). The Valsalva maneuver enhances contrast detection of the right-to-left shunt.

Transesophageal echocardiography is currently considered the reference standard for PFO diagnosis, allowing direct imaging of the interatrial septum and visualization of the right-to-left shunt. However, false-negative transesophageal echocardiograms are possible and may result from (1) inadequate visualization of the septum; (2) elevated left atrial pressures preventing right-to-left passage of contrast *(34,35)*; (3) blood flow directed from the inferior vena cava along (i.e., in parallel to) the interatrial septum, thus preventing impingement of the anticubital bubbles against the interatrial septum; or (4) an improperly performed Valsalva maneuver. On the other hand, a false-positive transesophageal contrast study may be caused by a pulmonary arteriovenous shunt *(36)*.

Transcranial Doppler ultrasound is also used for PFO diagnosis and it is based on the detection of air microbubbles in the right or left middle cerebral artery after peripheral application of agitated saline. This method is established in clinical routine and provides direct evidence of paradoxical cerebral echo contrast embolization *(37)*.

CLINICAL AND PROGNOSTIC RELEVANCE OF PFO IN ACUTE PE

Hypoxemia

The cause of hypoxemia is often multifactorial and the contribution of a right-to-left shunt through a PFO may be overlooked when more obvious pulmonary or cardiac causes of hypoxemia are present. PFO-related hypoxemia may complicate the course of right ventricular infarction *(38–41)*, tricuspid valve disease *(42–44)*, or right ventricular hypertension *(45–47)*, with increased right atrial pressure predisposing to a right-to-left shunt through the PFO. Similarly, positive-pressure ventilation and positive end expiratory pressure may exacerbate hypoxemia by enhancing right-to-left shunt *(48)*.

Although the pathophysiological mechanisms leading to arterial hypoxemia in patients with acute PE are incompletely understood *(49–51)*, pulmonary hypertension with an elevated right atrial pressure as a result of submassive or massive PE may exacerbate right-to-left shunt through a PFO, thus causing a further decrease of arterial oxygenation *(52,53)* beyond that caused by PE itself.

In a prospective study published in 1992, we investigated the clinical relevance of right-to-left shunt through a PFO in 85 patients with acute PE *(16)*. Significant differences were observed in the arterial oxygen tension depending on the presence or absence of a PFO. Under room air, patients with echocardiographically-diagnosed PFO had significantly lower arterial oxygen tension compared to those without a PFO *(16)* (Fig. 3). On the other hand, no differences were observed regarding the arterial carbon dioxide tension. The presence of an intracardiac right-to-left shunt should therefore always be taken into account when encountering a dramatic drop in partial arterial oxygen pressure in patients with PE *(51)*.

Paradoxical Embolism

As explained above, definite confirmation of paradoxical embolism requires direct visualization of a right atrial thrombus crossing the foramen ovale, but observation of this phenomenon during life is very rare *(54–56)* (Fig. 4). Therefore, the diagnosis of paradoxical embolism is presumptive in the vast majority of cases and relies on (1) the occurrence of an arterial thromboembolic event in the absence of atrial fibrillation, disease of the left side of the heart, or severe artherosclerosis of the thoracic aorta; (2) the detection of right-to-left shunt, usually through a PFO or an atrial septal defect; and (3) the presence of venous thrombosis or PE *(5,9)*.

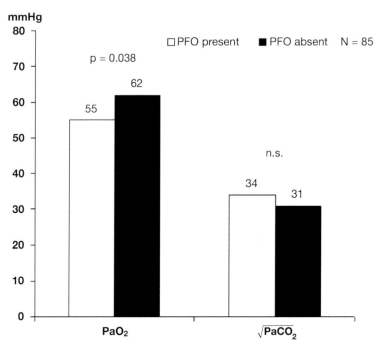

Fig. 3. Influence of a PFO on arterial hypoxemia in patients with PE and right ventricular dysfunction.

Several clinical studies, most of them performed in young patients with stroke, yielded data to support the clinical relevance of a PFO *(13–15,57)*. Patients with PFO were at risk for recurrent arterial thromboembolic events, with a combined stroke and transient ischemic attack rate of 3.4 to 3.8% per year *(58,59)*. A large PFO size *(60–62)* and presence of an atrial septal aneurysm *(63,64)* were identified as morphological characteristics portending a high risk for paradoxical embolism. At present, percutaneous PFO closure appears to be a promising technique for secondary prevention of recurrent systemic thromboembolism *(65)*.

The clinical relevance of a PFO in patients with acute PE and right ventricular dysfunction (elevated right-sided cardiac pressures) was investigated in a prospective study by our own group. The end points of the study were overall mortality and complicated clinical course during the hospital stay defined as death, cerebral or peripheral arterial thromboembolism, major bleeding, or need for endotracheal intubation or cardiopulmonary resuscitation *(26)*. The results provided a clear confirmation of the hypothesis that patients with PE and PFO may frequently suffer paradoxical embolism, which in turn has a substantial impact on their in-hospital morbidity and mortality. Right-to-left shunt through a PFO was diagnosed in 48 patients (35%), and patients with a PFO had significantly higher incidence of ischemic stroke (13 vs 2.2%; $p = 0.02$) and peripheral arterial embolism (15 vs 0%; $p < 0.001$; Table 2). Overall, the risk of a complicated in-hospital course was 5.2 times higher in patients with a PFO.

In-Hospital Mortality and Complications

Accurate risk stratification remains a major challenge in patients with acute PE (*see* Chapters 4 and 5). Two large prospective registries demonstrated that beside clinical and hemodynamic instability, at present, acute right ventricular dysfunction is a major

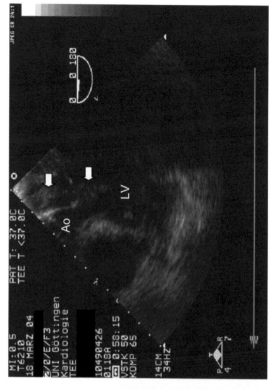

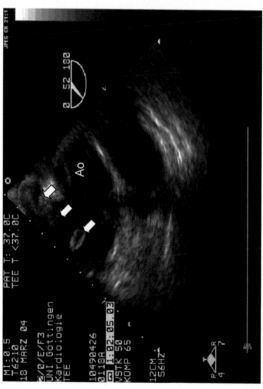

Fig. 4. Transesophageal echocardiographic visualization of a right atrial thrombus crossing the foramen ovale, a direct indicator of impending paradoxical embolism. Left panel: at the beginning of the examination, a large serpentine floating thrombus (arrows) was detected in the right atrium, being partly trapped in the PFO. Right panel: a few minutes later, the largest part of the floating thrombus had crossed the PFO and now was in the left atrium, protruding through the mitral valve into the left ventricle. During the examination, the thrombus disappeared from the cardiac cavities. Within minutes, the patient developed a painful, cold upper-left extremity. Emergency surgery was performed, and the embolus was retrieved from the brachial artery. Ao, aortic valve; LV, left ventricle.

85

Table 2
In-Hospital Clinical Events in Patients
With Acute Massive or Submassive PE Depending on the Presence of PFO

	Patients with PFO (n = 48)	Patients without PFO (n = 91)	P
Event			
Ischemic stroke	6 (13%)	2 (2.2%)	0.02
Peripheral arterial embolism	7 (15%)	0	<0.001
Cerebral bleeding	2 (4.2%)	1 (1.1%)	0.27
Other major bleeding	8 (17%)	19 (21%)	0.66
Endotracheal intubation	17 (35%)	15 (16%)	0.02
Cardiopulmonary resuscitation	9 (19%)	10 (11%)	0.30
Death	16 (33%)	13 (14%)	0.015

PFO, patent foramen ovale. From Konstantinides et al. *(26)*.

determinant of outcome during the in-hospital course *(66,67)*. By detecting right ventricular enlargement and hypokinesis, echocardiography can identify high-risk patients with overt or impending right ventricular failure *(68,69)* and possibly those who may benefit from thrombolytic treatment *(70,71)*. Furthermore, ECG abnormalities, or elevation of cardiac biomarkers such as troponin I, troponin T, or natriuretic peptides, are useful tools for risk stratification and the optimization of management in patients with acute PE *(72–75)*. In addition to these predictors of an adverse outcome, we tested the hypothesis that PFO is an important prognostic indicator regarding mortality and the occurrence of cardiovascular complications in patients with acute PE and RV dysfunction. Patients with a PFO detected by contrast echocardiography had a death rate of 33%, as opposed to 14% in those with a negative echo-contrast examination *(26)*. In fact, PFO was associated with more than a 10-fold increase in death risk. Logistic regression analysis demonstrated that the only independent predictors of mortality were a PFO and arterial hypotension at presentation. Similarly, the frequency of serious in-hospital complications such as arterial thromboembolism, major bleeding, need for endotracheal intubation, or cardiopulmonary resuscitation was very high in patients with a PFO. These results strongly support the prognostic impact of a PFO as an independent prognostic predictor of adverse outcome in patients with acute PE.

REFERENCES

1. Hagen PT, Scholz DG, Edwards WD. Incidence and size of patent foramen ovale during the first 10 decades of life: an autopsy study of 965 normal hearts. Mayo Clin Proc 1984;59:17–20.
2. Meister SG, Grossman W, Dexter L, Dalen JE. Paradoxical embolism: diagnosis during life. Circulation 1972;53:292–298.
3. Cheng TO. Paradoxical embolism: a diagnostic challenge and its detection during life. Circulation 1976; 53:565–568.
4. Cohnheim J. Thrombose und Embolie: Vorlesung über allgemeine Pathologie. Berlin Germany. Hirschwald 1877;1:134.
5. Johnson BJ. Paradoxical embolism. J Clin Pathol 1951;4:316–332.
6. Nellessen U, Daniel WG, Matheis G, Oelert H, Depping K, Lichtlen PR. Impending paradoxical embolism from atrial thrombus: correct diagnosis by transesophageal echocardiography and prevention by surgery. J Am Coll Cardiol 1985;5:1002–1004.

7. Nelson CW, Snow FR, Barnett M, McRoy L, Wechsler AS, Nixon JV. Impending paradoxical embolism: echocardiographic diagnosis of an intracardiac thrombus crossing a patent foramen ovale. Am Heart J 1991;122:859–862.

8. Inoue T, Tadehara F, Hinoi T, et al. Paradoxical peripheral embolism coincident with acute pulmonary thromboembolism. Intern Med 2005;44(3):243–245.

9. Hales CA, Johnson RA. Pulmonary thromboembolism and non-thromboembolic pulmonary vascular disease. In: Eagle KA, Haber E, DeSanctis RW, Austen WG, eds. Practice of Cardiology. 2nd ed. Little, Brown and Co, Boston, MA, 1989, pp. 1299–1301.

10. Kronik G, Mösslacher H. Positive contrast echocardiography in patients with patent foramen ovale and normal right heart hemodynamics. Am J Cardiol 1982;49(7):1806–1809.

11. Lynch JJ, Schuchard GH, Gross CM, Wann LS Prevalence of right-to-left atrial shunting in a healthy population: detection by Valsalva maneuver contrast echocardiography. Am J Cardiol 1984;53(10):1478–1480.

12. Webster MW, Chancellor AM, Smith HJ, et al. Patent foramen ovale in young stroke patients. Lancet 1988;2(8601):11–12.

13. Lechat P, Mas JL, Lascault G, et al. Prevalence of patent foramen ovale in patients with stroke. N Engl J Med 1988;318(18):1148–1152.

14. Hausmann D, Mugge A, Becht I, Daniel WG. Diagnosis of patent foramen ovale by transesophageal echocardiography and association with cerebral and peripheral embolic events. Am J Cardiol 1992;70(6):668–672.

15. Di Tullio M, Sacco RL, Gopal A, Mohr JP, Homma S. Patent foramen ovale as a risk factor for cryptogenic stroke. Ann Intern Med 1992;117(6):461–465.

16. Kasper W, Geibel A, Tiede N, Just H. Patent foramen ovale in patients with haemodynamically significant pulmonary embolism. Lancet 1992;340(8819):561–564.

17. Dethy S, Manto M, Kentos A, et al. PET findings in a brain abscess associated with a silent atrial septal defect. Clin Neurol Neurosurg 1995;97(4):349–353.

18. Moon RE, Camporesi EM, Kisslo JA. Patent foramen ovale and decompression sickness in divers. Lancet 1989;1(8637):513–514.

19. Germonpre P, Dendale P, Unger P, Balestra C. Patent foramen ovale and decompression sickness in sports divers. J Appl Physiol 1998;84(5):1622–1626.

20. Cartoni D, De Castro S, Valente G, et al. Identification of professional scuba divers with patent foramen ovale at risk for decompression illness. Am J Cardiol 2004;94:270–273.

21. Seward JB, Hayes DL, Smith HC, et al. Platypnea-orthodeoxia: clinical profile, diagnostic workup, management, and report of seven cases. Mayo Clin Proc 1984;59(4):221–231.

22. Pell AC, Hughes D, Keating J, Christie J, Busuttil A, Sutherland GR. Fulminating fat embolism syndrome caused by paradoxical embolism through a patent foramen ovale. N Engl J Med 1993;329:926–929.

23. Dubourg O, Bourdarias JP, Farcot JC, et al. Contrast echocardiographic visualization of cough-induced right to left shunt through a patent foramen ovale. J Am Coll Cardiol 1984;4(3):587–594.

24. Langholz D, Louie EK, Konstadt SN, Rao TL, Scanlon PJ. Transesophageal echocardiographic demonstration of distinct mechanisms for right to left shunting across a patent foramen ovale in the absence of pulmonary hypertension. J Am Coll Cardiol 1991;18(4):1112–1117.

25. Keidar S, Grenadier E, Binenboim C, Palant A. Transient right to left atrial shunt detected by contrast echocardiography in the acute stage of pulmonary embolism. J Clin Ultrasound 1984;12(7):417–419.

26. Konstantinides S, Geibel A, Kasper W, Olschewski M, Blumel L, Just H. Patent foramen ovale is an important predictor of adverse outcome in patients with major pulmonary embolism. Circulation 1998;97(19):1946–1951.

27. Thompson T, Evans W. Paradoxical embolism. Q J Med 1930;23:135–152.

28. Nemec JJ, Marwick TH, Lorig RJ, et al. Comparison of transcranial Doppler ultrasound and transesophageal contrast echocardiography in the detection of interatrial right-to-left shunts. Am J Cardiol 1991;68(15):1498–1502.

29. de Belder MA, Tourikis L, Griffith M, Leech G, Camm AJ. Transesophageal contrast echocardiography and color flow mapping: methods of choice for the detection of shunts at the atrial level? Am Heart J 1992;124(6):1545–1550.

30. Karnik R, Stollberger C, Valentin A, Winkler WB, Slany J. Detection of patent foramen ovale by transcranial contrast Doppler ultrasound. Am J Cardiol 1992;69(5):560–562.

31. Belkin RN, Pollack BD, Ruggiero ML, Alas LL, Tatini U. Comparison of transesophageal and transthoracic echocardiography with contrast and color flow Doppler in the detection of patent foramen ovale. Am Heart J 1994;128(3):520–525.

32. Job FP, Ringelstein EB, Grafen Y, et al. Comparison of transcranial contrast Doppler sonography and transesophageal contrast echocardiography for the detection of patent foramen ovale in young stroke patients. Am J Cardiol 1994;74(4):381–384.

33. Van Camp G, Franken P, Melis P, Cosyns B, Schoors D, Vanoverschelde JL. Comparison of transthoracic echocardiography with second harmonic imaging with transesophageal echocardiography in the detection of right to left shunts. Am J Cardiol 2000;86(11):1284–1287, A9.

34. Siostrzonek P, Lang W, Zangeneh M, et al. Significance of left-sided heart disease for the detection of patent foramen ovale by transesophageal contrast echocardiography. J Am Coll Cardiol 1992;19(6):1192–1196.

35. Movsowitz HD, Movsowitz C, Jacobs LE, Kotler MN. Negative air-contrast test does not exclude the presence of patent foramen ovale by transesophageal echocardiography. Am Heart J 1993;126(4):1031–1032.

36. Van Camp G, Cosyns B, Vandenbossche JL. Non-smoke spontaneous contrast in left atrium intensified by respiratory manoeuvres: a new transoesophageal echocardiographic observation. Br Heart J 1994;72(5):446–451.

37. Teague SM, Sharma MK. Detection of paradoxical cerebral echo contrast embolization by transcranial Doppler ultrasound. Stroke 1991;22(6):740–745.

38. Wendel CH, Dianzumba S, Joyner CR. Right-to-left interatrial shunt secondary to an extensive right ventricular myocardial infarction. Clin Cardiol 1985;8(4):230–232.

39. Bansal RC, Marsa RJ, Holland D, Beehler C, Gold PM. Severe hypoxemia due to shunting through a patent foramen ovale: a correctable complication of right ventricular infarction. J Am Coll Cardiol 1985;5(1):188–192.

40. Uppstrom EL, Kern MJ, Mezei L, Mrosek D, Labovitz A. Balloon catheter closure of patent foramen ovale complicating right ventricular infarction: improvement of hypoxia and intracardiac venous shunting. Am Heart J 1988;116(4):1092–1097.

41. Fessler MB, Lepore JJ, Thompson BT, Semigran MJ. Right-to-left shunting through a patent foramen ovale in right ventricular infarction: improvement of hypoxemia and hemodynamics with inhaled nitric oxide. J Clin Anesth 2003;15(5):371–374.

42. Turek MA, Karovitch A, Aaron SD, Brais M. Persistent hypoxemia occurring as a complication of tricuspid valve endocarditis. J Am Soc Echocardiogr 2000;13(5):412–414.

43. Bier A, Jones J, Lazar E, Factor S, Keefe D. Endocarditis of a tricuspid prosthesis causing valvular stenosis and shunting through a patent foramen ovale. Chest 1986;90(2):293–295.

44. Movsowitz C, Podolsky LA, Meyerowitz CB, Jacobs LE, Kotler MN. Patent foramen ovale: a nonfunctional embryological remnant or a potential cause of significant pathology? J Am Soc Echocardiogr 1992;5(3):259–270.

45. Laine JF, Slama M, Petitpretz P, Girard P, Motte G. Danger of vasodilator therapy for pulmonary hypertension in patent foramen ovale. Chest 1986;89(6):894–895.

46. Begin R, Gervais A, Guerin L, Bureau MA. Patent foramen ovale and hypoxia in chronic obstructive pulmonary disease. Eur J Respir Dis 1981;62(6):373–375.

47. Dewan NA, Gayasaddin M, Angelillo VA, O'Donohue WJ, Mohiuddin S. Persistent hypoxemia due to patent foramen ovale in a patient with adult respiratory distress syndrome. Chest 1986;89(4):611–613.

48. Moorthy SS, Losasso AM. Patency of the foramen ovale in the critically ill patient. Anesthesiology 1974;41(4):405–407.

49. D'Alonzo GE, Bower JS, DeHart P, Dantzker DR. The mechanisms of abnormal gas exchange in acute massive pulmonary embolism. Am Rev Respir Dis 1983;128(1):170–172.

50. Jardin F, Gurdjian F, Desfonds P, Fouilladieu JL, Margairaz A. Hemodynamic factors influencing arterial hypoxemia in massive pulmonary embolism with circulatory failure. Circulation 1979;59(5):909–912.

51. Wilson JE, Pierce AK, Johnson RL Jr, et al. Hypoxemia in pulmonary embolism, a clinical study. J Clin Invest 1971;50(3):481–491.

52. Hale GS, Clarebrough JK, Fox P, Blair N, McDonald IG, Chestermann C. Severe pulmonary embolism complicated by right-to-left shunting: diagnosis and implications in management. Aust NZ J Med 1979;9:953.

53. Lang I, Steurer G, Weissel M, Burghuber OC. Recurrent paradoxical embolism complicating severe thromboembolic pulmonary hypertension. Eur Heart J 1988;9(6):678–681.

54. Loscalzo J. Paradoxical embolism: clinical presentation, diagnostic strategies, and therapeutic options. Am Heart J 1986;112(1):141–145.

55. Kavarana MN, Boice T, Gray LA. Impending paradoxical embolism across a patent foramen ovale: case report. Heart Surg Forum 2005;8(1):E47–E48.

56. Delvigne M, Vermeersch P, van den Heuvel P. Thrombus-in-transit causing paradoxical embolism in cerebral and coronary arterial circulation. Acta Cardiol 2004;59(6):669–672.

57. Gabelmann M, Hetzel A, Geibel A. Das offene Foramen ovale – ein Risikofaktor oder ein Nebenbefund bei Patienten mit cerebralen Ischämien? Intensivmed 1998;35:607–614.

58. de Belder MA, Tourikis L, Leech G, Camm AJ. Risk of patent foramen ovale for thromboembolic events in all age groups. Am J Cardiol 1992;69(16):1316–1320.

59. Mas JL, Zuber M. Recurrent cerebrovascular events in patients with patent foramen ovale, atrial septal aneurysm, or both and cryptogenic stroke or transient ischemic attack. French Study Group on Patent Foramen Ovale and Atrial Septal Aneurysm. Am Heart J 1995;130(5):1083–1088.

60. Kerut EK, Norfleet WT, Plotnick GD, Giles TD. Patent foramen ovale: a review of associated conditions and the impact of physiological size. J Am Coll Cardiol 2001;38(3):613–623.

61. Hausmann D, Mugge A, Daniel WG. Identification of patent foramen ovale permitting paradoxic embolism. J Am Coll Cardiol 1995;26(4):1030–1038.

62. Stone DA, Godard J, Corretti MC, et al. Patent foramen ovale: association between the degree of shunt by contrast transesophageal echocardiography and the risk of future ischemic neurologic events. Am Heart J 1996;131(1):158–161.

63. Mas JL, Arquizan C, Lamy C, et al; Patent Foramen Ovale and Atrial Septal Aneurysm Study Group. Recurrent cerebrovascular events associated with patent foramen ovale, atrial septal aneurysm, or both. N Engl J Med 2001;345(24):1740–1746.

64. Mugge A, Daniel WG, Angermann C, et al. Atrial septal aneurysm in adult patients. A multicenter study using transthoracic and transesophageal echocardiography. Circulation 1995;91(11):2785–2792.

65. Windecker S, Wahl A, Chatterjee T, et al. Percutaneous closure of patent foramen ovale in patients with paradoxical embolism: long-term risk of recurrent thromboembolic events. Circulation 2000;101(8):893–898.

66. Goldhaber SZ, Visani L, De Rosa M. Acute pulmonary embolism: clinical outcomes in the International Cooperative Pulmonary Embolism Registry (ICOPER) Lancet 1999;353(9162):1386–1389.

67. Kasper W, Konstantinides S, Geibel A, et al. Management strategies and determinants of outcome in acute major pulmonary embolism: results of a multicenter registry. J Am Coll Cardiol 1997;30(5):1165–1171.

68. Kasper W, Konstantinides S, Geibel A, Tiede N, Krause T, Just H. Prognostic significance of right ventricular afterload stress detected by echocardiography in patients with clinically suspected pulmonary embolism. Heart 1997;77(4):346–349.

69. Quiroz R, Kucher N, Schoepf UJ, et al. Right ventricular enlargement on chest computed tomography: prognostic role in acute pulmonary embolism. Circulation 2004;109(20):2401–2404.

70. Konstantinides S, Geibel A, Olschewski M, et al. Association between thrombolytic treatment and the prognosis of hemodynamically stable patients with major pulmonary embolism: results of a multicenter registry. Circulation 1997;96(3):882–888.

71. Konstantinides S, Geibel A, Heusel G, Heinrich F, Kasper W; Management Strategies and Prognosis of Pulmonary Embolism-3 Trial Investigators. Heparin plus alteplase compared with heparin alone in patients with submassive pulmonary embolism. N Engl J Med 2002;347(15):1143–1150.

72. Geibel A, Zehender M, Kasper W, Olschewski M, Klima C, Konstantinides S. Prognostic value of the ECG on admission in patients with acute major pulmonary embolism. Eur Respir J 2005;25(5):843–848.

73. Giannitsis E, Lehrke S, Wiegand UK, et al. Risk stratification in patients with inferior acute myocardial infarction treated by percutaneous coronary interventions: the role of admission troponin T. Circulation 2000;102(17):2038–2044.

74. Konstantinides S, Geibel A, Olschewski M, et al. Importance of cardiac troponins I and T in risk stratification of patients with acute pulmonary embolism. Circulation 2002;106(10):1263–1268.

75. Kucher N, Printzen G, Goldhaber SZ. Prognostic role of brain natriuretic peptide in acute pulmonary embolism. Circulation 2003;107(20):2545–2547.

7

Contemporary Diagnostic Algorithm for the Hemodynamically Stable Patient With Suspected Pulmonary Embolism

Arnaud Perrier, MD

CONTENTS

SUMMARY

No single diagnostic test has sufficient accuracy when used alone to confirm or rule out pulmonary embolism (PE). This even applies to pulmonary angiography, the historical gold standard in PE diagnosis. Therefore, modern diagnostic strategies for PE rely on combinations of noninvasive tests such as plasma D-dimer measurement, lower limb venous compression ultrasonography, ventilation-perfusion lung scan, and/or helical computed tomography, the results of which should be interpreted in the context of the clinical likelihood of PE. Pulmonary angiography is rarely necessary. Clinical probability of PE can be assessed with fair accuracy, either implicitly or by clinical prediction rules. Management studies, in which patients deemed not to have PE are left untreated and followed up to assess their 3-mo thromboembolic risk, have become the benchmark for validation of diagnostic algorithms. Cost-effectiveness analysis allows the evaluation and comparison of the various diagnostic sequences. The existing evidence shows that implementation of evidence-based diagnostic algorithms is feasible and may increase quality of care.

Key Words: Deep venous thrombosis; D-dimer; lower limb venous ultrasonography; ventilation-perfusion scintigraphy; helical computed tomography; pulmonary angiography; clinical assessment; diagnosis; cost-effectiveness.

From: *Contemporary Cardiology: Management of Acute Pulmonary Embolism*
Edited by: S. Konstantinides © Humana Press Inc., Totowa, NJ

INTRODUCTION

Over the past 15 yr, an increasing number of tests have become available to diagnose pulmonary embolism (PE). For example, the North American Prospective Investigation On Pulmonary Embolism Diagnosis (PIOPED) study definitively established the criteria for interpreting the results of ventilation-perfusion (V/Q) scintigraphy *(1)*. Plasma D-dimer measurement is now a validated and widely accepted first-line test for ruling out PE, provided it is used in combination with clinical probability and in the appropriate clinical setting *(2–4)*. Lower limb venous compression ultrasonography is a useful adjunct because of its high specificity for proximal deep venous thrombosis (DVT), the most frequent source of PE *(5)*. Finally, the development of helical computed tomography (CT) represents, without question, a revolution in our diagnostic armamentarium *(6,7)*.

The recent technical advances in imaging of the pulmonary vasculature probably permit correct diagnosis of PE in numerous centers not equipped with nuclear medicine facilities, because these institutions no longer need to transfer patients with clinically suspected PE for further diagnostic evaluation. In addition, thoracic imaging itself may be less frequently required owing to preselection of patients by means of clinical probability and D-dimer testing (*see* Chapter 1). On the other hand, a less favorable consequence is the increasing number and complexity of proposed diagnostic algorithms for PE, which make it very difficult for the clinician to understand and adopt a clear management strategy. In fact, this confusion may even result in the use of inappropriate criteria for diagnosing or ruling out PE *(3,8–10)*, therefore entailing the risk of unnecessarily submitting some patients to the risks of anticoagulant treatment or others to the mortality of untreated PE. Moreover, the diagnostic tests themselves are in constant change and evolution. For example, the large number of D-dimer assays currently available may lead some clinicians to believe that all tests possess similar diagnostic sensitivity and specificity, which is clearly not the case *(11)*. Helical CT has evolved from 3- to 5-mm-thick slices, using first-generation single-row detectors *(12)*, to 1-mm-thin slices with contemporary multirow CT scanners *(13)*, and the diagnostic performance of CT keeps improving at a rapid pace, generating the need for frequent updating of the clinical algorithms based on this procedure.

The characteristics of the individual diagnostic tests for PE are reviewed in Chapters 1, 2, and 3 of this book. The aim of the present chapter is to provide a guide for combining those tests in a rational and cost-effective manner, reviewing validated diagnostic strategies. Importantly, suspected PE in patients with shock or hemodynamic instability is a distinct clinical situation, and it warrants a specific diagnostic approach, which will be discussed in the following chapter. The strategies discussed in this chapter are thus restricted to the hemodynamically stable patient.

ARE DIAGNOSTIC STRATEGIES FOR PE NECESSARY?

Characteristics of Noninvasive Tests

The individual characteristics of diagnostic tests for PE are summarized in Table 1. Pulmonary angiography has been considered to have almost ideal sensitivity and specificity for PE. Therefore, it was, until recently, the only test capable of both ruling in and ruling out PE as a single procedure. However, it is invasive *(14)*, costly *(15)*, and, because it is rarely performed, the expertise for interpreting angiographic findings is rapidly decreasing except in specialized centers. Moreover, it cannot even be considered a true

Table 1
Performance of Diagnostic Tests in Suspected Nonmassive PE

Test	Sensitivity, %	Specificity, %
Pulmonary angiogram (1,50)	97	98
Ventilation-perfusion lung scan		
Normal (1,30,35,51)	99	–
Nondiagnostic (1)	–	–
High-probability (1)	–	91
D-dimer testing		
Rapid ELISA assay (17,24,45,52)	99	41
Immunoturbidimetric assays (53,54)	98	40
Whole blood agglutination assay (18,55)	85	68
Lower limb venous compression ultrasonography (5,30,56,57)	50	97
Helical CT		
Single-detector row (26,27)	70	90
Multidetector-row (58)	90	95

ELISA, enzyme-linked immunosorbent assay.

"gold standard", because animal (16) and clinical studies showed that certain pulmonary clots visible on CT are not visualized by angiography. On the other hand, no single non-invasive test allows reaching a definite diagnosis in all patients suspected of having PE, and it is therefore necessary to combine them. Multidetector-row CT (13) may serve that purpose, but even if this is established by further studies, it will still be more cost-effective to combine D-dimer to CT in order to spare unnecessary imaging studies.

Prevalence of PE

The prevalence of PE is decreasing among patients presenting with symptoms compatible with this disorder. Indeed, in the early 1990s, the prevalence of PE was approx 35% in most series (1). In other words, a clinician suspecting PE would confirm the disease in one of every three patients. In recent European series, the prevalence of PE remained stable at approx 20 to 25% (17). In contrast, in certain North American series, that figure has dropped to approx 10% (18). Clearly, the threshold of clinical suspicion has become lower, but there is no proof that this has increased the absolute number of PEs detected annually. Instead, it is more likely that a number of patients are unnecessarily submitted to a cascade of potentially costly tests, again highlighting the need for cost-effective diagnostic strategies.

Diagnostic Algorithms for PE and Quality of Care

Recent utilization reviews have shown that the adherence to accepted diagnostic standards for PE is extremely poor (19,20). Importantly, a recent French multicenter utilization review (21) provided evidence that using inappropriate criteria for ruling out PE has unfavorable clinical consequences. In that series, diagnostic management was inappropriate in 43% of the 1529 patients, and the majority of erroneous diagnoses were in those patients in whom PE was ruled out (626/1100, 57%). A thromboembolic event occurred during follow-up in 1.2% of patients who were appropriately managed compared with 7.7% of those in whom PE was (erroneously) ruled out based on inappropriate diagnostic criteria (absolute risk difference, 6.5%; 95% confidence interval [CI], 4.0 to 9.1) (21). On the other hand, actively implementing a validated diagnostic algorithm undoubtedly improves the management of suspected PE. In a recent Dutch study, only 11% of patients with a nondiagnostic V/Q scan underwent further testing and 55% of patients were treated despite an uncertain diagnosis, but these figures improved significantly after implementation of an algorithm (19). That experience demonstrates that implementing a diagnostic strategy can significantly reduce the proportion of patients inappropriately treated with anticoagulants and potentially submitted to bleeding complications. Diagnostic algorithms are therefore a distinct necessity and may help increase quality of care.

Is There a Single Valid Diagnostic Algorithm for PE?

There are several (and not just one) valid diagnostic algorithms for suspected PE. Each center has its particular logistics, and not all tests are available in every hospital, except perhaps in large teaching hospitals. In general, in smaller centers, access to D-dimer testing and helical CT is more widespread compared to venous ultrasound and V/Q scintigraphy. One center may be using a highly sensitive enzyme-linked immunosorbent (ELISA) D-dimer assay, whereas another selects a less sensitive bedside test. Therefore, it is important to adapt management algorithms to local logistics.

VALIDATION OF DIAGNOSTIC STRATEGIES FOR PE

There is no ideal reference procedure for diagnosing PE. The invasive character of pulmonary angiography is not its only limitation; interobserver agreement is poor, especially at the subsegmental arterial level. In the PIOPED study (1), expert readers agreed in 92% of cases for ruling in PE, and in only 83% of cases for ruling it out. At the subsegmental level, concordance fell to 60%. A recent systematic review of series in which patients with an angiogram negative for PE did not receive anticoagulation treatment and were followed over a 3-mo period demonstrated that 1 to 2% of these patients had DVT or PE during that period (22). Given the high recurrence risk of untreated PE, this finding is generally interpreted as indirect but strong evidence that PE was missed by the initial diagnostic procedure.

Further evidence against the use of pulmonary angiography as the sole reference standard in diagnostic algorithms for PE comes from a number of observations that suggest that not all angiographically detected PEs may need to be treated. For instance, in series including clinical follow-up, the 3-mo thromboembolic risk in patients left untreated based on the negative result of a highly sensitive negative D-dimer assay was below 1% (17,23,24). This is in apparent contradiction with the results of another study, in which all patients underwent both a highly sensitive D-dimer test and pulmonary angiography. In that study, 50% of patients with subsegmental PE (20% of the cohort) had a falsely negative D-dimer result (25). A plausible explanation is that small emboli that are associated with negative D-dimer results may be clinically unimportant. Data based on single-detector CT point to the same conclusion. In two studies that adhered to strict methodological criteria, the sensitivity of CT was only 70% (26,27). Combining lower limb venous ultrasonography with CT increased the overall diagnostic yield to 80%, which implies that such a combination would still miss 20% of all PE (26). Nevertheless, outcome studies established that patients left untreated based on a negative CT and lower limb venous ultrasound had a 3-mo thromboembolic risk below 2%, similar to that of those with negative pulmonary angiograms (17,28,29). This implies that the small clots missed by the combina-

Table 2
Three-Month Thromboembolic Risk
Associated With Ruling Out PE by Various Diagnostic Criteria

Diagnostic criterion	Patients tested, n	Thromboembolic risk, % (95% CI)
Normal pulmonary angiogram *(22)*	1050	1.7 (1.0 to 2.7)
Normal perfusion lung scan *(34–36)*	1031	0.7 (0.3 to 1.4)
D-dimer		
Negative highly sensitive D-dimer and low or moderate clinical probability of PE *(17,24,45)*	671	0 (0 to 0.6)
Less sensitive negative D-dimer and low clinical probability of PE *(18)*	437	0.2 (0 to 1.3)
Nondiagnostic lung scintigraphy and absence of proximal DVT and low clinical probability of PE *(46,47)*	864	2.3 (1.5 to 3.5)
Negative single-detector CT scan and absence of proximal DVT and low or moderate clinical probability of PE *(17,48)*	975	1.7 (1.2 to 2.6)
Negative multidetector-row CT scan and low-moderate clinical probability of PE *(45)*	318	1.7 (0.7 to 3.9)

PE, pulmonary embolism; DVT, deep vein thrombosis.

tion of CT and ultrasound may be left untreated without entailing unfavorable consequences for patients. Therefore, the reference standard for judging the safety of a procedure (or strategy) used to exclude PE is no longer the comparison with the results of pulmonary angiography, but the results of clinical follow-up. The clinical outcome should be at least as good as that associated with a negative pulmonary angiogram, i.e., a 1 to 2%, 3-mo thromboembolic risk in patients left untreated, with an upper limit of the 95% CI below 4%. A rule-out criterion (whether a single test or a combination of tests) satisfying that condition does not exclude a small PE, but it ensures a safe outcome of the patient despite withholding anticoagulant treatment. Such studies are called "outcome" or "management" trials. Exclusion criteria validated in outcome studies performed to date are summarized in Table 2.

In contrast to the validation of rule-out strategies, outcome (management) studies are not appropriate for verifying the accuracy of "rule-in" diagnostic criteria for PE, because patients with a positive criterion are usually treated with anticoagulants without performing a pulmonary angiogram. This raises the question of the posttest probability threshold above which the diagnosis of PE should be considered satisfactorily established. For instance, the prevalence of angiographically proven PE in patients with high clinical probability and a high-probability V/Q scan was 96% in the PIOPED study *(1)*, but it dropped to 88% in patients with intermediate clinical probability, and further down to 56% in patients with low clinical probability. For clinical purposes, current recommendations accept a high probability scan as sufficient proof of PE regardless of clinical probability, although the Canadian algorithm requires confirmation by angiography in low-clinical-probability patients *(30)*. Arguably, the only technique that allows a rational definition of decision thresholds is decision analysis, because decision models incorporate all the significant elements: the characteristics of the diagnostic tests, the risks associated with invasive testing, the risks due to anticoagulant treatment (for both true and false positives) and treatment efficacy. In addition to the posttest probability value, it also takes into account the risk of untreated PE, the effectiveness and the risks of anticoagulant treatment, and the risk of invasive diagnostic testing. Using standard decision models (31), it can be demonstrated that the posttest probability of PE (after a single test or a sequence of tests), above which the outcome (so-called expected utility) associated with performing an angiogram is poorer than treating the patient, is approx 60%.

Finally, management studies do not address the question of cost-effectiveness of diagnostic algorithms. Two equally safe management strategies may have vastly different cost-effectiveness ratios. For instance, V/Q scintigraphy followed, if nondiagnostic, by pulmonary angiography is highly effective, but this strategy is 30% more costly than performing D-dimer and, if positive, lower limb venous ultrasound (15,31,32). Thus, it becomes evident that management studies are only a step in the process of validating a new diagnostic test, or sequence of tests. Randomized trials are also appropriate for comparing two diagnostic strategies. A recent example is provided by a Canadian study comparing two algorithms for diagnosing DVT (33), and similar studies are underway for suspected PE.

VALIDATED DIAGNOSTIC STRATEGIES IN PE

V/Q Scintigraphy Followed by Angiography

This earliest rational diagnostic strategy for PE was based on the results of the PIOPED study (1). That series which established the performance of V/Q scintigraphy in comparison with pulmonary angiography showed that a normal perfusion lung scan had an almost 100% negative predictive value for PE. The safety of this rule-out criterion was subsequently verified by several outcome studies (34–36). At the other end of the spectrum, a so-called "high-probability" scintigraphic pattern has a high specificity and positive predictive value for PE (Table 1) and is generally considered as an adequate rule-in criterion. On the other hand, other scintigraphic results, such as a low- or intermediate-probability scan according to the PIOPED interpretation criteria, do not allow a definitive conclusion and should be reported as nondiagnostic. Therefore, starting the diagnostic workup with a V/Q lung scan and performing an angiogram in patients with a nondiagnostic result is a reasonable strategy. However, although well validated, this approach is no longer widely used because of the high proportion (50 to 70%) of nondiagnostic scintigraphic results. Nevertheless, it is still the benchmark to which the costs and effectiveness of newer diagnostic algorithms have to be compared (15,31,32,37–40).

Clinical Probability Assessment Prior to Imaging Studies

Despite the fact that the "scintigraphy-angiography" strategy has been endorsed by numerous consensus conferences in the past, empirical observations have shown that only a minority of patients with a nondiagnostic V/Q scan underwent pulmonary angiography (41,42). Indeed, most clinicians were reluctant to demand this invasive procedure, particularly in patients with a low clinical probability. Although clinical assessment was made mostly on implicit grounds at the time of the PIOPED study (1), its usefulness and validity was confirmed by the results of diagnostic tests. Thus, in a patient with a low clinical (pretest) probability, the posttest probability of PE after a nondiagnostic V/Q scan is only approx 4%. This is probably acceptable for ruling out PE. In contrast, the posttest probability of PE is higher in patients with intermediate or high clinical probability and a similar scintigraphic result, which makes it an unreliable rule-out criterion. Interestingly, physicians

Table 3

Appropriateness of Diagnostic Criteria for PE According to Clinical Probability

Diagnostic criterion	Clinical probability of PE		
	Low	Moderate	High
PE absent			
Pulmonary angiogram negative	+	+	+
Normal perfusion lung scan	+	+	+
Negative D-dimer			
ELISA or other highly sensitive assay	+	+	–
Less-sensitive assay or whole blood agglutination assay	+	–	–
Nondiagnostic lung scintigram and absence of proximal DVT	+	–	–
Negative single- or multidetector-row CT and absence of proximal DVT	+	+	–
Negative single-detector CT	+	–	–
Negative multidetector-row CT[a]	+	+	–
PE present			
Pulmonary angiogram positive	+	+	+
High-probability ventilation-perfusion lung scan	+	+	+
Proximal DVT (and symptoms of PE)	+	+	+
Positive single- or multidetector-row CT	+	+	+

PE, pulmonary embolism; ELISA, enzyme-linked immunosorbent assay; DVT, deep vein thrombosis. +, valid diagnostic criterion; –, invalid criterion. [a]preliminary evidence.

in the PIOPED study assigned each patient to one of three clinical probability categories (low, intermediate, or high), allowing the determination of the true prevalence of PE in each of these subgroups. The results showed that for each scintigraphic result category (low, intermediate, and high scintigraphic probability), the prevalence of PE increased according to the clinical probability of the disease. This is one of the rare empiric demonstrations of Bayes' rule *(43)*. Taken together, these data demonstrate that clinical probability is essential for interpreting the results of lung scintigraphy. However, clinical probability assessment is also necessary to interpret D-dimer results. Less sensitive (sensitivity approx 85 to 90%) bedside assays allow ruling out PE only in patients with a low clinical probability, because the negative predictive value approaches 100% only in that subgroup. On the other hand, highly sensitive ELISA assays (sensitivity greater than 95%) may also be applied to patients with a moderate clinical probability. The safety of highly sensitive D-dimer assays for ruling out PE even in patients with a high clinical probability is not established, but the prevalence of PE could be as high as 10 to 15% in such patients according to Bayes' rule. The efficacy of various diagnostic criteria for ruling out PE according to clinical probability is shown in Table 3. Clinical probability can be validly assessed either implicitly or by prediction rules (*see* Chapter 1) *(18,44)*.

D-Dimer Testing Combined With Clinical Probability

Plasma D-dimer is a product of the degradation of cross-linked fibrin and its measurement by a biological test is inexpensive. Acute venous thromboembolism results in an elevation of plasma D-dimer concentrations in almost all patients because of the activation of coagulation and fibrinolysis. Therefore, this parameter carries a high diagnostic sensitivity and is a good rule-out instrument. On the other hand, its specificity is poor, and an elevated D-dimer level does not rule in PE. Because most patients with suspected PE will not eventually have the disease, it is reasonable to use D-dimer as a first-line test after having assessed the clinical probability of PE. As explained previously and as shown by several outcome studies, a negative result allows safely ruling out PE in patients with low or moderate clinical probability when using a highly sensitive ELISA assay *(17,24, 45)*. Less sensitive assays should be restricted to patients with low clinical probability (Table 3). Of note, D-dimer rules out PE in approximately one out of three patients suspected of having the disease in the emergency department. Thus, whatever the diagnostic tests and sequence selected in patients with an elevated D-dimer, its use is highly cost-effective, reducing costs by approx 20% *(15)*.

Lower Limb Venous Compression Ultrasonography

Most PEs originate from clots located in the deep veins of the lower limbs, especially the proximal veins. Therefore, finding DVT in a patient admitted because of thoracic symptoms suggestive of PE may be considered diagnostic of acute venous thromboembolism and warrants anticoagulant treatment. Whether thoracic imaging is still necessary in these patients is the subject of debate. On one hand, it needs to be considered that, if the diagnosis is established exclusively by the clinical symptoms of PE and the detection of DVT, no baseline thoracic imaging will be available for comparison in the event of suspected PE recurrence. However, this limitation is theoretical and rarely poses clinical problems in our experience. Because 40 to 50% of patients with PE are found to have proximal DVT on ultrasound, performing ultrasonography before thoracic imaging allows a definite diagnosis in approx 1 patient out of 10 (given an overall prevalence of PE of 20%).

Dutch and North American groups reserve compression ultrasonography for patients with a negative CT or nondiagnostic V/Q scintigraphy *(8)*. The diagnostic yield of ultrasonography in such patients is much lower. However, lower limb ultrasonography must be performed in patients with a negative single-detector CT because of the low (70%) sensitivity of first-generation CT scans. In fact, the only well-validated rule-out criterion in well-designed outcome studies using single-detector CT is the combination of negative ultrasound and a negative CT scan in a patient with a low or moderate clinical probability of PE. Ultrasonography is probably no longer necessary in patients with a negative multidetector row CT because of the high sensitivity of the latter test (*see* Diagnostic Strategy Based On Helical CT). However, even in centers equipped with multidetector row CT, ultrasound may still be useful to reduce costs and avoid unnecessary irradiation in patients with suspected PE and DVT *(15)*.

DIAGNOSTIC STRATEGY BASED ON V/Q LUNG SCAN

The diagnostic algorithm illustrated in Fig. 1 is derived from the "scintigraphy-angiography" strategy described in the previous section. Measuring D-dimer as the initial test allows ruling out PE in approx 30% of patients in the emergency department. In an outcome study by the Geneva group *(24)*, D-dimer was measured regardless of the clinical probability, and it was negative in only 10% of patients with a high clinical probability. As only 10% of all patients had a high clinical likelihood of PE, the overall diagnostic yield of measuring D-dimer in such patients was negligible (approx 1%), and the absolute number of patients with that combination was too low to establish the safety of this rule-out criterion. Therefore, D-dimer measurement is *not* recommended in patients with a

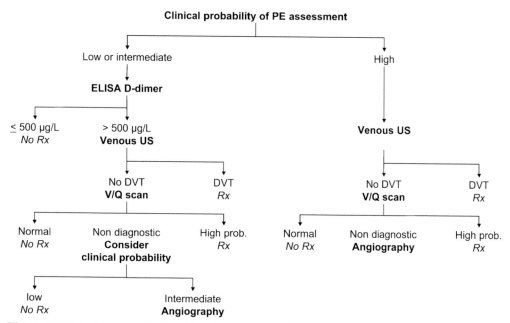

Fig. 1. Validated diagnostic algorithm for suspected PE including V/Q scan. Note that ELISA D-dimer is not useful in high-probability patients. Also, venous ultrasound must be performed either before or after scintigraphy when the V/Q scan is nondiagnostic. Rx, treatment.

high clinical probability. A negative D-dimer is an adequate rule-out criterion in patients with a low or moderate clinical probability when using a highly sensitive assay, and in patients with a low clinical probability with a less sensitive assay.

Lower limb venous compression ultrasonography is the second-line test in patients with an elevated D-dimer level and the initial test in patients with a high clinical probability. It detects DVT in approx 10% of patients, and thus V/Q scan needs to be performed in only 50 to 60% of the patients with suspected PE, establishing a definite diagnosis in approx 15% of the entire cohort. The 3-mo thromboembolic risk is less than 2% in patients with a low clinical probability, a nondiagnostic V/Q scan, and absence of proximal DVT on ultrasound *(46,47)*. This combination is found in approx 20% of patients and is considered an adequate rule-out criterion. In an outcome study evaluating this algorithm, pulmonary angiography was required in only 10% of patients and the 3-mo thromboembolic risk in patients left untreated based on the rule-out criteria of the strategy was approx 1% *(24)*. Depending on test availability, D-dimer measurement may be forfeited without compromising patient safety, although global costs and the number of necessary angiograms will be increased. In contrast, lower limb venous ultrasound is required to rule out PE in case of a nondiagnostic V/Q scan and a low clinical probability. Despite the growing utilization of CT, this algorithm remains practicable in centers with easier access to scintigraphy than to CT, and, possibly, in patients with contraindications to CT (mainly renal failure and allergy to contrast dye).

DIAGNOSTIC STRATEGY BASED ON HELICAL CT

This algorithm is illustrated in Fig. 2. The initial steps are the same as those of the algorithm based on V/Q scan (Fig. 1), but CT is performed instead in patients with an elevated

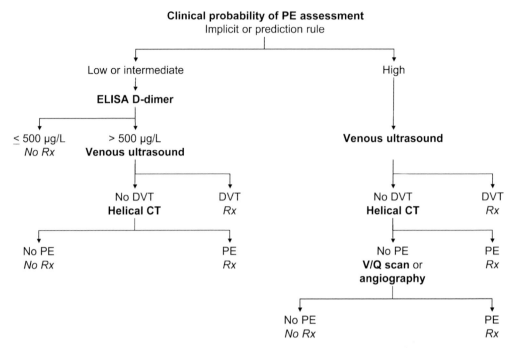

Fig. 2. Validated diagnostic algorithm for suspected pulmonary embolism (PE) including helical CT. Note that ELISA D-dimer is not useful in high-probability patients. Venous ultrasound needs to be performed when using single-detector helical CT, but it can be done either before or after the CT if the latter is negative. Venous ultrasound is probably unnecessary when using multidetector CT. Rx, treatment.

D-dimer level and a negative lower limb venous ultrasound. CT is required in 50 to 60% of patients. Because of its relatively low sensitivity, a negative single-detector CT does not allow ruling out PE, whereas the combination of a negative CT, a negative lower limb ultrasound, and low or moderate clinical probability safely rules out PE, as shown by recent outcome studies *(17,29,48)*. For high clinical probability patients who have a negative CT and negative ultrasound, further testing by V/Q scan and/or pulmonary angiography may still be recommended. However, this combination is rare: in the French multicenter "Evaluation du Scanner Spiralé dans l'Embolie Pulmonaire" (ESSEP) study, only 76 of the 1041 patients (7%) had this constellation of findings, and 4 of them had PE *(48)*. In the CTEP2 study, a three-center outcome study by the Geneva group validating the algorithm shown in Fig. 2, an angiogram was required in only 2% of patients *(17)*. Data on multidetector row CT are still scarce and well-designed prospective outcome studies are lacking. In the latest study from the Geneva group, all patients with elevated D-dimer levels or a high clinical probability underwent both multidetector row CT and lower limb ultrasonography *(45)*. The main study hypothesis was that if multidetector row CT has nearly ideal sensitivity, (1) the proportion of patients with a negative CT in the presence of proximal DVT on ultrasound and (2) the 3-mo thromboembolic risk in all patients with a negative CT, should be very low. CT and ultrasonography were negative in 318 patients, 3 of whom had a definite thromboembolic event and 2 died of possible PE during follow-up (3-mo risk of thromboembolism, 1.7%; 95% CI, 0.7 to 3.9). Only two patients had proximal DVT and a negative CT scan (0.6%; 95% CI, 0.2 to 2.2). Therefore, the overall 3-mo risk of thromboembolism in patients with "exclusion" of PE would have been 1.5% (95% CI, 0.8 to 3.0), if D-dimer and multidetector row CT had been the only tests used to rule out PE and ultrasonography had not been performed. However, this was not a true outcome study because all patients had both a CT scan and a lower limb venous ultrasound. The CHRISTOPHER study investigators *(49)* have just published a large-scale outcome study in a cohort of 3306 patients (including 18% inpatients) that evaluated a simple scheme based on clinical assessment, D-dimer, and multidetector row CT. Patients in whom PE was considered unlikely and in whom D-dimer was negative (n = 1057, 32%) were not treated and had a low 0.5% 3-mo thromboembolic risk. Patients in whom PE was likely or with an abnormal D-dimer result had a CT scan and were managed according to the CT result. PE was ruled out by CT in 1505 patients and the 3-mo thromboembolic risk was similarly low in patients left untreated (1.3%, 95% CI: 0.7 to 2.0%). Taken together, the CTEP2 and the CHRISTOPHER study provide strong support for a simple algorithm including clinical assessment, D-dimer, and multidetector row CT for suspected PE.

CONCLUSIONS

Numerous algorithms now exist for suspected nonmassive PE. Clinical probability assessment has become an undisputable first step, generally followed by plasma D-dimer measurement. Venous ultrasound may precede or follow thoracic imaging, which may consist of V/Q scintigraphy or helical CT. In both cases, a negative venous ultrasound is required to rule out PE in patients with a nondiagnostic lung scan or a negative single-detector CT. Pulmonary angiography is now rarely, if ever, necessary.

REFERENCES

1. The PIOPED Investigators. Value of the ventilation-perfusion scan in acute pulmonary embolism. JAMA 1990;263:2753–2759.
2. Stein PD, Hull RD, Patel KC, et al. D-Dimer for the exclusion of acute venous thrombosis and pulmonary embolism: a systematic review. Ann Intern Med 2004;140:589–602.
3. Kruip MJ, Leclercq MG, van der Heul C, Prins MH, Buller HR. Diagnostic strategies for excluding pulmonary embolism in clinical outcome studies. A systematic review. Ann Intern Med 2003;138:941–951.
4. Bounameaux H, Perrier A. D-dimer in the diagnosis of venous thromboembolism. In: Dalen JE, ed. Venous Thromboembolism. Marcel Dekker Inc, New York, NY, 2003, pp. 133–148.
5. Kearon C, Ginsberg JS, Hirsh J. The role of venous ultrasonography in the diagnosis of suspected deep venous thrombosis and pulmonary embolism. Ann Intern Med 1998;129:1044–1049.
6. Rathbun SW, Raskob GE, Whitsett TL. Sensitivity and specificity of helical computed tomography in the diagnosis of pulmonary embolism: a systematic review. Ann Intern Med 2000;132:227–232.
7. Mullins MD, Becker DM, Hagspiel KD, Philbrick JT. The role of spiral volumetric computed tomography in the diagnosis of pulmonary embolism. Arch Intern Med 2000;160:293–298.
8. Fedullo PF, Tapson VF. Clinical practice. The evaluation of suspected pulmonary embolism. N Engl J Med 2003;349:1247–1256.
9. Goldhaber SZ. Pulmonary embolism. Lancet 2004;364:244.
10. British Thoracic Society guidelines for the management of suspected acute pulmonary embolism. Thorax 2003;58:470–483.
11. Perrier A. D-dimer for suspected pulmonary embolism: whom should we test? Chest 2004;125:807–809.
12. Rémy-Jardin M, Rémy J, Wattinne L, Giraud F. Central pulmonary thromboembolism: diagnosis with spiral volumetric CT with the single-breath-hols technique. Comparison with pulmonary angiography. Radiology 1992;185:381–387.
13. Schoepf UJ, Costello P. CT angiography for diagnosis of pulmonary embolism: state of the art. Radiology 2004;230:329–337.
14. Stein PD, Athanasoulis C, Alavi A, et al. Complications and validity of pulmonary angiography in acute pulmonary embolism. Circulation 1992;85:462–468.

15. Perrier A, Nendaz MR, Sarasin FP, Howarth N, Bounameaux H. Cost-effectiveness of diagnostic strategies for suspected pulmonary embolism including helical computed tomography. Am J Respir Crit Care Med 2003;167:39–44.
16. Baile EM, King GG, Muller NL, et al. Spiral computed tomography is comparable to angiography for the diagnosis of pulmonary embolism. Am J Respir Crit Care Med 2000;161:1010–1015.
17. Perrier A, Roy PM, Aujesky D, et al. Diagnosing pulmonary embolism in outpatients with clinical assessment, D-dimer measurement, venous ultrasound, and helical computed tomography: a multicenter management study. Am J Med 2004;116:291–299.
18. Wells PS, Anderson DR, Rodger M, et al. Excluding pulmonary embolism at the bedside without diagnostic imaging: management of patients with suspected pulmonary embolism presenting to the emergency department by using a simple clinical model and d-dimer. Ann Intern Med 2001;135:98–107.
19. Berghout A, Oudkerk M, Hicks SG, Teng TH, Pillay M, Buller HR. Active implementation of a consensus strategy improves diagnosis and management in suspected pulmonary embolism. QJM 2000;93: 335–340.
20. Hagen PJ, van Strijen MJ, Kieft GJ, Graafsma YP, Prins MH, Postmus PE. The application of a Dutch consensus diagnostic strategy for pulmonary embolism in clinical practice. Neth J Med 2001;59:161–169.
21. Roy PM, Meyer G, Vielle B, et al. Appropriateness and outcomes of diagnostic management of suspected pulmonary embolism in emergency departments. Ann Intern Med 2006;144:157–164.
22. van Beek EJ, Brouwerst EM, Song B, Stein PD, Oudkerk M. Clinical validity of a normal pulmonary angiogram in patients with suspected pulmonary embolism—a critical review. Clin Radiol 2001;56:838–842.
23. Kruip MJ, Slob MJ, Schijen JH, van der Heul C, Buller HR. Use of a clinical decision rule in combination with D-dimer concentration in diagnostic workup of patients with suspected pulmonary embolism: a prospective management study. Arch Intern Med 2002;162:1631–1635.
24. Perrier A, Desmarais S, Miron MJ, et al. Non-invasive diagnosis of venous thromboembolism in outpatients. Lancet 1999;353:190–195.
25. De Monye W, Sanson BJ, Mac Gillavry MR, et al. Embolus location affects the sensitivity of a rapid quantitative D-dimer assay in the diagnosis of pulmonary embolism. Am J Respir Crit Care Med 2002; 165:345–348.
26. Perrier A, Howarth N, Didier D, et al. Performances of helical computed tomography in unselected outpatients with suspected pulmonary embolism. Ann Intern Med 2001;135:88–97.
27. Van Strijen MJ, De Monye W, Kieft GJ, Pattynama PM, Prins MH, Huisman MV. Accuracy of single-detector spiral CT in the diagnosis of pulmonary embolism: a prospective multicenter cohort study of consecutive patients with abnormal perfusion scintigraphy. J Thromb Haemost 2005;3:17–25.
28. Musset D, Rosso J, Petitpretz M, et al. Acute pulmonary embolism: diagnostic value of digital subtraction angiography. Radiology 1988;166:455–459.
29. Van Strijen MJ, De Monye W, Schiereck J, et al. Single-detector helical computed tomography as the primary diagnostic test in suspected pulmonary embolism: a multicenter clinical management study of 510 patients. Ann Intern Med 2003;138:307–314.
30. Wells PS, Ginsberg JS, Anderson DR, et al. Use of a clinical model for safe management of patients with suspected pulmonary embolism. Ann Intern Med 1998;129:997–1005.
31. Perrier A, Buswell L, Bounameaux H, et al. Cost-effectiveness of noninvasive diagnostic aids in suspected pulmonary embolism. Arch Intern Med 1997;157:2309–2316.
32. Oudkerk M, van Beek JR, van Putten WLJ, Büller HR. Cost-effectiveness analysis of various strategies in the diagnostic management of pulmonary embolism. Arch Intern Med 1993;153:947–954.
33. Wells PS, Anderson DR, Rodger M, et al. Evaluation of D-dimer in the diagnosis of suspected deep-vein thrombosis. N Engl J Med 2003;349:1227–1235.
34. Hull RD, Raskob GE, Coates G, Panju AA. Clinical validity of a normal perfusion lung scan in patients with suspected pulmonary embolism. Chest 1990;97:23–26.
35. Kipper MS, Moser KM, Kortman KE, Ashburn WL. Long-term follow-up of patients with suspected pulmonary embolism and a normal lung scan. Chest 1982;82:411–415.
36. van Beek EJR, Kuyer PMM, Schenk BS, Brandjes DPM, ten Cate JW, Büller HR. A normal perfusion lung scan in patients with clinically suspected pulmonary embolism. Frequency and clinical validity. Chest 1995;108:170–173.
37. Hull RD, Pineo GF, Stein PD, Mah AF, Butcher MS. Cost-effectiveness of currently accepted strategies for pulmonary embolism diagnosis. Semin Thromb Hemost 2001;27:15–23.
38. Hull RD, Feldstein W, Stein PD, Pineo GF. Cost-effectiveness of pulmonary embolism diagnosis. Arch Intern Med 1996;156:68–72.

39. Michel BC, Seerden RJ, Rutten FF, Van Beek EJ, Buller HR. The cost-effectiveness of diagnostic strategies in patients with suspected pulmonary embolism. Health Econ 1996;5:307–318.

40. van Erkel AR, van Rossum AB, Bloem JL, Kievit J, Pattynama PM. Spiral CT angiography for suspected pulmonary embolism: a cost-effectiveness analysis. Radiology 1996;201:29–36.

41. Henschke CI, Mateescu I, Yankelevitz DF. Changing practice patterns in the workup of pulmonary embolism. Chest 1995;107:940–945.

42. Sostman HD, Ravin CE, Sullivan DC, Mills SR, Glickman MG, Dorfman GS. Use of pulmonary angiography for suspected pulmonary embolism: influence of scintigraphic diagnosis. AJR 1982;139:673–677.

43. Sackett DL, Haynes RB, Guyatt GH, Tugwell P, eds. Clinical Epidemiology: A Basic Science for Clinical Medicine, Second Edition. Lippincott, Williams & Wilkins, Boston, 1991.

44. Wicki J, Perneger TV, Junod A, Bounameaux H, Perrier A. Assessing clinical probability of pulmonary embolism in the emergency ward: a simple score. Arch Intern Med 2001;161:92–97.

45. Perrier A, Roy PM, Sanchez O, et al. Multidetector-row computed tomography in suspected pulmonary embolism. N Engl J Med 2005;352:1760–1768.

46. Wells PS, Anderson DR, Bormanis J, Guy F, Mitchell M, Lewandowski B. SimpliRED D-dimer can reduce the diagnostic tests in suspected deep vein thrombosis [letter]. Lancet 1998;351:1405–1406.

47. Perrier A, Miron MJ, Desmarais S, et al. Using clinical evaluation and lung scan to rule out suspected pulmonary embolism: is it a valid option in patients with normal results of lower-limb venous compression ultrasonography? Arch Intern Med 2000;160:512–516.

48. Musset D, Parent F, Meyer G, et al. Diagnostic strategy for patients with suspected pulmonary embolism: a prospective multicentre outcome study. Lancet 2002;360:1914–1920.

49. van Belle A, Buller HR, Huisman MV, et al. Effectiveness of managing suspected pulmonary embolism using an algorithm combining clinical probability, D-dimer testing, and computed tomography. JAMA 2006;295:172–179.

50. Carson JL, Kelley MA, Duff A, Palevitch M. The clinical course of pulmonary embolism. N Engl J Med 1992;326:1240–1245.

51. Hull RD, Raskob GE, Ginsberg JS, et al. A noninvasive strategy for the treatment of patients with suspected pulmonary embolism. Arch Intern Med 1994;154:289–297.

52. de Moerloose P, Desmarais S, Bounameaux H, et al. Contribution of a new, rapid, individual and quantitative automated D-dimer ELISA to exclude pulmonary embolism. Thromb Haemost 1996;75:11–13.

53. Oger E, Leroyer C, Bressollette L, et al. Evaluation of a new, rapid, and quantitative D-dimer test in patients with suspected pulmonary embolism. Am J Respir Crit Care Med 1998;158:65–70.

54. Bates SM, Grand'Maison A, Johnston M, Naguit I, Kovacs MJ, Ginsberg JS. A latex D-dimer reliably excludes venous thromboembolism. Arch Intern Med 2001;161:447–453.

55. Ginsberg JS, Wells PS, Kearon C, et al. Sensitivity and specificity of a rapid whole-blood assay for D-dimer in the diagnosis of pulmonary embolism. Ann Intern Med 1998;129:1006–1011.

56. Turkstra F, Kuijer PMM, van Beek EJR, Brandjes DPM, ten Cate JW, Büller HR. Diagnostic utility of ultrasonography of leg veins in patients suspected of having pulmonary embolism. Ann Intern Med 1997;126:775–781.

57. Perrier A, Bounameaux H. Ultrasonography of leg veins in patients suspected of having pulmonary embolism. Ann Intern Med 1998;128:243.

58. Schoepf UJ, Goldhaber SZ, Costello P. Spiral computed tomography for acute pulmonary embolism. Circulation 2004;109:2160–2167.

8

Contemporary Diagnostic Algorithm for the Hemodynamically Unstable Patient With Suspected Massive Pulmonary Embolism

Stavros V. Konstantinides, MD

SUMMARY

Massive pulmonary embolism (PE) with overt hemodynamic compromise and cardiogenic shock is a life-threatening situation with an extremely poor prognosis. Management of the unstable, hypotensive patient with suspected massive PE poses a great challenge to the skills of the clinician in the intensive care unit or the emergency room, and it should direct the focus on rapid institution of treatment rather than absolute diagnostic certainty. Although not directly validated in large prospective management studies, a fast, simple diagnostic algorithm is recommended, based on confirmation of right ventricular dysfunction and, possibly, detection of large intracardiac or proximal pulmonary thrombi by transthoracic bedside echocardiography (echo). This approach minimizes time loss, helps avoid unnecessary patient transportation, and permits rapid therapeutic aspiration. Helical computed tomography may, alternatively, be used if echo is not immediately available or yields nondiagnostic findings.

Key Words: Massive pulmonary embolism; cardiogenic shock; right ventricular dysfunction; echocardiography; helical computed tomography.

INTRODUCTION

The previous chapter (Chapter 7) discussed the diagnostic workup of the hemodynamically stable patient with suspected pulmonary embolism (PE) and presented contemporary algorithms that have been validated in prospective management studies. In contrast, in the patient presenting with hemodynamic compromise and shock, the management strategy is based on the individual physician's experience and clinical judgement rather than on a solid body of evidence and/or widely accepted guidelines.

From: *Contemporary Cardiology: Management of Acute Pulmonary Embolism*
Edited by: S. Konstantinides © Humana Press Inc., Totowa, NJ

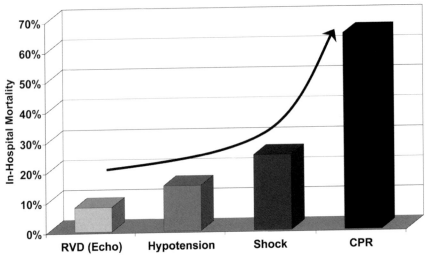

Fig. 1. Escalation of in-hospital mortality with increasing severity of hemodynamic instability at presentation. Data from the Management Strategies and Prognosis in Pulmonary Embolism Registry *(1)*. RVD, right ventricular dysfunction.

Massive PE is undoubtedly a life-threatening situation with an extremely poor prognosis. In the 1,001-patient Management Strategies and Prognosis of Pulmonary Embolism (MAPPET) registry, in-hospital mortality was 8% in initially normotensive patients who exhibited signs of right ventricular dysfunction on echocardiography, but it doubled (15%) in patients who presented with persistent arterial hypotension, defined as systolic arterial pressure of less than 90 mmHg or a drop in systolic pressure by at least 40 mmHg for at least 15 min *(1)*. Mortality rose to 25% in patients with cardiogenic shock (clinical signs of tissue hypoperfusion and hypoxia) at presentation, and it was as high as 65% in those who underwent cardiopulmonary resuscitation before or shortly after admission (Fig. 1). These results on a large population of patients with PE confirmed the findings of earlier series, which had reported a 32% mortality rate in patients with massive PE and cardiogenic shock *(2)*. More recently, a retrospective analysis of the International Cooperative Pulmonary Embolism Registry (ICOPER) showed that, among 2392 patients with acute PE and known systolic arterial blood pressure at presentation, massive PE was diagnosed in 108 (4.5%) and was associated with a 52.4% 90-d mortality rate as opposed to the 14.7% mortality rate of patients with nonmassive PE *(3)*.

Clinical suspicion of acute massive PE in a hemodynamically unstable patient is based on the symptoms, signs, and predisposing factors discussed in Chapter 1, but, clearly, there is no rationale for performing a D-dimer test in this emergency situation. No further time should be lost, and a bedside echocardiogram should be performed immediately, because it is the fastest and thus most appropriate initial test for confirming the presence of acute right ventricular failure (Fig. 2). The echocardiographic criteria for the diagnosis of right ventricular dysfunction were reviewed in Chapter 4. Although their limitations always need to be kept in mind, these criteria are relatively easy to learn and apply, and this fact explains the popularity of echocardiography among physicians involved in emergency medicine and intensive care. Additional valuable information that can be obtained from ultrasound imaging includes the presence of large floating worm-like intracardiac thrombi *(4–6)*, which signify an imminent threat of recurrent massive PE and should

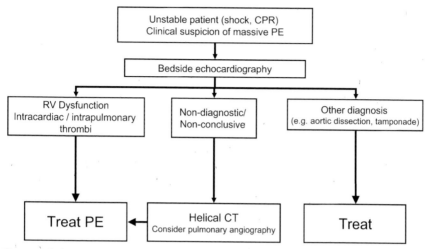

Fig. 2. Proposed algorithm for the management of the hemodynamically stable patient with suspected massive PE.

prompt emergency surgical embolectomy (Chapter 12) or, alternatively, thrombolysis, if surgery is not immediately available.

Despite the lack (and nonfeasibility) of a "formal" validation of cardiac ultrasound in the diagnosis of massive PE, a recent review of the available studies confirmed its usefulness in the presence of hemodynamic instability (7). Moreover, contemporary guidelines recommend echocardiography for the diagnostic workup of every patient with acute right or left ventricular cardiac failure (8), because it is not only capable of diagnosing (or excluding) massive PE, but may also provide alternative explanations for the patient's hypotension and shock, such as cardiomyopathy, large myocardial infarction, valvular or congenital disease, pericardial tamponade, or aortic dissection.

Patients with massive PE who present with refractory hypoxemia and/or neurological abnormalities may have right-to-left shunt or paradoxical thromboembolism through a patent foramen ovale (6,9,10); this condition is promptly detected by echocardiography, with or without echo contrast injection, and is associated with a particularly poor prognosis (see Chapter 6).

Finally, in mechanically ventilated patients, transesophageal echocardiography is a valuable alternative to transthoracic imaging, permitting not only assessment of cardiac function but also direct visualization of possible thrombi in the right atrium, foramen ovale, right ventricle, or the proximal segments of the common and right pulmonary artery (11).

As indicated in the proposed algorithm displayed in Fig. 2, the presence of right ventricular failure on echocardiography, with or without evidence of intracardiac or intrapulmonary thrombi, should prompt immediate treatment of massive PE without seeking confirmation of the diagnosis by further imaging procedures. As discussed in Chapters 10 and 11, there is, at present, consensus that thrombolysis is the treatment of choice for the majority of these hemodynamically unstable patients (12,13), despite the absence (and, perhaps, nonfeasibility) of large randomized trials to prove its efficacy and support this recommendation (14). Surgical embolectomy, if immediately available on site, is a reasonable alternative to thrombolysis (15,16), particularly in case of contraindications to the use of thrombolytic agents (see Chapter 12).

If echocardiography fails to confirm the clinical suspicion of massive PE or suggest an alternative diagnosis, spiral computed tomography (*see* Chapter 3) is the next fastest and the most reliable diagnostic method, although it does require transportation of the unstable patient to the radiology department. Alternatively, pulmonary angiography can be considered, especially if catheter-based aspiration of thrombus is a treatment option in the particular institution (*see* Chapter 13).

CONCLUSION

Management of the unstable patient with suspected massive PE poses a great challenge to the skills of the clinician in the intensive care unit or the emergency room, and it should direct the focus on rapid institution of treatment rather than absolute diagnostic certainty. Although not directly validated in large prospective management studies, the two-step algorithm presented in Fig. 2 is based on the well-documented and widely accepted value of echocardiography in this setting. This approach minimizes time loss and permits rapid therapeutic measures including thrombolysis, surgical embolectomy, or catheter-based thrombus aspiration.

REFERENCES

1. Kasper W, Konstantinides S, Geibel A, et al. Management strategies and determinants of outcome in acute major pulmonary embolism: results of a multicenter registry. J Am Coll Cardiol 1997;30:1165–1171.
2. Alpert JS, Smith R, Carlson J, Ockene IS, Dexter L, Dalen JE. Mortality in patients treated for pulmonary embolism. JAMA 1976;236:1477–1480.
3. Kucher N, Rossi E, De Rosa M, Goldhaber SZ. Massive pulmonary embolism. Circulation 2006;113: 577–582.
4. Konstantinides S, Geibel A, Kasper W. Role of cardiac ultrasound in the detection of pulmonary embolism. Semin Resp Crit Care Med 1996;17:39–49.
5. Chartier L, Bera J, Delomez M, et al. Free-floating thrombi in the right heart: diagnosis, management, and prognostic indexes in 38 consecutive patients. Circulation 1999;99:2779–2783.
6. Torbicki A, Galie N, Covezzoli A, Rossi E, De Rosa M, Goldhaber SZ. Right heart thrombi in pulmonary embolism: results from the International Cooperative Pulmonary Embolism Registry. J Am Coll Cardiol 2003;41:2245–2251.
7. ten Wolde M, Sohne M, Quak E, Mac Gillavry MR, Buller HR. Prognostic value of echocardiographically assessed right ventricular dysfunction in patients with pulmonary embolism. Arch Intern Med 2004; 164:1685–1689.
8. Nieminen MS, Bohm M, Cowie MR, et al. Executive summary of the guidelines on the diagnosis and treatment of acute heart failure: the Task Force on Acute Heart Failure of the European Society of Cardiology. Eur Heart J 2005;26:384–416.
9. Kasper W, Geibel A, Tiede N, Just H. Patent foramen ovale in patients with haemodynamically significant pulmonary embolism. Lancet 1992;340:561–564.
10. Konstantinides S, Geibel A, Kasper W, Olschewski M, Blumel L, Just H. Patent foramen ovale is an important predictor of adverse outcome in patients with major pulmonary embolism [see comments]. Circulation 1998;97:1946–1951.
11. Pruszczyk P, Torbicki A, Kuch-Wocial A, Szulc M, Pacho R. Diagnostic value of transoesophageal echocardiography in suspected haemodynamically significant pulmonary embolism. Heart 2001;85:628–634.
12. British Thoracic Society. Guidelines for the management of suspected acute pulmonary embolism. Thorax 2003;58:470–483.
13. European Society of Cardiology TFoPE. Guidelines on diagnosis and management of acute pulmonary embolism. Eur Heart J 2000;21:1301–1336.
14. Jerjes-Sanchez C, Ramírez-Rivera A, de Lourdes G, et al. Streptokinase and heparin versus heparin alone in massive pulmonary embolism: a randomized controlled trial. J Thromb Thrombolysis 1995;2: 227–229.
15. Aklog L, Williams CS, Byrne JG, Goldhaber SZ. Acute pulmonary embolectomy: a contemporary approach. Circulation 2002;105:1416–1419.
16. Dauphine C, Omari B. Pulmonary embolectomy for acute massive pulmonary embolism. Ann Thorac Surg 2005;79:1240–1244.

II TREATMENT AND SECONDARY PROPHYLAXIS OF VENOUS THROMBOEMBOLISM

9

Heparin Anticoagulation

Graham F. Pineo, MD, FRCPC, FACP
and Russell D. Hull, MBBS, MSc, FRCPC, FACP

SUMMARY

In the initial treatment of patients presenting with acute pulmonary embolism (PE), anticoagulation is based either on unfractionated heparin (UFH) by continuous intravenous infusion and activated partial thromboplastin time monitoring, or on low-molecular-weight heparin (LMWH) given by once- or twice-daily subcutaneous injections. There have been several studies comparing the use of UFH and LMWH for the treatment of deep vein thrombosis (DVT), all demonstrating that LMWH is at least as effective and safe as UFH by continuous intravenous infusion. Fewer studies have compared the use of UFH and LMWH for the treatment of acute PE, but the evidence is that, as in DVT, LMWH is equally effective and safe compared to UFH. Furthermore, LMWH offers the convenience of out-of-hospital treatment for hemodynamically stable patients with nonmassive PE without the need for laboratory monitoring. Therefore, in the recent guidelines of the American College of Chest Physicians, either LMWH or UFH is recommended for the initial treatment of venous thromboembolism. In patients with advanced renal insufficiency, the recommendation is to use UFH rather the LMWH.

Key Words: Venous thromboembolism; heparin; low-molecular-weight heparin; fondaparinux.

From: *Contemporary Cardiology: Management of Acute Pulmonary Embolism*
Edited by: S. Konstantinides © Humana Press Inc., Totowa, NJ

INTRODUCTION

Deep venous thrombosis (DVT) and pulmonary embolism (PE) can be considered as manifestations of a single disease entity that is commonly referred to as venous thrombo-embolism (VTE). There is some evidence that patients who present with symptomatic PE have a worse prognosis in terms of recurrent VTE and death than do those who present with symptomatic DVT alone *(1)*. Furthermore, patients who present with symptomatic PE may have a higher risk of suffering recurrent PE rather than recurrent DVT in the future *(2,3)*. Nonetheless, the initial and long-term treatment of patients with either DVT or PE is essentially the same, as recommended in the Evidence-Based Guidelines recently released at the American College of Chest Physicians VII Conference on Antithrombotic and Thrombolytic Therapy *(4)*.

The objectives of the treatment of patients with VTE are: (1) to prevent death from acute PE; (2) to prevent recurrent PE or DVT; and (3) to prevent the postthrombotic syndrome. With regard to the latter goal, the use of graduated compression stockings has been shown to significantly decrease the incidence of the postthrombotic syndrome *(5)*. On the other hand, treatment and secondary prevention of PE is based on effective anticoagulation, which initially consists of either intravenous unfractionated heparin (UFH) or subcutaneous low-molecular-weight heparin (LMWH). Long-term oral anticoagulation with a Vitamin K antagonist (discussed in Chapter 14) commences in conjunction with these therapies. This chapter will review the current state of the art in the initial anticoagulation of patients presenting with DVT and PE, focusing on the use of UFH and LMWH.

UFH FOR THE INITIAL TREATMENT OF VTE AND PE

The anticoagulant activity of UFH depends on a unique pentasaccharide that binds to antithrombin (AT) and potentiates its inhibiting effects on thrombin and activated factor X (Xa) *(6)*. Approximately one-third of all heparin molecules contain this pentasaccharide sequence, regardless of whether they are low- or high-molecular-weight fractions *(6–8)*. It is the pentasaccharide sequence that confers the molecular high affinity of heparins for AT *(6–8)*. Heparin also catalyzes the inactivation of thrombin by another plasma cofactor (cofactor II), which acts independently of AT *(8)*. Moreover, heparin exerts a number of thrombin-unrelated effects that include the release of tissue factor pathway inhibitor, the binding to numerous plasma and platelet proteins, endothelial cells, and leukocytes *(6)*, the suppression of platelet function, and an increase in vascular permeability *(8)*.

An established approach to anticoagulant therapy for VTE is the combination of continuous intravenous infusion of UFH with oral warfarin. The length of the recommended initial intravenous heparin therapy has gradually been reduced to 5 d, thus shortening the hospital stay and leading to significant cost saving *(9,10)*. The early start (e.g., on the second hospital day) of warfarin treatment overlapping with heparin administration has become standard practice for the majority of patients with VTE who are hemodynamically stable. Exceptions include patients who require immediate medical or surgical intervention, such as thrombolysis or insertion of a vena cava filter, or patients at very high risk of bleeding. Heparin is continued until the international normalized ratio has been within the therapeutic range (2.0–3.0) for two consecutive days *(4)*.

Heparin is cleared by a rapid saturable mechanism involving its binding to endothelial cell receptors and macrophages, and also by a slower clearance that occurs primarily through the renal tract. Heparin clearance is dose-dependent, becoming slower with increasing doses of intravenously administered heparin. Clearance following subcutaneous injection is even longer. Therefore, the anticoagulant response to a standard dose of heparin varies widely among patients, and thus individual anticoagulant monitoring with the use of the activated partial thromboplastin time (APTT), or of heparin levels, is mandatory, so that the heparin dosage can be titrated to the individual patient *(8)*. There is wide variability in the APTT and heparin blood levels with different reagents and even with different batches of the same reagent. It is, therefore, vital for each laboratory to establish the minimal therapeutic level of heparin, as measured by the APTT, that will provide a heparin blood level of 0.3 to 0.7 IU/mL, as assessed by factor Xa inhibition, for each batch of thromboplastin reagent being used, particularly if the reagents are provided by different manufacturers *(8)*.

It has been established from experimental studies and clinical trials that the efficacy of heparin therapy depends on achieving a critical therapeutic level of anticoagulation within the first 24 h of treatment *(10–12)*. In fact, data from rigorous clinical trials indicate that failure to achieve the therapeutic APTT threshold by 24 h is associated with an unacceptable frequency of recurrent VTE in the long-term *(11,13–16)*. For example, a recently published study compared subcutaneous adjusted-dose UFH with fixed-dose LMWH for the initial treatment of VTE, including those patients (16% of the study population) who presented with symptomatic PE. The investigators reported that, in the UFH therapeutic arm, recurrent VTE occurred in 2.7% of the patients who reached an APTT therapeutic threshold within 24 h as compared to 8.2% of those who failed to do so ($p =$ 0.02) *(13)*. The recurrences occurred throughout the 3-mo follow-up period and could not be attributed to inadequate oral anticoagulant therapy *(13)*. These data strongly support the need for meticulous monitoring of the APTT in patients receiving UFH. On the other hand, for patients with apparent heparin resistance, that is those who require very high doses of intravenous UFH to achieve therapeutic levels of APTT, measurement of heparin blood levels has been used for more effective and reliable monitoring *(8)*. Another alternative is the use of LMWH, discussed later.

Although a strong correlation exists between subtherapeutic APTT values and recurrent VTE, the relationship between supratherapeutic APTT (i.e., an APTT ratio of 2.5 or higher) and bleeding is less clear *(11)*. Indeed, bleeding during heparin therapy appears to be more closely related to underlying clinical risk factors than to APTT elevation above the therapeutic range *(11)*. Recent studies confirm that excess body weight and age greater than 65 yr are independent risk factors for heparin-related bleeding *(8)*.

Numerous audits of heparin therapy indicate that administration of intravenous heparin is fraught with difficulty, and that the clinical practice of using an *ad hoc* approach to heparin dose-titration frequently results in inadequate therapy. Consequently, the use of a prescriptive approach or protocol for administering intravenous heparin therapy has been evaluated in prospective studies of patients with VTE *(11,14,17)*.

In one clinical trial that focused on the treatment of DVT, patients were given either intravenous heparin alone followed by warfarin, or intravenous heparin and simultaneous warfarin (heparin/warfarin) *(10)*. The heparin nomogram used is summarized in Tables 1 and 2. Only 1 and 2% of the patients in the heparin-only and the heparin/warfarin group, respectively, were undertreated for more than 24 h. Recurrent VTE (objectively documented) occurred rather infrequently in both groups (7%). Thus, subtherapeutic levels could be avoided in most patients, and the proposed heparin nomogram resulted in effective administration of heparin therapy in both treatment groups.

Table 1
Suggested Protocol for Continuous Intravenous Heparin Infusion

1. Administer initial intravenous heparin bolus: 5000 U.
2. Administer continuous intravenous heparin infusion: commence at 1680 U/h (24-h heparin dose of 40,320 U), except in the following patients, in whom heparin infusion is commenced at a rate of 1240 U/h (24-h dose of 29,760 U):
   a) patients who have undergone surgery within the previous 2 wk;
   b) patients with a previous history of peptic ulcer disease or gastrointestinal or genitourinary bleeding;
   c) patients with recent (ischemic) stroke within the previous 2 wk;
   d) patients with a platelet count >150 × 10⁹/L;
   e) patients with miscellaneous reasons for a high risk of bleeding (e.g., hepatic failure, renal failure, or vitamin K deficiency).
3. Adjust heparin dose by use of the APTT. The APTT test is performed in all patients as follows:
   a) 4–6 h after commencing heparin; the heparin dose is then adjusted;
   b) 4–6 h after the first dosage adjustment;
   c) then, as indicated by the nomogram for the first 24 h of therapy;
   d) thereafter once daily, unless the APTT is subtherapeutic[a], in which case the test is repeated 4–6 h after the heparin dose has been increased.

APTT, activated partial thromboplastin time.
[a]Subtherapeutic implies that APTT is less than 1.5 times the mean normal control value for the thromboplastin reagent being used.

Table 2
Intravenous Heparin Dose Titration Nomogram According to the APTT

APTT (s)	Rate change (mL/h)	Dose change (IU/24 h)[a]	Additional action
≤45	+6	+5760	Repeated APTT[b] in 4–6 h
46–54	+3	+2880	Repeated APTT in 4–6 h
55–85	0	0	None[c]
86–110	−3	−2880	Stop heparin treatment for 1 h; repeat APTT 4–6 h after restarting heparin treatment
>110	−6	−5760	Stop heparin treatment for 1 h; repeat APTT 4–6 h after restarting heparin treatment

[a]Heparin sodium concentration 20,000 IU in 500 mL = 40 IU/mL.
[b]With the use of Actin-FS thromboplastin reagent (Dade, Mississauga, Ontario, Canada).
[c]During the first 24 h, repeat APTT in 4–6 h. Thereafter, the APTT will be determined once daily, unless subtherapeutic.
Adapted from ref. 11 with permission.

In another clinical trial, a weight-based heparin dosage nomogram (Table 3) was compared with a standard-care nomogram (14). Patients on the weight-adjusted heparin nomogram received a starting dose of 80 U/kg as a bolus and 18 U/(kg / h) as an infusion. The heparin dose was adjusted to maintain an APTT of 1.5 to 2.3 times control. In the weight-adjusted group, 97% of patients achieved the therapeutic range within 24 h compared with 77% in the standard-care group. Recurrent VTE was more frequent in the standard-care group, supporting the previous observation that subtherapeutic heparin during the initial 24 h is associated with a higher incidence of recurrences. This study included

Table 3
Weight-Based Nomogram for Initial Intravenous Heparin Therapy
(Numbers in Parentheses Show Comparison with Control)

	Dosage (in IU/kg)
Initial dose	80 as bolus, then 18 U/h
APTT <35 s (<1.2 times)	80 as bolus, then 4 U/h
APTT 35–45 s (1.2 1.5 times)	40 as bolus, then 2 U/h
APTT 46–70 s (1.5–2.3 times)	No change
APTT 71–90 s (2.3–3.0 times)	Decrease infusion rate by 2 U/h
APTT >90 s (>3.0 times)	Hold infusion 1 h, then decrease infusion rate by 3 U/h

APTT, activated partial thromboplastin time. (Adapted from ref. *14*, with permission.)

patients with unstable angina and arterial thromboembolism in addition to VTE, which suggests that the principles applied to a heparin nomogram for the treatment of VTE may be extrapolated to other clinical conditions. Continued use of the weight-based nomogram has been similarly effective *(17)*.

Adjusted-dose *subcutaneous UFH* has also been tested in the initial treatment of VTE. In an early study, patients presenting with proximal DVT were randomized to receive either 15,000 U of heparin every 12 h by subcutaneous injection or 30,000 units of heparin by continuous IV infusion following an initial bolus of 5000 U *(16)*. Therapeutic heparin levels and APTT levels were achieved at 24 h in 37% of the patients who received subcutaneous heparin compared with 71% of those receiving intravenous heparin. These findings were disappointing in view of the fact that, as emphasized previously, recurrent VTE occurs more frequently in patients who fail to achieve therapeutic heparin levels in terms of APTT values within the first 24 to 48 h of therapy as compared to those who achieve therapeutic levels quickly *(12)*. Nonetheless, there has been some interest in the use of UFH by the subcutaneous route for the initial treatment of VTE. A meta-analysis comparing subcutaneous with intravenous UFH in the setting of the initial treatment of DVT suggested that twice-daily subcutaneous heparin might be more effective in terms of recurrent DVT, and it was at least as safe *(18)*. The authors proposed that subcutaneous UFH could simplify treatment and permit out-of-hospital management for many of these patients. Efforts have been made to develop treatment nomograms for the optimal dosing of subcutaneous heparin *(19,20)*, and four randomized clinical trials compared the efficacy of subcutaneous UFH with subcutaneous LMWH in patients with proven VTE *(13,21–23)*. The largest of these trials, which was recently published, demonstrated that subcutaneous dose-adjusted UFH using a weight-based algorithm and APTT monitoring was as effective and safe as fixed-dose LMWH for the initial treatment of patients with VTE, of whom approx 16% presented with PE. The authors concluded that, for patients in whom UFH is chosen as initial treatment of PE, the use of the subcutaneous route might be a viable option that would permit out-of-hospital treatment *(13)*.

At present, UFH given by continuous intravenous infusion is, at least in the United States, the treatment of choice for the majority of patients presenting with acute PE. In other countries, including Canada, these patients are frequently treated with LMWH, unless they are hemodynamically unstable, thus necessitating emergency thrombolysis or surgical/interventional recanalization procedures (*see* Chapters 10–13), or at high risk for bleeding. In the latter case, correction of the anticoagulant effect of UFH by stopping the intravenous infusion and/or giving protamine sulfate is more effective when heparin is given by the intravenous route, as compared to the use of subcutaneous LMWH, which exhibits a longer half-life and can only be incompletely antagonized by protamine sulfate.

COMPLICATIONS OF HEPARIN THERAPY

The main adverse effects of heparin therapy include bleeding, thrombocytopenia, and osteoporosis. Osteoporosis has been reported in patients receiving UFH in dosages of 20,000 U/d (or more) for more than 6 mo. Demineralization can progress to the fracture of vertebral bodies or long bones, and the defect may not be entirely reversible *(8)*.

Patients at particular risk of bleeding while on heparin treatment are those who have had recent surgery or trauma, or who have other clinical factors predisposing to bleeding such as peptic ulcer, occult malignancy, liver disease, hemostatic defects, excess body weight, and age greater than 65 yr. Female gender also apears to predispose to bleeding *(8)*. The management of heparin-related bleeding depends on the location and severity of bleeding, the risk of recurrent VTE, and the APTT levels. Heparin should be discontinued temporarily or permanently. Patients with recent VTE may be candidates for insertion of an inferior vena cava filter. If urgent reversal of the heparin effect is required, protamine sulphate can be administered *(8)*.

Heparin-induced thrombocytopenia is a well-recognized complication of heparin therapy, usually occurring within 5 to 10 d after heparin treatment has started *(24–28)*. Approximately 1 to 2% of patients receiving UFH experience a fall in platelet count to less than the normal range or a 50% fall in the platelet count within the normal range. In the majority of these cases, mild to moderate thrombocytopenia appears to be a direct effect of heparin on platelets and is of no consequence. However, approx 0.1 to 0.2% of the patients receiving heparin will develop an immune thrombocytopenia mediated by immunoglobulin G antibody directed against a complex of platelet factor 4 (PF4) and heparin *(25)*. The development of heparin-induced thrombocytopenia may be accompanied by arterial or venous thrombosis, which may lead to serious consequences such as death or limb amputation *(27,28)*. Importantly, the diagnosis of heparin-induced thrombocytopenia, with or without thrombosis, must be made on clinical grounds, because the assays with the highest sensitivity and specificity are not readily available and have a slow turn-around time.

When the diagnosis of heparin-induced thrombocytopenia is made, heparin in all forms must be stopped immediately. Because continuation of anticoagulation will be required in most cases, alternative agents need to be considered *(26–28)*. The agents most extensively tested include lepirudin *(26–28)*, danaparoid sodium *(27,28)* and, more recently, the specific thrombin inhibitor argatroban *(28)*. Danaparoid is available for limited use on compassionate grounds, whereas hirudin and argatroban have been approved for use in the United States and Canada. Warfarin should not be started until one of the previously mentioned agents has been used for 3 or 4 d to suppress thrombin generation. Insertion of an inferior vena cava filter is rarely indicated.

LMWH FOR THE INITIAL
AND LONG-TERM TREATMENT OF VTE

The UFH currently in use clinically is polydispersed unmodified heparin with a mean molecular weight ranging from 10 to 16 kDa. In recent years, low-molecular-weight derivatives of commercial heparin have been prepared that have a mean molecular weight of

4–6 kDa *(29,30)*. The LMWHs commercially available are made by different processes (such as nitrous acid, alkaline, or enzymatic depolymerization) and they differ chemically and pharmacokinetically *(29,30)*. The clinical significance of these differences, however, remains unclear, and there have been very few studies directly comparing different LMWHs with respect to clinical outcomes *(30)*. Of note, the doses of the different LMWHs have been established empirically and these agents are not necessarily interchangeable. Therefore, at this time, the effectiveness and safety of each of the LMWHs must be tested separately *(30)*.

The LMWHs differ from UFH in numerous ways. Of particular importance are the following properties: (1) increased bioavailability (>90% after subcutaneous injection); (2) prolonged half-life; (3) predictable clearance, enabling once- or twice-daily injection; and (4) predictable AT response based on body weight, permitting treatment without laboratory monitoring *(8,29,30)*. Other possible advantages are their ability to inactivate platelet-bound factor Xa, resistance to inhibition by PF4, and their decreased effect on platelet function and vascular permeability, possibly accounting for less hemorrhagic effects than UFH at comparable AT doses *(8)*.

There has been hope that the LMWHs could have fewer serious complications such as bleeding *(29,30)*, heparin-induced thrombocytopenia *(25,27)*, and osteoporosis *(31)* when compared with UFH. Evidence is accumulating that these complications are indeed less frequent with the use of LMWH. Moreover, although LMWH has not been approved for the prevention and treatment of VTE in pregnancy, these drugs do not cross the placenta and case series indicate they are both effective and safe in this setting (*see* Chapter 17). On the other hand, all LMWHs cross-react with UFH and therefore *cannot* be used as alternative therapy in patients who develop heparin-induced thrombocytopenia.

Several LMWHs are available for the prevention and treatment of VTE in various countries. Four LMWHs have been approved for clinical use in Canada and two LMWHs have been approved for use in the United States.

In a number of early clinical trials (some of which were dose-finding), LMWH given by subcutaneous or intravenous injection was compared with continuous intravenous UFH, with repeat venography at d 7–10 being the primary end point. These studies demonstrated that LMWH was at least as effective as UFH in preventing extension or increasing resolution of thrombi on repeat venography. Subsequently, subcutaneous unmonitored LMWH was compared with continuous intravenous heparin in a number of clinical trials for the treatment of proximal DVT using long-term follow-up as an outcome measure *(32–39)* (Table 4). These studies showed that LMWH was at least as effective and safe as UFH in the treatment of proximal DVT. Three of these studies indicated that LMWH used predominantly out-of-hospital was as effective and safe as intravenous UFH given in-hospital *(37–39)*. Pooling of the most methodologically sound studies indicates a significant advantage for LMWH in the reduction of major bleeding and mortality *(40)*. Moreover, economic analysis of treatment with LMWH vs intravenous heparin demonstrated that LMWH was cost-effective for treatment in-hospital as well as out-of-hospital *(41)*.

Long-term LMWH has been compared with oral anticoagulant (warfarin) therapy in patients presenting with proximal DVT *(42)*. Although these studies differ in their design and the dosage of LMWH, they do indicate that LMWH is a useful alternative to warfarin therapy. Long-term LMWH treatment has been used in patients who have recurrence of VTE while on therapeutic doses of warfarin. More recently, long-term LMWH was compared with long-term warfarin for the treatment of a broad spectrum of patients and in

Table 4
LMWH vs UFH for the Treatment of Proximal DVT: Study Overview

Reference	Treatment	Mortality [no.(%)]	Recurrent VTE [no.(%)]	Major bleeding [no.(%)]
Hull et al. (32)	Tinzaparin	10/213 (4.7)[a]	6/213 (2.8)	1/213 (0.5)[a]
	Heparin	21/219 (9.6)	15/219 (6.8)	11/219 (5.0)
Prandoni et al. (33)	Nadroparin	6/85 (7.1)	6/85 (7.1)	1/85 (1.2)
	Heparin	12/85 (14.1)	12/85 (14.1)	3/85 (3.8)
Lopaciuk et al. (34)[b]	Nadroparin	0/74	0/74 (0)	0/74
	Heparin	1/72 (1.4)	3/72 (4.2)	1/72 (1.4)
Simonneau et al. (35)	Enoxaparin	3/67 (4.5)	0/67	0/67
	Heparin	2/67 (3.0)	0/67	0/67
Lindmarker et al. (36)[c]	Dalteparin	2/101 (2.0)	5/101 (5.0)	1/101 (1.0)
	Heparin	3/103 (2.9)	3/103 (2.9)	0/103
Koopman et al. (37)	Nadroparin	14/202 (6.9)	14/202 (6.9)	1/202 (0.5)
	Heparin	16/198 (8.1)	17/198 (8.6)	4/198 (2.0)
Levine et al. (38)	Enoxaparin	11/247 (4.5)	13/247 (5.3)	5/247 (2.0)
	Heparin	17/253 (6.7)	17/253 (6.7)	3/253 (1.2)
Columbus	Clivarin	36/510 (7.1)	27/510 (5.3)	16/510 (3.1)
Investigators (39)	Heparin	39/511 (7.6)	25/511 (4.9)	12/511 (2.3)

[a]p < 0.05 vs heparin (mortality and major bleeding).
[b]19.5% had calf vein DVT and/or involvement of the popliteal.
[c]42.6% distal DVT only.
LMWH, low-molecular-weight heparin; UFH, unfractionated heparin; DVT, deep vein thrombosis.

patients with cancer presenting with proximal DVT (43,44). Based on these results, long-term LMWH has been recommended for a period of at least 6 mo for patients presenting with DVT or PE and cancer (4).

LMWH TREATMENT FOR PATIENTS PRESENTING WITH PE

Evidence is accumulating that LMWH can be safely used to treat acute nonmassive PE. In a dose-finding study, three doses of nadroparin were compared with continuous intravenous UFH for the initial treatment of patients presenting with PE (45). After d 8, improvement in pulmonary vascular obstruction and major bleeding rates were similar in the UFH and the LMWH group receiving the lowest dose of nadroparin. In an open randomized clinical trial, the LMWH dalteparin, given at the dosage of 120 anti-Xa U/kg twice daily for 10 d, was compared with UFH, given by continuous intravenous infusion for 10 d, in patients with nonmassive PE (46). There were no episodes of recurrent PE and no major bleeding in either group during the treatment period, and the decrease in pulmonary vascular obstruction on perfusion lung scans between d 0 and d 10 was similar in the two groups.

The Columbus study compared the use of the LMWH reviparin given according to a fixed weight-based schedule twice daily, compared with UFH given by intravenous infusion, for approx 5 d prior to starting warfarin in patients presenting with DVT or PE (27% of the patients presented with PE) (39). Patients were stratified according to whether they presented with DVT or PE. During both the initial hospitalization and the follow-up period, no difference was observed between the two treatment groups with regard to the

Table 5
Heparin Anticoagulation for PE:
Outcome Events in the LMWH vs UFH Treatment Group

	Heparin	LMWH	p Value
Recurrent VTE	7/103 (6.8%)	0/97 (0.0%)	0.014[a] 0.009[b]
Major bleeding (initial therapy)	2/103 (1.9%)	1/97 (1.0%)	
Minor bleeding	3/103 (2.9%)	1/97 (1.0%)	
Death	9/103 (8.7%)	6/97 (6.2%)	

[a]Fisher's exact test.
[b]Log rank analysis.
PE, pulmonary embolism; LMWH, low-molecular-weight heparin; UFH, unfractionated heparin; VTE, venous thromboembolism.
Adapted from ref. 48 with permission.

incidence of recurrent VTE or death, or in the occurrence of major bleeding. Overall, the therapeutic efficacy of LMWH in patients with PE was similar to that in patients presenting with DVT only. It was concluded that fixed-dose subcutaneous LMWH was as effective and safe as adjusted-dose intravenous UFH for the initial management of patients presenting with PE.

In the only randomized clinical trial focusing on patients with PE to date (47), 612 patients with symptomatic PE, who were considered not to require thrombolytic therapy or embolectomy, received either the LMWH tinzaparin, given by once-daily, weight-adjusted subcutaneous injection, or UFH given by APTT-adjusted continuous intravenous infusion. Patients in the tinzaparin arm received 175 anti-Xa U/Kg per day for an average of 7 d, with warfarin starting on d 1–3 and continued for 3 mo. The remaining patients received UFH for an average of 7 d, with warfarin also starting on d 1–3 and continued for 3 mo. Of the 1482 consecutive patients who met the entry criteria, 766 (52%) were excluded. Of these, 177 (23.1%) required thrombolytic therapy and 55 (7.2%) had interruption of the inferior vena cava. Neither the incidence of recurrent VTE or death over the initial and follow-up period nor the incidence of major bleeding differed between the two treatment groups. The authors concluded that LMWH was as effective and as safe as intravenous UFH in the treatment of acute PE. They pointed out, however, that their selection criteria excluded a number of patients at high risk of death, recurrent thrombosis, or bleeding. In these high-risk groups, the efficacy and safety of LMWH remains to be determined.

Data from an earlier randomized clinical trial also support the use of LMWH in the treatment of patients with PE (32). In a double-blind prospective trial of patients presenting with proximal DVT, the LMWH tinzaparin, given at the dosage of 175 anti-Xa U/kg per day for 6 d, was compared with UFH given by continuous intravenous infusion and monitored by a heparin-APTT nomogram for at least 6 d. Warfarin was started in both arms on d 2 and continued for 3 mos. Within 48 h of entry into the study, all patients had a ventilation-perfusion lung scan and chest X-ray performed. Of the 219 patients receiving UFH, 103 (47.0%) had high probability for PE, whereas of the 213 LMWH patients, 97 (45.5%) had high-probability perfusion lung scan findings (48) (Table 5). Patients with PE were well-matched in terms of clinical characteristics. Recurrent VTE occurred in 7 (6.8%) of 103 patients receiving intravenous heparin as opposed to none of the 97 patients who received LMWH. Major bleeding associated with initial therapy occurred in one patient (1%) who was given LMWH and in two patients (1.9%) given intravenous heparin. Death occurred during the 3-mo interval of the trial in 6 (6.2%) of patients on LMWH and 9 (8.7%) of patients on UFH. One patient in the UFH died of acute PE on d 1 *(48)*.

The data from the previously described studies *(47,48)*, which used the same LMWH (tinzaparin) at the same dosage, were pooled for patients who had both documented proximal DVT and PE. Recurrent VTE occurred in 2 of 254 (0.8%) patients who received LMWH vs 10 (3.9%) of 255 patients who received UFH (odds ratio, 0.20; 95% confidence interval [CI], 0.042–0.92; $p = 0.022$) *(49)*. Major bleeding occurred in 3 (1.2%) patients on LMWH compared to 5 (1.96%) patients on UFH. The mortality rate for patients on LMWH was 12 (4.7%) vs 17 (6.7%) for those on UFH. Thus, this analysis suggests a decrease in the incidence of recurrent VTE in patients receiving LMWH as compared with UFH, with a similar risk for major bleeding.

In many centers, patients presenting with PE who are hemodynamically stable and have no other indications for hospital admission are increasingly being treated out of hospital. This practice is supported by several cohort studies *(50,51)*, including one small randomized trial that compared LMWH for 90 d with UFH and warfarin according to the usual regimen *(52)*. Outcomes in terms of recurrent VTE and bleeding were similar in both groups, but the median hospital length of stay was shorter in the enoxaparin group (4 vs 6 d; $p = 0.001$).

SPECIAL CONSIDERATIONS
FOR THE USE OF LMWH IN THE TREATMENT OF VTE

The LMWHs differ in their pharmacological properties and are therefore considered to be distinct entities by the regulatory bodies *(8)*. There are, for example, differences regarding the effect of severe renal impairment on the metabolism and clearance of some of the LMWHs such as enoxaparin and nadroparin *(53,54)*. Furthermore, there is some evidence that the LMWH tinzaparin may not accumulate in patients with renal insufficiency down to a glomerular filtration rate of 25 mL/min, suggesting that, in elderly patients with renal insufficiency, excessive factor Xa inhibition could be less likely with this substance *(55, 56)*. Moreover, there are differences in the degree to which protamine sulfate can inhibit the anticoagulant effect of various LMWHs, with the reduction in Xa levels varying between 55 and 85% *(57)*. The activity by protamine sulfate is directly related to the number of sulfate radicals on the site chains of the LMWH *(57)*.

There has been concern that, in patients who are obese or morbidly obese, using LMWH at dosages based on weight adjustment may lead to excessively high anti-factor Xa levels. Regulatory agencies have, therefore, imposed a cap on the daily dose of LMWH at 18,000 U, corresponding to a maximal body weight of 108 kg. There is, however, recent evidence that anti-factor Xa levels remain in the therapeutic range when the LMWHs tinzaparin and dalteparin continue to be given at a weight-adjusted dosage in obese patients weighing more than 108 kg, even if this results in exceeding the proposed upper limit of 18,000 U/d *(58,59)*. In fact, there is concern that limiting the LMWH dosage in these patients may pose them at a higher risk of recurrent thrombosis.

There has been considerable debate about the need for measurement of factor Xa levels as a means of monitoring therapy with LMWH. Such levels are justified in the treatment of VTE in pregnancy or in childhood, but there is little justification for measurement of

Xa levels in other settings *(8)*. Furthermore, little correlation seems to exist between factor Xa levels and severe bleeding or thrombosis *(60)*. Most of the LMWHs are given by twice-daily injection, but there is no evidence that this is either more effective or safer than once-daily injection *(61)*. Finally, concern has been raised regarding the use of subcutaneous LMWH in patients who are on pressor agents as, for example, in intensive care units. These reservations appear to be justified, since anti-Xa levels were lower following subcutaneous injection of LMWH in patients who were on pressor agents as compared to age-matched controls *(62)*.

SUBCUTANEOUS FONDAPARINUX FOR THE INITIAL TREATMENT OF PE

The pentasaccharide fondaparinux, given by subcutaneous injection at three different dosages depending on body weight, was compared with continuous intravenous UFH monitored by APTT measurements in patients presenting with symptomatic PE *(63)*. Recurrent VTE was observed in 1.3% of patients on fondaparinux vs 1.7% on UFH. Major bleeding was seen in 1.3% of patients on fondaparinux compared to 1.1% on UFH. Mortality rates at 3 mo were similar in the two groups. In the fondaparinux group, 14.5% of the patients received the drug in part on an outpatients basis. It was concluded that once-daily subcutaneous fondaparinux without laboratory monitoring was as effective and safe as adjusted-dose intravenous UFH for the initial treatment of hemodynamically stable patients with PE *(63)*.

CONCLUSIONS

For the initial treatment of patients presenting with PE, UFH by continuous intravenous infusion, or LMWH by once- or twice-daily subcutaneous injection, are the recommended treatment choices at present. The meta-analyses of numerous studies comparing LMWH by subcutaneous injection to intravenous UFH for patients presenting with DVT have shown a comparable incidence of recurrent VTE and bleeding, and a decreased incidence of mortality in favor of LMWH. Although fewer studies have compared LMWH and UFH for the initial treatment of patients with PE, the existing evidence suggests that LMWH is equally effective and safe and offers the convenience of out-of-hospital treatment without laboratory monitoring apart from measurement of platelet counts. Therefore, the recently updated ACCP guidelines endorse both LMWH and UFH for the initial treatment of VTE, but it is recommended to prefer LMWH to UFH in patients with DVT who can be treated on an outpatient basis, and in hemodynamically stable patients with non-massive PE. On the other hand, in patients with advanced renal failure (glomerular filtration rate less than 25 mL/min), it appears to be safer to use UFH.

REFERENCES

1. Douketis JD, Foster GA, Crowther MA, et al. Clinical risk factors and timing of recurrent venous thromboembolism during the initial 3 months of anticoagulant. Arch Intern Med 2000;160(22):3431–3436.
2. Douketis JD, Kearon C, Bates B, et al. Risk of fatal pulmonary embolism in patients with treated venous thromboembolism. JAMA 1998;279(6):458–462.
3. Heit JA, Mohr DN, Silverstein MD, et al. Predictors of recurrence after deep vein thrombosis and pulmonary embolism. A population-based cohort study. Arch Intern Med 2000;160:761–768.
4. Buller HR, Agnelli G, Hull RD, et al. Antithrombotic therapy for venous thromboembolic disease; The Seventh ACCP Conference on Antithrombotic and Thrombolytic Therapy. Chest 2004;126(3):401S–428S.

5. Brandjes DPM, Buller HR, Heijboer H, et al. Randomised trial of effect of compression stockings in patients with symptomatic proximal-vein thrombosis. Lancet 1997;349:759–762.

6. Lane DA. Heparin binding and neutralizing protein. In: Lane DA, Lindahl U, eds. Heparin, chemical and biological properties, clinical applications. Edward Arnold, London, 1989, pp. 363–391.

7. Rosenberg RD, Lam L. Correlation between structure and function of heparin. Proc Natl Acad Sci USA 1979;76:1218–1222.

8. Hirsh J, Raschke R. Heparin and low-molecular-weight heparin: The Seventh ACCP Conference on antithrombotic and thrombolytic therapy. Chest 2004;126(3):188S–204S.

9. Gallus A, Jackaman J, Tillett J, et al. Safety and efficacy of warfarin started early after submassive venous thrombosis or pulmonary embolism. Lancet 1986;2:1293–1296.

10. Hull RD, Raskob GE, Rosenbloom D, et al. Heparin for 5 days as compared with 10 days in the initial treatment of proximal venous thrombosis. N Engl J Med 1990;322:1260–1264.

11. Hull RD, Raskob GE, Rosenbloom DR, et al. Optimal therapeutic level of heparin therapy in patients with venous thrombosis. Arch Intern Med 1992;152:1589–1595.

12. Hull RD, Raskob GE, Brant RF, et al. The importance of initial heparin treatment on long-term clinical outcomes of antithrombotic therapy. Arch Intern Med 1997;157:2317–2321.

13. Writing Committee for the Galilei Investigators. Subcutaneous adjusted-dose UFH vs fixed-dose low-molecular-weight heparin in the initial treatment of venous thromboembolism. Arch Intern Med 2004; 164:1077–1083.

14. Raschke RA, Reilly BM, Guidry JR, et al. The weight based heparin dosing nomogram compared with a 'standard care' nomogram. Ann Intern Med 1993;119:874–881.

15. Hull RD, Raskob GE, Brant RF, Pineo GF, Valentine KA. Relation between the time to achieve the lower limit of the APTT therapeutic range and recurrent venous thromboembolism during heparin treatment for deep vein thrombosis. Arch Intern Med 1997;157:2562–2568.

16. Hull RD, Raskob GE, Hirsh J, et al. Continuous intravenous heparin compared with intermittent subcutaneous heparin in the initial treatment of proximal-vein thrombosis. N Engl J Med 1986;315:1109–1114.

17. Raschke R, Hirsh J, Guidry JR. Suboptimal monitoring and dosing of UFH in comparative studies with low-molecular-weight heparin. Ann Intern Med 2003;138(9):720–723.

18. Hommes DW, Bura A, Mazzolai L, et al. Subcutaneous heparin compared with continuous intravenous heparin administration in the initial treatment of DVT. A meta-analysis. Annals Intern Med 1992;116: 279–284.

19. Prandoni P, Bagatella P, Bernardi E, et al. Use of an algorithm for administering subcutaneous heparin in the treatment of deep vein thrombosis. Ann Intern Med 1998;129:299–302.

20. Kearon C, Harrison L, Crowther M, et al. Optimal dosing of subcutaneous heparin for the treatment of DVT. Thromb Res 2000;97:395–403.

21. Faivre R, Neuhart Y, Kieffer Y, et al. Un nouveau traitement des thromboses vein euses profondes: les fractions d'heparine de bas poids moleculaire. Etude randomisee. Presse Medicale 1988;17:197–200.

22. Lopaciuk S, Meissner AJ, Filipecki S, et al. Subcutaneous low molecular weight heparin versus subcutaneous UFH in the treatment of DVT: a Polish multicenter trial. Thromb Haemost 1992;68:14–18.

23. Belcaro G, Nicolaides AN, Cesarone MR, et al. Comparison of low-molecular-weight heparin, administered primarily at home, with UFH, administered in hospital, and subcutaneous heparin, administered at home for deep-vein thrombosis. Angiology 1999;50(10):781–787.

24. Kelton JG. Heparin-induced thrombocytopenia. Haemostasis 1986;16:173–186.

25. Greinacher A, Warkentin TE. Treatment of heparin-induced thrombocytopenia: an overview. In: Warkentin TE, Greinacher A, eds. Heparin-induced thrombocytopenia, 2nd edition. Marcel Dekker, Inc., New York, 2001.

26. Greinacher A, Eichler P, Lubenow N, et al. Heparin-induced thrombocytopenia with thromboembolic complications: meta-analysis of two prospective trials to assess with value of parenteral treatment with lepirudin and its therapeutic aPTT range. Blood 2000;96:846–851.

27. Warkentin TE, Chong BH, Greinacher A. Heparin-induced thrombocytopenia: towards consensus. Thromb Haemost 1998;79:1–7.

28. Warkentin TE. Review. Heparin-induced thrombocytopenia: pathogenesis and management. Br J Haematol 2003;121:535–555.

29. Barrowcliffe TW, Curtis AD, Johnson EA, et al. An international standard for low molecular weight heparin. Thromb Haemost 1988;60:1–7.

30. Weitz JI. Low molecular weight heparins. N Engl J Med 1997;337:688–698.

31. Shaugnessy SG, Young E, Deshamps P, et al. The effects of low molecular weight and standard heparin on calcium loss from fetal rat calvaria. Blood 1995;86:1368–1373.

32. Hull RD, Raskob GE, Pineo GF, et al. Subcutaneous low molecular weight heparin compared with continuous intravenous heparin in the treatment of proximal vein thrombosis. N Engl J Med 1992;326:975–988.

33. Prandoni P, Lensing AW, Buller HR, et al. Comparison of subcutaneous low molecular weight heparin with intravenous standard heparin in proximal deep vein thrombosis. Lancet 1992;339:441–445.

34. Lopaciuk S, Meissner AJ, Filipecki S, et al. Subcutaneous low molecular weight heparin in the treatment of deep vein thrombosis. a Polish multicentre trial. Thromb Haemost 1992;68:14–18.

35. Simonneau G, Charbonier B, Decousus H, et al. Subcutaneous low molecular weight heparin compared with continuous intravenous UFH in the treatment of proximal deep vein thrombosis. Arch Intern Med 1993;153:1541–1546.

36. Lindmarker P, Holmstrom M, Granqvist S, et al. Comparison of once-daily subcutaneous Fragmin with continuous intravenous unfractionated heparin in the treatment of deep venous thrombosis. Thromb Haemost 1994;72:186–190.

37. Koopman MMW, Prandoni P, Piovelia F, et al. Treatment of venous thrombosis with intravenous UFH administered in the hospital as compared with subcutaneous low molecular weight heparin administered in the hospital as compared with subcutaneous low molecular weight heparin administered at home. N Engl J Med 1996;334:682–687.

38. Levine M, Gent M, Hirsh J, et al. A comparison of low molecular weight heparin administered primarily at home with UFH administered in the hospital for proximal deep vein thrombosis. N Engl J Med 1996; 334:667–681.

39. The Columbus Investigators. Low molecular weight heparin in the treatment of patients with venous thromboembolism. N Engl J Med 1997;337:657–662.

40. Gould MK, Dembitzer AD, Doyle RL, et al. Low-molecular-weight heparins compared with UFH for treatment of acute deep venous thrombosis. A meta-analysis of randomized, controlled trials. Ann Intern Med 1999;130:800–809.

41. Hull RD, Raskob GE, Rosenbloom D, et al. Treatment of proximal vein thrombosis with subcutaneous low molecular weight heparin vs. intravenous heparin. An economic perspective. Arch Intern Med 1997; 157:289–294.

42. van der Heijden JF, Hutten BA, Buller HR, et al. Vitamin K antagonists or low-molecular-weight heparin for the long term treatment of symptomatic venous thromboembolism. The Cochrane Database of Systematic Reviews 2002;(1):CD002001.

43. Lee AY, Levine MN, Baker BI, et al. Low-molecular-weight heparin versus coumarin for the prevention of recurrent venous thromboembolism in patients with cancer. N Engl J Med 2003;349:146–153.

44. Hull R, Pineo GF, Mah A, et al. A randomized trial evaluating long-term low-molecular-weight heparin therapy for three months versus intravenous heparin followed by warfarin sodium [abstract]. Blood 2002;100:148a.

45. Thery C. Simonneau G, Meyer G, et al. Randomized trial of subcutaneous low-molecular-weight heparin CY 216 (Fraxiparine) compared with intravenous UFH in the curative treatment of submassive pulmonary embolism. A dose-ranging study. Circulation 1992;85(4):1380–1389.

46. Meyer G, Brenot F, Pacouret G, et al. Subcutaneous low-molecular-weight heparin Fragmin versus intravenous UFH in the treatment of acute non massive pulmonary embolism: an open randomized pilot study. Thromb Haemost 1995;74(6):1432–1435.

47. Simonneau G, Sors H, Charbonnier B, et al. A comparison of low-molecular-weight heparin with UFH for acute pulmonary embolism. N Engl J Med 1997;337:663–669.

48. Hull RD, Raskob GE, Brant RF, et al. Low-molecular-weight heparin vs heparin in the treatment of patients with pulmonary embolism. Arch Intern Med 2000;160:229–236.

49. Hull RD, Pineo GF. A meta-analysis of a once daily regimen using tinzaparin for the treatment of patients with proximal deep-vein thrombosis and complicating objectively documented pulmonary embolism. Abstract. Chest 2000;118(4 Suppl):81S.

50. Kovacs MJ, Anderson D, Morrow B, et al. Outpatient treatment of pulmonary embolism with dalteparin. Thromb Haemost 2000;83(2):209–211.

51. Kher A, Samama MM. Primary and secondary prophylaxis of venous thromboembolism with low-molecular-weight heparins: prolonged thromboprophylaxis, an alternative to vitamin K antagonists. J Thromb Haemost 2005;3:473–481.

52. Beckman JA, Dunn K, Sasahara AA, et al. Enoxaparin monotherapy without oral anticoagulation to treat acute symptomatic pulmonary embolism. Thromb Haemost 2003;89(6):953–958.

53. Mismetti B, Laporta-Simitsidis S, Navarro C, et al. Aging and venous thromboembolism influence the pharmacodynamics of the anti-factor Xa and anti-thrombin activities of a low molecular weight heparin (nadroparin). Thromb Haemost 1998;79:1162–1165.

54. Nagge J, Crowther M, Hirsh J. Is impaired renal function a contraindication to the use of low-molecular-weight heparin? Arch Intern Med 2002;162:2605–2609.

55. Pautas E, Gouin I, Bellot O, et al. Safety profile of tinzaparin administered once daily at a standard curative dose in two hundred very elderly patients. Drug Saf 2002;25(10):725–733.

56. Siguret V, Pautas E, Fevrier M, et al. Elderly patients treated with tinzaparin (Innohep®) administered once daily (175 anti-Xa IU/kg): anti-Xa and anti-IIa activities over 10 days. Thromb Haemost 2000; 84(5):800–804.

57. Crowther MA, Berry LR, Monagle PT, et al. Mechanisms responsible for the failure of protamine to inactivate low-molecular-weight heparin. Br J Haemat 2002;116:178–186.

58. Hainer JW, Barrett JS, Assaid CA, et al. Dosing in heavy-weight/obese patients with the LMWH, tinzaparin: a pharmacodynamic study. Thromb Haemost 2002;87:817–823.

59. Al-Yaseen E, Wells PS, Anderson J, et al. The safety of dosing dalteparin based on actual body weight for the treatment of acute venous thromboembolism in obese patients. J Thromb Haemost 2005;3(1):100–102.

60. Rosenbloom D, Ginsberg JS. Arguments against monitoring levels of anti-factor Xa in conjunction with low-molecular-weight heparin therapy. Can J Hosp Pharm 2002;55:15–19.

61. Dolovich LR, Ginsberg JS, Douketis JD, et al. A meta-analysis comparing low-molecular-weight heparins with UFH in the treatment of venous thromboembolism: examining some unanswered questions regarding location of treatment, product type, and dosing frequency. Arch Intern Med 2000;160:181–188.

62. Dorffler-Melly J, de Jonge E, Pont AC, et al. Bioavailability of subcutaneous low-molecular-weight heparin to patients on vasopressors. Lancet 2002;359:849–850.

63. The Matisse Investigators. Subcutaneous fondaparinux versus intravenous UFH in the initial treatment of pulmonary embolism. N Engl J Med 2003;349(18):1695–1702.

10

Thrombolysis

Guy Meyer, MD

Contents

Summary

Clinically stable patients without major comorbidity, who receive anticoagulant treatment for pulmonary embolism (PE), have a low in-hospital mortality rate ranging between 1 and 2%. In contrast, more than 25% of patients with massive PE, defined by persistently low blood pressure or shock at presentation, die during the first 2 wk after diagnosis. Available evidence indicates that thrombolytic treatment reduces the mortality risk in these patients, who, however, represent only 4.5% of all patients admitted to the hospital for PE. Further data support the notion that normotensive patients with submassive PE, defined by the presence of right ventricular dysfunction detected on echocardiography or indicated by elevated cardiac biomarkers, may also have a higher mortality risk than patients with normal right ventricular function. These patients may represent more than 20% of all patients admitted to the hospital for acute PE. Indirect evidence suggests that thrombolytic treatment may reduce the mortality rate in these patients, but the available controlled studies were not powerful enough to confirm or refute this hypothesis. A large randomized controlled trial is urgently needed to resolve this issue. Recombinant tissue-type plasminogen activator, given as a 100-mg dose over 2 h, is the most systematically studied thrombolytic regimen for patients with acute PE. It acts faster than regimens using urokinase or streptokinase, and should be considered as the reference thrombolytic treatment for patients with PE.

Key Words: Thrombolysis; massive pulmonary embolism; submassive pulmonary embolism; tissue-type plasminogen activator.

From: *Contemporary Cardiology: Management of Acute Pulmonary Embolism*
Edited by: S. Konstantinides © Humana Press Inc., Totowa, NJ

INTRODUCTION

The overall hospital mortality rate of unselected patients with pulmonary embolism (PE) has been estimated at 9%, and it depends primarily on the hemodynamic status of the patient and the underlying disease *(1)*. Recent studies have shown that, for clinically stable patients without major comorbidity, the in-hospital mortality rate under effective anti-coagulant treatment is between 1 and 2% *(2,3)*. In contrast, more than 25% of patients presenting with low blood pressure die during the first 2 wk after diagnosis *(1,4,5)*. However, a number of studies also showed that a subgroup of patients with normal blood pressure who have right ventricular failure on admission as detected by echocardiography may have an increased mortality rate compared to patients with normal echocardiographic findings *(6)*. Recent data further suggest that cardiac biomarkers such as troponin and brain natriuretic peptide (BNP) can also help identify patients with an adverse outcome among those with normal blood pressure *(7,8)* *(see* Chapters 4 and 5). Accordingly, PE can be classified into the following categories: (1) massive PE defined by a systolic blood pressure no higher than 90 mmHg, or a pressure drop of at least 40 mmHg for at least 15 min; and (2) nonmassive PE *(9)*. In addition *submassive* PE is considered as a subcategory of nonmassive PE with evidence of right ventricular dysfunction *(9)*.

Thrombolytic treatment is generally recommended for unstable patients with massive PE, who, however, represent no more than 4.5% of all patients admitted to hospital for PE *(1)*. On the other hand, the use of thrombolytic treatment in patients with submassive PE remains controversial. Some indirect evidence supports the use of thrombolysis in these patients, but controlled studies could neither confirm nor exclude a significant reduction in mortality.

HEMODYNAMIC BENEFITS
OF THROMBOLYTIC TREATMENT IN PE

Thrombolytic treatment induces a rapid decline of pulmonary artery resistance in patients with acute PE and pulmonary hypertension. In the plasminogen activator Italian multi-center study 2 (PAIMS 2) study, alteplase given as a 100-mg dose over 2 hours reduced mean pulmonary artery pressure from 30.2 ± 7.8 mmHg to 21.0 ± 6.7 mmHg after 2 h, whereas no significant change was observed with heparin alone *(10)*. In the same study, the cardiac index increased from 2.1 ± 0.5 L/(min/m^2) to 2.4 ± 0.5 L/(min/m^2) in the alteplase group, whereas no change was observed in the heparin group. In the urokinase pulmonary embolism trial (UPET) study, no significant change in hemodynamic parameters was observed after 24 h of heparin infusion, whereas a significant 23% reduction in pulmonary artery mean pressure was observed in the patients who received urokinase *(11)*. Early reversal of right ventricular dysfunction has also been documented by serial ECG in patients receiving alteplase compared to those receiving heparin alone *(12)*.

REDUCTION OF PULMONARY VASCULAR OBSTRUCTION

Thrombolytic treatment produces a faster decrease in vascular obstruction compared to treatment with heparin. In the PAIMS 2 study, the severity of pulmonary vascular obstruction as assessed by the Miller index (an angiographic score of pulmonary vascular obstruction with a maximum value of 34) decreased significantly from 28.3 ± 2.9 to 24.8 ± 5.2 at the end of the alteplase infusion, whereas no significant difference was observed in patients who received heparin alone *(10)*. Using serial lung scanning, Goldhaber et al.

observed a greater reduction of vascular obstruction 24 h after the start of treatment with alteplase *(12)*. Importantly, however, studies also showed that the differences between the thrombolysis and the heparin group disappeared after 7 d of follow-up *(10)*. Thus, thrombolytic therapy restores pulmonary vascular patency and reduces pressure overload of the right ventricle more rapidly than heparin alone, but both types of treatment result in a similar extent of improvement after 1 wk.

HEMORRHAGIC COMPLICATIONS OF THROMBOLYSIS

A recent meta-analysis of controlled studies compared thrombolytic treatment with heparin in patients with PE *(13)*. The overall rate of major bleeding was 9.1% in the patients who were allocated to thrombolytic treatment compared to 6.1 % in those who received heparin. The relative risk for major bleeding associated with thrombolysis was 1.42 (95% confidence interval [CI], 0.81–2.46). Most of the bleeding events occurred in studies that used central venous access for angiography and hemodynamic monitoring. Notably, such invasive diagnostic procedures are rarely used in current clinical practice, and, accordingly, recent studies have shown that major bleeding rates are now much lower under either treatment. However, intracranial bleeding remains a major concern in patients receiving thrombolytic treatment. In thrombolysis studies focusing on patients with PE, the incidence of intracranial bleeding was estimated at 1.9% (95% CI, 0.7–4.1%), and thus appeared to be higher than in patients with myocardial infarction *(14)*. Risk factors include older age and invasive diagnostic procedures *(15)*.

EFFECTS OF THROMBOLYSIS
ON PE-RELATED MORTALITY AND PROGNOSIS

Patients With Massive PE

The definition of massive PE has long been based on the severity of angiographically detected pulmonary vascular obstruction. In fact, when vascular obstruction exceeds 50 to 60%, pulmonary vascular resistance increases sharply. Thus, this level of pulmonary vascular obstruction has been used to define massive PE *(16)*. However, recent data strongly suggest that PE-related mortality is not directly related to the degree of vascular obstruction itself, but rather to clinical findings at the time of diagnosis. For example, in the ICOPER registry, mortality was 58% in patients with hemodynamic instability compared to 15% in clinically stable patients *(1)*. In the same study, a systolic blood pressure less than 90 mmHg was independently associated with increased mortality (odds ratio [OR], 2.9; 95% CI, 1.7–5.0). Another large multicenter registry included 1001 patients with *major* PE, defined as right heart failure or pulmonary hypertension *(5)*. Four patient groups were prospectively defined: (1) patients with evidence of right ventricular pressure overload or pulmonary hypertension, but with normal blood pressure; (2) patients with arterial hypotension (systolic blood pressure less than 90 mmHg or a drop of at least 40 mmHg for more than 15 min), but without cardiogenic shock or need for catecholamine support (except for dopamine infusion at the rate of less than 5 µg/[kg/min]); (3) patients with arterial hypotension and cardiogenic shock and/or need for catecholamine administration to maintain adequate tissue perfusion; (4) patients with circulatory collapse who underwent cardiopulmonary resuscitation. Hospital mortality was 8.1% in group 1, 15.2% in group 2, 25% in group 3, and 62.5% in group 4 *(5)*. In view of these data, the diagnosis of *massive* PE is now based on clinical rather than angiographic parameters, and more specifically on the presence of hemodynamic instability (persistent arterial hypotension and/or cardiogenic shock) at presentation *(9)*.

One small randomized trial has compared streptokinase with heparin in patients with massive PE. Although 40 patients with massive or submassive PE were expected to be recruited, the trial was terminated early after only 8 patients were included. All patients had massive PE; four were allocated to streptokinase and survived, whereas four were allocated to heparin and died from cardiogenic shock during the 72 h following randomization *(17)*. These results prompted the ethics committee to stop the trial. In a recent meta-analysis of the controlled studies comparing thrombolytic therapy with heparin in patients with PE, a subgroup analysis was performed for the studies that included patients with massive PE and shock *(13)*. The mortality rate in these studies was 6.2% for the patients allocated to thrombolytic treatment and 12.7% for those allocated to heparin (OR, 0.47; 95% CI, 0.20–1.10). When recurrent PE and deaths were considered, the difference was significant, with a 9.4% event rate for patients allocated to thrombolytic treatment compared to 19% for those allocated to heparin treatment (OR, 0.45; 95% CI, 0.22–0.92) *(13)*. Importantly however, only a minority of the patients included in the prospective thrombolysis trials performed to date had massive PE with cardiogenic shock.

In contrast to the aforementioned (limited) data from prospective trials, the results of a retrospective case series covering a 10-yr period in a single center suggested that thrombolytic treatment might not reduce the mortality rate in unstable patients with severe shock. Either heparin alone or heparin plus thrombolytic therapy was given to 34 patients with massive PE and metabolic acidosis, according to the opinion of the physician in charge *(18)*. Of 20 patients who received heparin treatment, 60% died. Similarly, of 14 patients who received thrombolytic treatment, 57% died during the hospital stay. However, this retrospective study defined the presence of metabolic acidosis as one of its inclusion criteria. It may thus have selected patients with irreversible right ventricular myocardial damage who were possibly too sick to benefit from any effective recanalization therapy. In fact, the MAPPET study also suggested that *delayed* thrombolytic therapy of patients with PE may be associated with a worse clinical outcome *(5)*.

In conclusion, the body of evidence currently available largely supports the notion that thrombolytic therapy reduces mortality in patients with massive PE. In particular, the high mortality rate seen in patients with massive PE who receive heparin alone, the early hemodynamic improvement observed with thrombolytic therapy, the results of the small randomized study by Jerjes-Sanchez et al., and the recent meta-analysis all strongly suggest that thrombolytic therapy should be instituted as early as possible in patients with massive PE. Thus, most authorities recommend the use of thrombolytic therapy for patients with massive PE *(9,19)*.

Patients With Submassive PE

Patients who present in a stable hemodynamic condition and have no major underlying disease have a remarkably low death rate when receiving anticoagulant treatment for PE. For example, a recent meta-analysis comparing unfractionated heparin with low-molecular-weight heparin (LMWH) for the initial treatment of PE reported an in-hospital mortality rate of 1.4% for the former and 1.2% for the latter treatment group *(20)*. Several studies have tried to identify a subgroup of patients with (possibly) higher mortality rates among those with normal blood pressure. Some studies used echocardiography to select these patients. For example, Ribeiro et al. first showed that mortality rate was higher in patients

Table 1
Mortality of Patients Receiving Heparin for Submassive PE,
i.e., With Normal Blood Pressure and Right Ventricular Dysfunction on Echocardiography

Study	Criteria for RV failure	n	Mortality
Konstaninides (23)	RV dilatation	290	11.1%
Grifoni (22)	RV dysfunction	65	5%
Hamel (24)	RV/LV end diastolic diameter > 0.6	64	0
Vielliard-Baron (18)	RV/LV end diastolic surface > 0.6 and paradoxal septal motion	32	3%
Giannitsis (21)	Paradoxal septal motion, or RV end diastolic diameter > 30 mm, or RV hypokinesis, or tricuspid regurgitation > 2.5 m/s	26	7.7%
Pruszczyk (7)	RV/LV end diastolic diameter > 0.6 and RV hypokinesis or tricuspid gradient > 30 mmHg	64	12.5%
Kucher (25)	RV hypokinesis	19	10.5%
Pruszczyk (8)	RV/LV end diastolic diameter > 0.5	51	19.6%
Kucher (26)	RV hypokinesis	405	16.3%

PE, pulmonary embolism; RV, right ventricle; LV, left ventricle.

with right ventricular dysfunction (10 deaths among 70 patients; 14%) compared to those with normal findings on echocardiography (no death among 56 patients; $p = 0.002$), although patients with hemodynamic instability were not separately assessed (6). In the International Cooperative Pulmonary Embolism Registry (ICOPER) study, the in-hospital death rate of patients with right ventricular failure was 18%, although, again, the patients with shock were not separately analyzed (1). More recently, several studies assessed the outcome of patients with normal blood pressure and right ventricular dysfunction on echocardiography (7,8,18,21–26). The mortality rate in these studies varied between 0 and 20% (Table 1). When the results of all the previously described studies are critically reviewed, it needs to be considered that the exact definition of right ventricular dysfunction on echocardiography varied from one study to another (see Chapter 4), and that some investigators did not stratify the patients according to their clinical status, including both stable and unstable patients. Also, treatment was not controlled, and some patients had already received thrombolytic treatment prior to ultrasound imaging. These limitations may account for the discrepancies observed.

In recent years, cardiac biomarkers were evaluated to select patients with submassive PE. BNP, pro-BNP, and cardiac troponins T and I all were associated with an increased risk of death in patients with PE. However, most studies did not carry out separate analyses of patients in a stable hemodynamic condition and patients with shock (Table 2). In one series, the in-hospital mortality of patients with normal blood pressure, high troponin levels, and an enlarged right ventricle was 25% (7). Another study from the same group showed that clinically stable patients with high pro-BNP levels had a 17% mortality rate (8). Scridon et al. observed an overall 30-d mortality rate of 19.9% in a retrospective series of 141 patients with PE. Troponin I values were elevated in 52% of the patients and the combination of right ventricular enlargement and elevated troponin I, which was present in 32% of the subjects, was associated with a 38% mortality rate (27). These findings were obtained in small numbers of patients recruited in a single center and need to be confirmed on a larger scale. In the meantime, it has to be admitted that the exact definition of *submassive* PE remains unclear. The outcome of patients with normal blood pressure, ele-

Table 2
In-Hospital Mortality of Patients With PE and Elevated Cardiac Biomarkers

Study	n	Biomarker	Threshold	Frequency of positive tests (%)	Mortality (%)[a]
Kucher (43)	91	cTnI	0.06 pg/mL	31	14
Giannitsis (21)	56	cTnT	0.10 ng/mL	32	44
Janata (44)	106	cTnT	0.09 ng/mL	12	34
Pruszczyk (7)	64	cTnT	0.01 ng/mL	50	25
ten Wolde (45)	110	BNP	21.7 pmol/mL	33	17
Kucher (25)	73	BNP	50 pg/mL	55	12
Pruszczyk (8)	79	Pro-BNP	153–334 pg/mL	83	22

Studies included both stable and unstable patients (i.e., massive and submassive PE).

PE, pulmonary embolism; cTnI, cardiac troponin I; cTnT, cardiac troponin T; BNP, brain natriuretic peptide; pro-BNP, pro brain natriuretic peptide; PPV, positive predictive value.

[a]Mortality in patients with elevated cardiac biomarker.

vated cardiac biomarkers, and/or an enlarged (dysfunctional) right ventricle needs further studies.

To date, the largest randomized study assessing thrombolytic treatment for submassive PE included 256 patients with PE and normal blood pressure who were allocated to receive either heparin alone or both alteplase and heparin (28). The primary end point consisted of the combination of in-hospital death or clinical deterioration requiring escalation of treatment. This was reached in 11% of the patients in the alteplase/heparin group compared to 24.6% in the heparin group ($p = 0.006$). The difference was mainly due to secondary open-label thrombolytic therapy, which was more frequent in the patients assigned to receive heparin (23.2%) than in those receiving alteplase (7.6%; $p = 0.001$). Death rate was 3.4% for the alteplase group and 2.2% for the heparin group. The unexpected low mortality rate in patients receiving heparin may be related to the low (30%) proportion of patients with right ventricular dilatation on echocardiography, or to the early use of rescue thrombolytic treatment for those patients who did not improve with heparin. Of the 10 other controlled studies that were conducted to compare thrombolytic therapy with heparin in patients with PE, none focused on submassive PE. These and the previous study were included in a meta-analysis that analyzed the outcome of 748 patients (13). The overall death rate was 4.3% for the patients allocated to thrombolytic therapy compared to 5.9% for those assigned to receive heparin (OR, 0.70; 95% CI, 0.37–1.30). In the subset of studies that included only clinically stable patients, death rate was 3.3% for those receiving thrombolytic therapy compared to 2.4% for those allocated to heparin (OR, 1.16; 95% CI, 0.44–3.05). Major bleeding was reported in 2.4% of patients in the thrombolysis group and 3.2% of patients in the heparin-only group (OR, 0.67; 95% CI, 0.24–1.86). As mentioned previously, however, most of these latter studies included patients both with submassive and nonmassive PE. Thus, the current evidence from controlled studies does not appear to indicate that patients with submassive PE receiving thrombolytic treatment may have a lower in-hospital mortality risk.

Despite negative results from controlled studies, some indirect evidence does suggest that thrombolytic therapy may favorably affect the outcome of patients with submassive PE. Goldhaber et al. analyzed retrospectively a subgroup of 36 patients with right ventricular hypokinesis who were included in a controlled study comparing thrombolytic therapy

Table 3
Thrombolytic Regimens
for PE Evaluated in Prospective Controlled Studies

Streptokinase	250,000 IU over 15 min + 100,000 IU/h over 12–24 h
	1.5 million IU over 2 h
Urokinase	4400 IU/kg over 30 min + 4400 IU/(kg/h) over 12–24 h
	3 million IU over 2 h
rtPA	100 mg over 2 h
	0.6 mg/kg over 15 min

PE, pulmonary embolism; rtPA, recombinant tissue type plasminogen activator.

and heparin. They observed 5 PE recurrences (two of them fatal) among 18 patients who were treated with heparin. In contrast, no deaths or recurrent PE occurred among 18 patients who received thrombolytic treatment *(12)*. In the MAPETT study, the death rate was higher for patients receiving heparin only, and thrombolytic treatment was the only independent predictor of a favorable outcome *(23)*. However, this was an observational study and treatments were not randomly allocated.

In conclusion, the current evidence does not directly support the thesis that thrombolytic therapy decreases the mortality rate of patients with submassive PE. On the other hand, a recent meta-analysis of the randomized thrombolysis trials performed to date suggested that a clinically relevant reduction in death rate might exist. As a result, experts have expressed contradicting opinions and recommendations regarding the indications for thrombolytic therapy in these patients *(29–32)*. A large international randomized study comparing thrombolysis to heparin in 1000 patients with submassive PE defined by elevated troponin and right ventricular failure (assessed by echocardiography or spiral computed tomography) is currently being planned to clarify this issue.

WHICH IS THE OPTIMAL THROMBOLYTIC REGIMEN IN PE?

Different thrombolytic regimens have been evaluated in controlled trials (Table 3). In the USPET study, urokinase given as a bolus dose of 4400 IU/kg followed by a 12-h or 24-h maintenance infusion of 4400 IU/(kg/h) was compared to streptokinase given as a 250,000 IU bolus dose followed by a 100,000 IU/h infusion given over 24 h *(33)*. The three regimens produced the same degree of hemodynamic and angiographic improvement with no significant differences regarding major hemorrhage. A subsequent European study found no difference concerning safety or efficacy when the same dose of urokinase was administered over 12 or over 24 h *(34)*.

In two randomized controlled trials, recombinant tissue type plasminogen activator (rtPA) given as a 2-h, 100 mg infusion was compared with a 4400 IU/(kg/h) infusion of urokinase given over 12 or 24 h *(35,36)*. In both studies, rtPA led to a faster hemodynamic and angiographic improvement, but the two drugs yielded comparable hemodynamic results by the end of the urokinase infusion. A nonsignificant reduction in major bleeding was observed in both studies for the patients receiving rtPA, although they were not powerful enough to detect significant differences in major bleeding rates *(35,36)*. The same

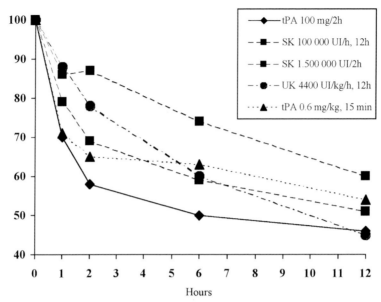

Fig. 1. Reduction of total pulmonary vascular resistance in response to different thrombolytic regimens evaluated in prospective randomized studies. TPR, total pulmonary resistance; tPA, tissue type plasminogen activator; SK, streptokinase; UK, urokinase.

rtPA regimen was subsequently compared with a shorter regimen of urokinase, given as a 3 million IU infusion over 2 h *(37)*. No differences were observed regarding hemodynamic improvement and bleeding between the groups, suggesting that when the two drugs are given over the same time period, they have similar efficacy and safety.

More recently, two randomized controlled trials compared rtPA with streptokinase given as a 12-h, 100,000 IU/h infusion or as 1.5 million IU given over 2 h *(38,39)*. Again, the 2-h regimen of rtPA resulted in faster hemodynamic improvement compared to the 12-h streptokinase infusion, whereas no difference was observed when the two drugs were given over the same 2-h period *(38,39)*. The rate of major bleeding was lower for patients receiving the 2-h streptokinase infusion than for those receiving rtPA, although this difference did not reach statistical significance *(38)*. Two further studies compared the efficacy and safety of a 0.6 mg/kg body weight of rtPA given over a period of 15 min with 100 mg given over a period of 2 h *(40,41)*. Hemodynamic improvement was slightly but significantly faster for the 2-h regimen, although the 0.6 mg/kg dosage was associated with a nonsignificant reduction in major bleeding *(40,41)*.

The reduction in total pulmonary vascular resistance produced by the fibrinolytic regimens evaluated in recent controlled studies is given in Fig. 1. Although a direct comparison of these various regimens is difficult, the 100 mg rtPA dosage given over 2 h seems to produce the fastest hemodynamic improvement and might be the preferred option in severely compromised patients.

It is difficult to compare the bleeding rates of different studies because the criteria for major bleeding varied from one study to another *(42)*. Keeping this limitation in mind, major bleeding rates were very similar in most of the recent studies using similar invasive diagnostic and monitoring procedures *(36,38,39,41)*. The bleeding rates observed under different thrombolytic regimens are given in Table 4.

Table 4
Major Bleeding in Recent Controlled Studies
Comparing Different Thrombolytic Regimens in Patients With PE

	n	Lytic agent	Regimen	Major bleeding rate (%)
Meyer (36)	29	UK	4400 IU/(kg/h) over 12 h	8 (28)
	34	rtPA	100 mg over 2 h	7 (21)
Sors (41)	36	rtPA	0.6 mg/kg over 15 min	4 (11)
	17	rtPA	100 mg over 2 h	4 (24)
Meneveau (39)	25	SK	100,000 IU/h over 12 h	3 (12)
	25	rtPA	100 mg over 2 h	4 (16)
Meneveau (38)	43	SK	1.5 million IU over 2 h	3 (7)
	23	rtPA	100 mg over 2 h	5 (22)

PE, pulmonary embolism; UK, urokinase; SK, streptokinase; rtPA, recombinant tissue type plasminogen activator.

Table 5
Contraindications to Thrombolytic Therapy in PE

Major contraindications
• Uncontrolled active bleeding
• Ischemic stroke within the last 2 mo
• Spontaneous intracranial bleeding
Minor contraindications
• Major surgery or delivery within the past 10 d
• Trauma within the past 15 d
• Neurosurgery or ophthalmologic surgery within the past month
• Severe hypertension (systolic, >180 mmHg; diastolic, >120 mmHg)
• Platelet count < 100,000 μL

CONTRAINDICATIONS TO THROMBOLYTIC THERAPY

For patients with hemodynamic compromise who do not improve with anticoagulation and pressure support, the benefit of thrombolytic treatment outweighs its bleeding risk even in the presence of minor contraindications. Alternative treatment options such as pulmonary embolectomy are presented in Chapter 12, but they may be associated with a high mortality risk. The main contraindications to thrombolytic therapy are given in Table 5.

ADDITIONAL MEASURES

As most of the bleeding episodes occur at the puncture site, it is essential to try to avoid invasive diagnostic procedures such as conventional pulmonary angiography to confirm PE when the use of thrombolytic treatment is considered. Thrombolytic therapy can be given via a peripheral vein, and central venous lines should be avoided. When rtPA is given as a 100-mg dose, or when urokinase or streptokinase are chosen, heparin should be interrupted during thrombolysis and resumed as soon as the activated partial thromboplastin time is within the target range. There are still no conclusive data regarding the combination of LMWH and thrombolytic therapy in PE, although the safety of such treatment has been documented for acute myocardial infarction. For patients receiving thrombolytic treatment for PE, there is no need for any other laboratory test than the activated partial thromboplastin time. Fibrinogen monitoring is of no help.

CONCLUSION

Patients who have PE with systemic hypotension and clinical evidence of poor tissue perfusion have a high mortality rate if they receive heparin alone. Available evidence strongly suggests the use of thrombolytic treatment in these patients. Recent data indicate that patients with so-called submassive PE may have a higher mortality risk than patients with normal right ventricular function. Indirect evidence suggests that thrombolytic treatment may also reduce the mortality rate in these patients, although the controlled studies available to date were not powerful enough to confirm or refute this hypothesis. A large randomized controlled trial is urgently needed to address this issue. Alteplase, given as a 100-mg dose over 2 h, is the most systematically evaluated thrombolytic regimen for patients with PE. It acts faster than regimens using urokinase or streptokinase and should be considered as the thrombolytic treatment of choice for patients with PE.

REFERENCES

1. Goldhaber SZ, Visani L, De Rosa M. Acute pulmonary embolism: clinical outcomes in the International Cooperative Pulmonary Embolism Registry (ICOPER). Lancet 1999;353:1386–1389.
2. Buller HR, Davidson BL, Decousus H, et al. Subcutaneous fondaparinux versus intravenous unfractionated heparin in the initial treatment of pulmonary embolism. N Engl J Med 2003;349:1695–1702.
3. Simonneau G, Sors H, Charbonnier B, et al. A comparison of low-molecular-weight heparin with unfractionated heparin for acute pulmonary embolism. The THESEE Study Group. Tinzaparine ou Heparine Standard: Evaluations dans l'Embolie Pulmonaire. N Engl J Med 1997;337:663–669.
4. Alpert JS, Smith R, Carlson J, Ockene IS, Dexter L, Dalen JE. Mortality in patients treated for pulmonary embolism. JAMA 1976;236:1477–1480.
5. Kasper W, Konstantinides S, Geibel A, et al. Management strategies and determinants of outcome in acute major pulmonary embolism: results of a multicenter registry. J Am Coll Cardiol 1997;30:1165–1171.
6. Ribeiro A, Lindmarker P, Juhlin-Dannfelt A, Johnsson H, Jorfeldt L. Echocardiography Doppler in pulmonary embolism: right ventricular dysfunction as a predictor of mortality rate. Am Heart J 1997;134:479–487.
7. Pruszczyk P, Bochowicz A, Torbicki A, et al. Cardiac troponin T monitoring identifies high-risk group of normotensive patients with acute pulmonary embolism. Chest 2003;123:1947–1952.
8. Pruszczyk P, Kostrubiec M, Bochowicz A, et al. N-terminal pro-brain natriuretic peptide in patients with acute pulmonary embolism. Eur Respir J 2003;22:649–653.
9. Guidelines on diagnosis and management of acute pulmonary embolism. Task Force on Pulmonary Embolism, European Society of Cardiology. Eur Heart J 2000;21:1301–1336.
10. Dalla-Volta S, Palla A, Santolicandro A, et al. PAIMS 2: alteplase combined with heparin versus heparin in the treatment of acute pulmonary embolism. Plasminogen activator Italian multicenter study 2. J Am Coll Cardiol 1992;20:520–526.
11. The urokinase pulmonary embolism trial. A national cooperative study. Circulation 1973;47:II1–108.
12. Goldhaber SZ, Haire WD, Feldstein ML, et al. Alteplase versus heparin in acute pulmonary embolism: randomised trial assessing right-ventricular function and pulmonary perfusion. Lancet 1993;341:507–511.
13. Wan S, Quinlan DJ, Agnelli G, Eikelboom JW. Thrombolysis compared with heparin for the initial treatment of pulmonary embolism: a meta-analysis of the randomized controlled trials. Circulation 2004;110:744–749.
14. Kanter DS, Mikkola KM, Patel SR, Parker JA, Goldhaber SZ. Thrombolytic therapy for pulmonary embolism. Frequency of intracranial hemorrhage and associated risk factors. Chest 1997;111:1241–1245.
15. Mikkola KM, Patel SR, Parker JA, Grodstein F, Goldhaber SZ. Increasing age is a major risk factor for hemorrhagic complications after pulmonary embolism thrombolysis. Am Heart J 1997;134:69–72.
16. Azarian R, Wartski M, Collignon MA, et al. Lung perfusion scans and hemodynamics in acute and chronic pulmonary embolism. J Nucl Med 1997;38:980–983.
17. Jerjes-Sanchez C, Ramirez-Rivera A, de Lourdes Garcia M, et al. Streptokinase and heparin versus heparin alone in massive pulmonary embolism: a randomized controlled trial. J Thromb Thrombolysis 1995;2:227–229.

18. Vieillard-Baron A, Page B, Augarde R, et al. Acute cor pulmonale in massive pulmonary embolism: incidence, echocardiographic pattern, clinical implications and recovery rate. Intensive Care Med 2001; 27:1481–1486.
19. Buller HR, Agnelli G, Hull RD, Hyers TM, Prins MH, Raskob GE. Antithrombotic therapy for venous thromboembolic disease: the Seventh ACCP Conference on Antithrombotic and Thrombolytic Therapy. Chest 2004;126:401S–428S.
20. Quinlan DJ, McQuillan A, Eikelboom JW. Low-molecular-weight heparin compared with intravenous unfractionated heparin for treatment of pulmonary embolism: a meta-analysis of randomized, controlled trials. Ann Intern Med 2004;140:175–183.
21. Giannitsis E, Muller-Bardorff M, Kurowski V, et al. Independent prognostic value of cardiac troponin T in patients with confirmed pulmonary embolism. Circulation 2000;102:211–217.
22. Grifoni S, Olivotto I, Cecchini P, et al. Short-term clinical outcome of patients with acute pulmonary embolism, normal blood pressure, and echocardiographic right ventricular dysfunction. Circulation 2000; 101:2817–2822.
23. Konstantinides S, Geibel A, Olschewski M, et al. Association between thrombolytic treatment and the prognosis of hemodynamically stable patients with major pulmonary embolism: results of a multicenter registry. Circulation 1997;96:882–888.
24. Hamel E, Pacouret G, Vincentelli D, et al. Thrombolysis or heparin therapy in massive pulmonary embolism with right ventricular dilation: results from a 128-patient monocenter registry. Chest 2001;120:120–125.
25. Kucher N, Printzen G, Goldhaber SZ. Prognostic role of brain natriuretic peptide in acute pulmonary embolism. Circulation 2003;107:2545–2547.
26. Kucher N, Rossi E, De Rosa M, Goldhaber SZ. Prognostic role of echocardiography among patients with acute pulmonary embolism and a systolic arterial pressure of 90 mm Hg or higher. Arch Intern Med 2005;165:1777–1781.
27. Scridon T, Scridon C, Skali H, Alvarez A, Goldhaber SZ, Solomon SD. Prognostic significance of troponin elevation and right ventricular enlargement in acute pulmonary embolism. Am J Cardiol 2005; 96:303–305.
28. Konstantinides S, Geibel A, Heusel G, Heinrich F, Kasper W. Heparin plus alteplase compared with heparin alone in patients with submassive pulmonary embolism. N Engl J Med 2002;347:1143–1150.
29. Konstantinides S. Thrombolysis in submassive pulmonary embolism? Yes. J Thromb Haemost 2003;1: 1127–1129.
30. Dalen JE. Thrombolysis in submassive pulmonary embolism? No. J Thromb Haemost 2003;1:1130–1132.
31. Thabut G, Logeart D. Thrombolysis for pulmonary embolism in patients with right ventricular dysfunction: con. Arch Intern Med 2005;165:2200–2203; discussion 2204–2205.
32. Goldhaber SZ. Thrombolytic therapy for patients with pulmonary embolism who are hemodynamically stable but have right ventricular dysfunction: pro. Arch Intern Med 2005;165:2197–2199; discussion 2204–2205.
33. Urokinase-streptokinase embolism trial. Phase 2 results. A cooperative study. JAMA 1974;229:1606–1613.
34. The UKEP study: multicentre clinical trial on two local regimens of urokinase in massive pulmonary embolism. The UKEP Study Research Group. Eur Heart J 1987;8:2–10.
35. Goldhaber SZ, Kessler CM, Heit J, et al. Randomised controlled trial of recombinant tissue plasminogen activator versus urokinase in the treatment of acute pulmonary embolism. Lancet 1988;2:293–298.
36. Meyer G, Sors H, Charbonnier B, et al. Effects of intravenous urokinase versus alteplase on total pulmonary resistance in acute massive pulmonary embolism: a European multicenter double-blind trial. The European Cooperative Study Group for Pulmonary Embolism. J Am Coll Cardiol 1992;19:239–245.
37. Goldhabern SZ, Kessler CM, Heit JA, et al. Recombinant tissue-type plasminogen activator versus a novel dosing regimen of urokinase in acute pulmonary embolism: a randomized controlled multicenter trial. J Am Coll Cardiol 1992;20:24–30.
38. Meneveau N, Schiele F, Metz D, et al. Comparative efficacy of a two-hour regimen of streptokinase versus alteplase in acute massive pulmonary embolism: immediate clinical and hemodynamic outcome and one-year follow-up. J Am Coll Cardiol 1998;31:1057–1063.
39. Meneveau N, Schiele F, Vuillemenot A, et al. Streptokinase vs alteplase in massive pulmonary embolism. A randomized trial assessing right heart haemodynamics and pulmonary vascular obstruction. Eur Heart J 1997;18:1141–1148.

40. Goldhaber SZ, Agnelli G, Levine MN. Reduced dose bolus alteplase vs conventional alteplase infusion for pulmonary embolism thrombolysis. An international multicenter randomized trial. The Bolus Alteplase Pulmonary Embolism Group. Chest 1994;106:718–724.

41. Sors H, Pacouret G, Azarian R, Meyer G, Charbonnier B, Simonneau G. Hemodynamic effects of bolus vs 2-h infusion of alteplase in acute massive pulmonary embolism. A randomized controlled multicenter trial. Chest 1994;106:712–717.

42. Meyer G, Gisselbrecht M, Diehl JL, Journois D, Sors H. Incidence and predictors of major hemorrhagic complications from thrombolytic therapy in patients with massive pulmonary embolism. Am J Med 1998; 105:472–477.

43. Kucher N, Wallmann D, Carone A, Windecker S, Meier B, Hess OM. Incremental prognostic value of troponin I and echocardiography in patients with acute pulmonary embolism. Eur Heart J 2003;24:1651–1656.

44. Janata K, Holzer M, Laggner AN, Mullner M. Cardiac troponin T in the severity assessment of patients with pulmonary embolism: cohort study. BMJ 2003;326:312–313.

45. ten Wolde M, Tulevski, II, Mulder JW, et al. Brain natriuretic peptide as a predictor of adverse outcome in patients with pulmonary embolism. Circulation 2003;107:2082–2084.

11

Management of the Patient With Fulminant Pulmonary Embolism Undergoing Cardiopulmonary Resuscitation

Fabian Spöhr, MD
and Bernd W. Böttiger, MD, DEAA

Contents

Summary

Patients with cardiac arrest after fulminant pulmonary embolism (PE) have a very poor prognosis. Conventional cardiopulmonary resuscitation (CPR) is frequently unsuccessful because it does not treat the underlying condition. Although thrombolysis is an effective therapeutic option for patients with acute PE, this treatment has traditionally been withheld during CPR because of the anticipated risk of severe hemorrhagic complications associated with chest compressions. This chapter focuses on the mechanisms of action of thrombolytic therapy during CPR after acute PE on the basis of experimental and clinical data. In fact, most data suggest a significant improvement of overall and neurological outcome in patients receiving thrombolysis during CPR after massive PE. Although the use of thrombolytics is indeed associated with an increased incidence of hemorrhagic complications in this setting, critical bleeding complications are rare and do not seem to outweigh the potential benefits of this therapeutic option. Therefore, thrombolytic therapy should not be withheld in patients suffering cardiac arrest after massive PE, particularly if conventional CPR has failed to show immediate success and other treatment options (e.g., surgical embolectomy) are not available.

From: *Contemporary Cardiology: Management of Acute Pulmonary Embolism*
Edited by: S. Konstantinides © Humana Press Inc., Totowa, NJ

Key Words: Cardiac arrest; cardiopulmonary resuscitation; massive pulmonary embolism; thrombolysis; outcome.

INTRODUCTION

Sudden cardiac arrest carries a very poor prognosis. Acute massive pulmonary embolism (PE) is the second most frequent cause of sudden cardiac arrest, accounting for up to 9.6% of the cases *(1,2)*. In fact, in patients suffering acute massive PE, the course of the disease is frequently rapid and fatal. Within 1–2 h after the onset of symptoms, 40–90% of these patients have been reported to require cardiopulmonary resuscitation (CPR) *(3,4)*.

Conventional CPR is often not effective in fulminant PE unless the thrombotic embolus itself can be removed immediately. However, therapeutic options such as surgical embolectomy or catheter-assisted techniques are not readily available in all hospitals or in the prehospital setting. In contrast, the use of thrombolytic drugs is established in most hospitals and has been shown to be effective in the treatment of patients without cardiac arrest suffering acute PE *(5)*. Nevertheless, mechanical CPR has historically been regarded as a contraindication to a thrombolytic therapy because of the anticipated risk of severe bleeding associated with potentially traumatic resuscitation procedures such as chest compressions. Therefore, thrombolysis has not become a standard treatment in this setting, even though clinical data suggested a benefit regarding survival and neurological outcome in patients receiving thrombolytic drugs for the treatment of cardiac arrest caused by acute PE *(6)*. Currently, CPR is no longer regarded as a contraindication to thrombolysis in patients suffering acute myocardial infarction *(7,8)*. Consequently, evidence for the use of thrombolytics during CPR in patients with acute PE needs to be discussed in the light of recent clinical data.

This chapter focuses on experimental and clinical results and on safety aspects of a novel or, rather, rediscovered therapeutic approach to patients with fulminant PE undergoing CPR.

THEORETICAL BACKGROUND SUPPORTING THROMBOLYSIS IN FULMINANT PE UNDER CPR

Cardiac failure in patients with fulminant PE occurs as a consequence of a vicious pathophysiologic circle with increased pressure load of the right ventricle causing an increased right ventricular volume and, consequently, a septal shift resulting in decreased left ventricular preload and cardiac output. Coronary ischemia and increased wall stress of the right ventricle precipitate right ventricular ischemia, which is thought to be the cause of right ventricular failure *(5)*. In view of these pathophysiological considerations, it is not surprising that the outcome of patients suffering cardiac arrest after massive PE is very poor, and that even return of spontaneous circulation (ROSC) is rarely achieved by conventional resuscitation *(2)*. Thrombolytic treatment during CPR in patients with fulminant PE aims at treating the underlying pathophysiological cause for cardiac arrest at an early stage.

There are at least two mechanisms that may contribute to the favorable effects of thrombolysis during CPR. The first, most intuitive mechanism, is direct and specific thrombolysis-mediated restoration of patency at the site of pulmonary occlusion. Chest compressions during mechanical resuscitation may amplify the effect of thrombolysis, because resolution of obstructing thrombi is supposed to be more effective after they have been mechanically fragmented *(9)*.

The second mechanism is at the level of microcirculatory reperfusion as suggested by experimental and clinical studies. After cardiac arrest, microcirculatory reperfusion failure is common and determines outcome (10). Although the pathophysiology of cerebral reperfusion disorders has not been completely understood, increased blood viscosity, endothelial cell swelling, leukocyte-endothelial interactions, and activation of coagulation with subsequent microcirculatory fibrin deposition and thrombosis have been reported to be important factors (11,12). The resulting cerebral "no reflow" phenomenon prolongs cerebral ischemia and reduces the chances of recovery after cardiac arrest. Experimental data have indeed shown that, within minutes after cardiac arrest, microthrombi are formed in cerebral microvessels (13). For example, cats receiving thrombolysis during resuscitation 15 min after cardiac arrest exhibited a significantly reduced cerebral "no reflow" in the entire forebrain compared to untreated control animals (14). Thus, it appears that the severity and extent of "no reflow" translates into neurological outcome.

It has been hypothesized that an imbalance between coagulation and fibrinolysis may lead to microcirculatory fibrin formation and microthrombosis during reperfusion after cardiac arrest. In fact, in an analysis of blood coagulation activity in patients with out-of-hospital cardiac arrest, we found marked activation of blood coagulation in all cases (15). This activated state was detectable until 8 to 48 h after ROSC. In contrast, the plasma levels of D-dimer, an indicator of endogenous fibrinolytic activity, were, in most cases, not markedly increased during CPR. From these data we concluded that, after cardiac arrest, a marked activation of blood coagulation may occur that is not counterbalanced by an appropriate activation of endogenous fibrinolysis. Massive fibrin generation with consecutive impairment of fibrinolysis during and after CPR in patients who suffered out-of-hospital cardiac arrest also was reported in another study (16). In addition, significant platelet activation was reported during and after CPR in humans (17,18). Evidence exists that the activation of coagulation during reperfusion after cardiac arrest may be caused by a combination of hypoxia, blood stasis, endothelial cell damage, and high levels of catecholamines in the blood (11).

In summary, the poor prognosis of patients suffering cardiac arrest after fulminant PE is caused by the underlying pathophysiological changes that are not influenced by conventional resuscitation efforts. Thrombolytic treatment may have two beneficial effects in patients with cardiac arrest after massive PE. Whereas the direct effects of thrombolytics on pulmonary thrombi are aimed at treating the underlying disease, the effect of thrombolytics on microcirculatory reperfusion after cardiac arrest may contribute to an improved neurological outcome of the patients even after prolonged resuscitation (9,11).

CLINICAL STUDIES
ON THROMBOLYSIS DURING CPR

The first report on thrombolysis in a patient with fulminant PE undergoing CPR was published more than 30 yr ago (22). Many other case reports followed, most of them demonstrating an exceptionally high rate of ROSC after thrombolysis following unsuccessful conventional treatment. Moreover, these case reports pointed to a surprisingly high number of neurologically intact survivors even after prolonged CPR. Although the success of thrombolysis as suggested by these reports may, in part, be attributed to selection bias in publication, the outcome data were viewed as particularly encouraging (19).

Apart from case reports, a number of case series and clinical studies on thrombolysis during CPR after massive PE exist in the literature (Table 1). In an early study, 20 patients

Table 1
Thrombolysis During CPR in Patients With Acute PE

Author	Study type	Number of patients	Thrombolytic agent	CPR-related bleeding	Number of survivors
Köhle 1984 (20)	prospective	20	SK	–	11
Scholz 1990 (21)	retrospective	9	SK/UK/ rt-PA	pectoral/ sternal hemorrhage; liver laceration	5
Horstkotte 1990 (41)	retrospective	17	UK	hemothorax (2 patients); liver hemorrhage	12
Siebenlist 1990 (42)	case series	2	rt-PA	–	2
Böttiger 1991 (43)	case series	2	UK	liver contusion	2
Hopf 1991 (44)	case series	7	rt-PA	–	6
Sigmund 1991 (45)	case series	2	SK / rt-PA	–	2
Westhoff-Bleck 1991 (46)	case series	5	rt-PA	–	3
Scheeren 1994 (47)	case series	3	rt-PA	–	2
Kürkciyan 2000 (2)	retrospective	21	rt-PA	hepatic rupture (2 patients); mediastinal bleeding	2
Ruiz-Bailèn 2001 (48)	case series	6	rt-PA	–	4
Total		94		9 (9.6%)	51 (54.3%)

CPR, cardiopulmonary resuscitation; PE, pulmonary embolism; rt-PA, recombinant tissue plasminogen activator (alteplase); SK, streptokinase; UK, urokinase.

requiring CPR underwent pulmonary angiography for diagnosis of fulminant PE. In these patients, streptokinase was administered locally, i.e., at the site of the PE. ROSC was achieved in 11 patients (55%) (20). A further study retrospectively analyzed a series of nine patients with acute PE proven by angiography. After administration of a thrombolytic drug during CPR (streptokinase, urokinase, or alteplase), seven patients were hemodynamically stabilized, and five patients survived. Of note, the duration of CPR to achieve ROSC was up to 90 min (21). Finally, another retrospective study compared a group of 21 patients presenting with cardiac arrest after massive PE who were treated with a bolus dose of recombinant tissue plasminogen activator (alteplase) during CPR, with a control group of 21 patients who received standard treatment. ROSC was achieved significantly more frequently in the thrombolysis group compared to the nonthrombolyis group (17 vs 9, $p <$ 0.05). Survival rates were, however, not significantly different between both groups (2 vs 1 survivor) (2).

Thus, clinical studies and case series suggest a significantly improved rate of ROSC in patients undergoing thrombolysis during cardiac arrest after massive PE. Compared to patients who receive standard in-hospital CPR, resulting in a survival rate of approx 15% (22,23), this strategy may translate into an improved long-term survival (54.3%; Table 1). In addition, and importantly, the neurological recovery of most survivors appeared to be complete after CPR in combination with thrombolysis, although the duration of resuscitation often exceeded 90 min.

OUT-OF-HOSPITAL THROMBOLYSIS

Out-of-hospital cardiac arrest is associated with a very poor prognosis. It has been estimated that only 5–14% of patients with out-of-hospital cardiac arrest survive without severe neurological impairment *(19,24)*. Acute myocardial infarction and massive PE are the two most common underlying diseases, being present in 50–70% of patients with out-of-hospital cardiac arrest *(25,26)*. In fact, fulminant PE is estimated to account for up to 9.6% of all cases *(1)*.

In all out-of-hospital studies on thrombolysis during CPR, an inclusion criterion was a suspected cardiac cause of cardiac arrest (i.e., acute myocardial infarction or massive PE). It is thus estimated that patients suffering cardiac arrest after acute massive PE represented 5–7% of all patients included in out-of-hospital studies on thrombolyis during CPR. Overall, 4 studies on out-of-hospital thrombolysis including a total 299 patients were performed (Table 2). Klefisch and colleagues administered "rescue" thrombolytic treatment to 34 out-of-hospital cardiac arrest patients refractory to conventional advanced cardiac life support. Five of these patients survived longer than 3 wk, and three of them were eventually neurologically intact *(27)*. In a prospective study which was performed at our institution, 40 patients with out-of-hospital cardiac arrest received thrombolytic treatment with alteplase and heparin during CPR, following unsuccessful resuscitation for more than 15 min. The study group was compared with a control group of 50 patients with similar baseline characteristics. Significantly more patients could be hemodynamically stabilized in the thrombolysis group (ROSC, 68% vs 44%) and were admitted to an intensive care unit (58% vs 30%). Moreover, 15% of the patients treated with alteplase were discharged from the hospital alive, whereas only 8% of patients of the control group could be discharged *(28)*. These results were confirmed by a retrospective chart review including 108 patients with out-of-hospital cardiac arrest who received alteplase during CPR and 216 control patients. Patients in the thrombolysis group showed a significant improvement in ROSC (70.4% vs 51.0%), survival after 24 h (48.1% vs 32.9%), and survival to discharge (25.0% vs 15.3%) *(29)*. Interestingly, PE was the suspected cause for cardiac arrest in 17.6% of the patients who received a thrombolytic agent compared to only 4.6% of those in the control group, suggesting a bias to administer thrombolytics to patients with suspected massive PE. On the other hand, and in contrast to these findings, the first randomized, double-blind, placebo-controlled trial of out-of-hospital thrombolysis during cardiac arrest did not show an improved survival of patients with pulseless electrical activity of the heart who were treated with alteplase *(30)*. However, the outcome of the control group that was treated with conventional advanced cardiac life support was extremely poor, because there was not a single survivor among the 116 patients of this group. In such a study population, even a therapeutic approach with proven efficiacy, such as hypothermia, would probably have failed *(31)*. Therefore, the clinical relevance of this latter study must be regarded with great caution. Currently, a large randomized, double-blind, placebo-controlled international multicenter trial is underway to assess the efficacy and safety of thrombolytic treatment during CPR in patients with out-of-hospital cardiac arrest of presumed cardiac origin *(32)*.

CLINICAL DIAGNOSIS OF MASSIVE PE
AS A CAUSE OF CARDIAC ARREST

The cause of cardiac arrest is often very difficult to confirm in the emergency setting. There is very little, if any, time to perform diagnostic tests. However, at least in some cases,

Table 2
Thrombolysis During CPR—Out-of-Hospital Studies

Reference	Study type	Number of patients	Thrombolytic agent	CPR-related bleeding	Number of survivors
Klefisch 1995 (27)	prospective	34	SK	hemothorax	5
Böttiger 2001 (28)	prospective, controlled	40	rt-PA	–	6
Lederer 2001 (29)	retrospective, controlled	108	rt-PA	pericardial tamponade (2 patients); hemothorax (1)	27
Abu-Laban 2002 (30)	prospective, randomized, controlled	117	rt-PA	pulmonary hemorrhage (1); major hemorrhage, not specified (1)	1
Total		**299**		**6 (2.0%)**	**39 (13.0%)**

CPR, cardiopulmonary resuscitation; rt-PA, recombinant tissue plasminogen activator (alteplase); SK, streptokinase.

a typical medical history, a recent ECG, a chest radiograph, or the blood gas analysis, which may have been performed at symptom onset, can help rule out other pathological conditions such as myocardial infarction, cardiac tamponade, tension pneumothorax, or aortic aneurysm (6). Pulseless electrical activity as the initial heart rhythm during cardiac arrest is associated with a high probability of massive PE, and may therefore be an important clinical sign in the pre-hospital setting, provided that an ECG is available (1). Moreover, even during resuscitation, an echocardiography may be a useful tool for the diagnosis of massive PE, because it may reveal the presence of acute right ventricular enlargement and hypokinesis (see Chapter 4).

Thrombolytic therapy will, of course, have no beneficial effect and may be harmful in patients with cardiac arrest owing to a ruptured aortic aneurysm or intracranial bleeding. However, these patients have an extremely bad prognosis a priori, which can probably not be further deteriorated by thrombolytic treatment (9). In contrast, because acute myocardial infarction is the major differential diagnosis to massive PE in a patient with cardiac arrest (25,26), thrombolytic therapy may be beneficial even if the underlying disease cannot be diagnosed exactly.

SAFETY OF THROMBOLYSIS DURING CPR AFTER MASSIVE PE

The major safety concern associated with the use of thrombolytics is the risk of severe hemorrhagic complications. Bleeding complications are indeed not unusual after conventional CPR (33). Among CPR-related bleeding complications, hemorrhage of the heart, the great vessels and the lung, and abdominal bleeding, are most common (34,35). Autopsy studies suggested an incidence of more than 15% for hemorrhagic complications in unselected patients after CPR (36). On the other hand, it is well established that thrombolysis itself increases the risk of bleeding. In a meta-analysis of nine large randomized trials on thrombolysis for treatment of acute myocardial infarction, the risk for major bleeding, defined as bleeding that required transfusion or was life-threatening, was 1.1% within the first 35 d after thrombolysis, compared to 0.4% in the control group. The incidence of intracranial bleeding after thrombolysis for acute myocardial infarction was

0.8% compared to 0.1% in the control group without thrombolysis *(37)*. In comparison, the incidence of intracranial bleeding after thrombolysis for massive PE may be up to 1.9%, one-third of these episodes being fatal *(39)*. Overall, the risk for severe bleeding in patients with acute MI or PE who receive thrombolytics and do *not* necessitate CPR can be estimated to be between 1.9% and 3.0% as compared to 0.5% in patients not receiving thrombolytics *(38)*.

The risk of severe bleeding caused by thrombolysis *during* CPR may be higher than by thrombolysis *after* CPR. Retrospective studies on thrombolysis shortly *after* CPR suggest that the incidence of severe CPR-related bleeding complications is similar to the incidence of severe hemorrhage reported in the large studies on thrombolysis for acute myocardial infarction or PE. An analysis of 8 retrospective studies including 379 patients who received thrombolysis either shortly before or shortly after CPR revealed a risk of 1.1% for severe CPR-related bleeding complications *(36)*. These results were confirmed by a recent retrospective cohort study in 265 patients with cardiac arrest. The authors evaluated the incidence of bleeding complications caused by thrombolysis after out-of-hospital cardiac arrest in patients with acute myocardial infarction. Although major bleeding was more frequent in patients receiving thrombolytics (10 vs 5%), this difference was not significant. It was thus concluded that CPR is no reason to withhold this effective therapy in selected patients *(39,40)*.

The incidence of bleeding complications when thrombolysis is given *during* CPR in patients with massive PE appears to be higher, as shown in Table 1. A total of 11 studies including 94 patients reported CPR-related bleeding complications in 9 cases (9.6%). Although these hemorrhagic events were severe, no patient died as a result of bleeding. All bleeding complications could be treated by blood transfusion or urgent surgical intervention *(2,21)*. No fatal CPR-related bleedings have been reported in any of the in-hospital studies on thrombolysis during CPR in patients suffering massive PE.

Under *out-of-hospital* conditions, a significantly higher incidence of bleeding following the use of thrombolytics during CPR may be expected, as history taking and physical examination of the patient are often limited. The overall incidence of severe bleeding complications related to CPR, however, was 2.0% in the out-of-hospital studies on thrombolysis during CPR (Table 2). In the study by Klefisch et al., one of the five surviving patients showed a hemothorax after prolonged resuscitation (75 min) *(27)*. Lederer et al. reported 6 severe bleeding episodes confirmed at autopsy in a subgroup of 45 nonsurviving patients; 3 of these were considered to be directly related to CPR. In the corresponding control group of patients, there were seven cases of severe bleeding. Therefore, the incidence of severe hemorrhagic events was not significantly different between the two groups *(29)*. Finally, the study of Abu-Laban et al. reported pulmonary hemorrhage in the only surviving patient treated with alteplase, and one more major hemorrhage that was not specified *(30)*. None of these severe bleeding complications in patients with out-of-hospital cardiac arrest was fatal.

In summary, the overall incidence of CPR-related bleeding complications reported in the studies on thrombolysis during CPR does not support the notion that thrombolysis during out-of-hospital resuscitation could contribute to an unacceptable bleeding risk.

CONCLUSION

Because conventional resuscitation is often unsuccessful in patients with cardiac arrest after fulminant PE, thrombolysis during CPR may be an appropriate therapeutic option to improve overall and neurological outcome of these patients. Thrombolytic drugs can effectively treat the underlying pathophysiological condition by directly dissolving PEs, and they are likely to improve the microcirculatory reperfusion after cardiac arrest. Clinical studies provide increasing evidence for a beneficial effect of thrombolytic therapy during CPR in patients who suffer massive PE. The favorable neurological outcome of surviving patients may result from an improvement in the microcirculatory perfusion by thrombolytics. Importantly, although thrombolysis during CPR may increase the incidence of bleeding events, currently available data suggest that these potential risks probably do not outweigh the benefits of thrombolysis during cardiac arrest. A large randomized multicenter trial testing thrombolysis during resuscitation for out-of-hospital cardiac arrest is currently underway, and it is hoped that it will provide definitive answers regarding the effects and potential risks of this treatment form in the emergency setting.

REFERENCES

1. Courtney DM, Sasser HC, Pincus CL, Kline JA. Pulseless electrical activity with witnessed arrest as a predictor of sudden death from massive pulmonary embolism in outpatients. Resuscitation 2001;49: 265–272.
2. Kürkciyan I, Meron G, Sterz F, et al. Pulmonary embolism as a cause of cardiac arrest: presentation and outcome. Arch Intern Med 2000;160:1529–1535.
3. Böttiger BW, Bach A, Böhrer H, Martin E. Acute thromboembolism of the lung. Clinical picture—pathophysiology—diagnosis—therapy. Anaesthesist 1993;42:55–73.
4. Stein PD, Henry JW. Prevalence of acute pulmonary embolism among patients in a general hospital and at autopsy. Chest 1995;108:978–981.
5. Wood KE. Major pulmonary embolism: review of a pathophysiologic approach to the golden hour of hemodynamically significant pulmonary embolism. Chest 2002;121:877–905.
6. Böttiger BW, Böhrer H, Bach A, Motsch J, Martin E. Bolus injection of thrombolytic agents during cardiopulmonary resuscitation for massive pulmonary embolism. Resuscitation 1994;28:45–54.
7. Antman EM, Anbe DT, Armstrong PW, et al. ACC/AHA guidelines for the management of patients with ST-elevation myocardial infarction—executive summary: a report of the American College of Cardiology/American Heart Association Task Force on Practice Guidelines (Writing Committee to Revise the 1999 Guidelines for the Management of Patients With Acute Myocardial Infarction). Circulation 2004; 110:588–636.
8. Van de Werf F, Ardissino D, Betriu A, et al. Management of acute myocardial infarction in patients presenting with ST-segment elevation. The Task Force on the Management of Acute Myocardial Infarction of the European Society of Cardiology. Eur Heart J 2003;24:28–66.
9. Padosch SA, Motsch J, Böttiger BW. Thrombolysis during cardiopulmonary resuscitation. Anaesthesist 2002;51:516–532.
10. Hossmann KA. Ischemia-mediated neuronal injury. Resuscitation 1993;26:225–235.
11 Böttiger BW, Martin E. Thrombolytic therapy during cardiopulmonary resuscitation and the role of coagulation activation after cardiac arrest. Curr Opin Crit Care 2001;7:176–183.
12. Gando S, Nanzaki S, Morimoto Y, Kobayashi S, Kemmotsu O. Out-of-hospital cardiac arrest increases soluble vascular endothelial adhesion molecules and neutrophil elastase associated with endothelial injury. Intensive Care Med 2000;26:38–44.
13. Mossakowski MJ, Lossinsky AS, Pluta R, Wisniewski HM. Abnormalities of the blood-brain barrier in global cerebral ischemia in rats due to experimental cardiac arrest. Acta Neurochir Suppl (Wien) 1994; 60:274–276.
14. Fischer M, Böttiger BW, Popov-Cenic S, Hossmann KA. Thrombolysis using plasminogen activator and heparin reduces cerebral no-reflow after resuscitation from cardiac arrest: an experimental study in the cat. Intensive Care Med 1996;22:1214–1223.
15. Böttiger BW, Motsch J, Böhrer H, et al. Activation of blood coagulation after cardiac arrest is not balanced adequately by activation of endogenous fibrinolysis. Circulation 1995;92:2572–2578.
16. Gando S, Kameue T, Nanzaki S, Nakanishi Y. Massive fibrin formation with consecutive impairment of fibrinolysis in patients with out-of-hospital cardiac arrest. Thromb Haemost 1997;77:278–282.

17. Böttiger BW, Böhrer H, Böker T. Platelet Factor 4 release in patients undergoing cardiopulmonary resuscitation: can reperfusion be impaired by platelet aggregation? Acta Anaesthesiol Scand 1996;40: 631–635.

18. Gando S, Kameue T, Nanzaki S, Igarashi M, Nakanishi Y. Platelet activation with massive formation of thromboxane A2 during and after cardiopulmonary resuscitation. Intensive Care Med 1997;23:71–76.

19. Newman DH, Greenwald I, Callaway CW. Cardiac arrest and the role of thrombolytic agents. Ann Emerg Med 2000;35:472–480.

20. Köhle W, Pindur G, Stauch M, Rasche H. Hochdosierte Streptokinasetherapie bei fulminanter Lung-enarterienembolie. Anaesthesist 1984;33:469.

21. Scholz KH, Hilmer T, Schuster S, Wojcik J, Kreuzer H, Tebbe U. Thrombolysis in resuscitated patients with pulmonary embolism. Dtsch Med Wochenschr 1990;115:930–935.

22. Ballew KA, Philbrick JT, Caven DE, Schorling JB. Predictors of survival following in-hospital cardiopulmonary resuscitation. A moving target. Arch Intern Med 1994;154:2426–2432.

23. Bedell SE, Delbanco TL, Cook EF, Epstein FH. Survival after cardiopulmonary resuscitation in the hospital. N Engl J Med 1983;309:569–576.

24. Böttiger BW, Grabner C, Bauer H, et al. Long term outcome after out-of-hospital cardiac arrest with physician staffed emergency medical services: the Utstein style applied to a midsized urban/suburban area. Heart 1999;82:674–679.

25. Silfvast T. Cause of death in unsuccessful prehospital resuscitation. J Intern Med 1991;229:331–335.

26. Spaulding CM, Joly LM, Rosenberg A, et al. Immediate coronary angiography in survivors of out-of-hospital cardiac arrest. N Engl J Med 1997;336:1629–1633.

27. Klefisch F, Gareis R, Störk T, Möckel M, Danne O. Pröklinische ultima-ratio Thrombolyse bei therapierefraktörer kardiopulmonaler Reanimation. Intensivmedizin 1995;32:155–162.

28. Böttiger BW, Bode C, Kern S, et al. Efficacy and safety of thrombolytic therapy after initially unsuccessful cardiopulmonary resuscitation: a prospective clinical trial. Lancet 2001;357:1583–1585.

29. Lederer W, Lichtenberger C, Pechlaner C, Kroesen G, Baubin M. Recombinant tissue plasminogen activator during cardiopulmonary resuscitation in 108 patients with out-of-hospital cardiac arrest. Resuscitation 2001;50:71–76.

30. Abu-Laban RB, Christenson JM, Innes GD, et al. Tissue plasminogen activator in cardiac arrest with pulseless electrical activity. N Engl J Med 2002;346:1522–1528.

31. Böttiger BW, Padosch SA, Wenzel V, et al. Tissue plasminogen activator in cardiac arrest with pulseless electrical activity. N Engl J Med 2002;17:1281–1282.

32. Spöhr F, Arntz HR, Bluhmki E, et al. International multicentre trial protocol to assess the efficacy and safety of tenecteplase during cardiopulmonary resuscitation in patients with out-of-hospital cardiac arrest: the Thrombolysis in Cardiac Arrest (TROICA) Study. Eur J Clin Invest 2005;35:315–323.

33. Krischer JP, Fine EG, Davis JH, Nagel EL. Complications of cardiac resuscitation. Chest 1987;92: 287–291.

34. Bedell SE, Fulton EJ. Unexpected findings and complications at autopsy after cardiopulmonary resuscitation (CPR). Arch Intern Med 1986;146:1725–1728.

35. Nagel EL, Fine EG, Krischer JP, Davis JH. Complications of CPR. Crit Care Med 1981;9:424.

36. Spöhr F, Böttiger BW. Safety of thrombolysis during cardiopulmonary resuscitation. Drug Saf 2003;26: 367–379.

37. Indications for fibrinolytic therapy in suspected acute myocardial infarction: collaborative overview of early mortality and major morbidity results from all randomised trials of more than 1000 patients. Fibrinolytic Therapy Trialists' (FTT) Collaborative Group. Lancet 1994;343:311–322.

38. Kanter DS, Mikkola KM, Patel SR, Parker JA, Goldhaber SZ. Thrombolytic therapy for pulmonary embolism. Frequency of intracranial hemorrhage and associated risk factors. Chest 1997;111:1241–1245.

39. Böttiger BW, Spöhr F. The risk of thrombolysis in association with cardiopulmonary resuscitation: no reason to withhold this causal and effective therapy. J Intern Med 2003;253:99–101.

40. Kürkciyan I, Meron G, Sterz F, et al. Major bleeding complications after cardiopulmonary resuscitation: impact of thrombolytic treatment. J Intern Med 2003;253:128–135.

41. Horstkotte D, Heintzen M, Strauer B. Combined mechanical and thrombolytic reopening of the lung-stream-track with massive lung-arterial-embolism. Intensivmedizin 1990;27:124–132.

42. Siebenlist D, Gattenlöhner W. Fibrinolysis with rt-PA for fulminant pulmonary thromboembolism. Intensivmedizin 1990;27:302–305.

43. Böttiger BW, Reim SM, Diezel G. Successful treatment of a fulminant pulmonary embolism using a high-dose bolus injection of urokinase during cardiopulmonary resuscitation. Anasthesiol Intensivmed Notfallmed Schmerzther 1991;26:29–36.

44. Hopf HB, Flossdorf T, Breulmann M. Rekombinanter Gewebeplasminogenaktivator (rt-PA) zur Notfall-behandlung der perioperativen lebensbedrohlichen Lungenembolie (Stadium IV). Anaesthesist 1991;40: 309–314.

45. Sigmund M, Rubart M, Vom Dahl J, Uebis R, Hanrath P. Successful treatment of massive pulmonary embolism by combined mechanical and thrombolytic therapy. J Interv Cardiol 1991;4:63–68.

46. Westhoff-Bleck M, Gulba D, Claus G, Rafflenbeul W, Lichtlein P. Lysetherapie bei protrahierter kardio-pulmonaler Reanimation: Nutzen und Komplikationen. Z Kardiol 1991;80:139.

47. Scheeren TW, Hopf HB, Peters J. Intraoperative thrombolysis with rt-PA in massive pulmonary embo-lism during venous thrombectomy. Anösthesiol Intensivmed Notfallmed Schmerzther 1994;29:440–445.

48. Ruiz-Bailen M, Aguayo-de-Hoyos E, Serrano-Corcoles MC, et al. Thrombolysis with recombinant tissue plasminogen activator during cardiopulmonary resuscitation in fulminant pulmonary embolism. A case series. Resuscitation 2001;51:97–101.

12

Surgical Pulmonary Embolectomy

Ani C. Anyanwu, MD and Lishan Aklog, MD

SUMMARY

Pulmonary embolectomy is one of the oldest cardiac operations, dating back to the early 20th century. Initially performed blindly as a closed cardiac procedure, the operation is now performed on cardiopulmonary bypass with clots extracted from the opened pulmonary arteries under direct vision. Surgery was the mainstay of therapy for pulmonary emboli in the 1960s and 1970s. Presently, however, with the advent of effective nonsurgical therapy, pulmonary embolectomy is largely reserved for anatomically extensive central emboli with hemodynamic compromise or right ventricular strain, or for cases in which medical therapy has failed or is contraindicated. The results of surgery have improved greatly in recent years, with contemporary series reporting mortality rates below 10%. Patient selection and surgical management are the key to minimizing the mortality of this operation. If patients are operated on at an early stage, before the onset of irreversible right ventricular dysfunction or protracted cardiogenic shock, then the mortality risk is low. On the other hand, preoperative cardiac arrest leads to a fivefold increase in mortality. Modern intraoperative management includes cardiopulmonary bypass, avoidance of cardiac ischemia, extraction of clots under direct vision only, and placement of cava filters. Some patients are not suitable for pulmonary embolectomy, including those undergoing cardiopulmonary resuscitation, those with predominantly peripheral emboli, and patients who do not have immediate access to cardiac surgery (thrombolysis is preferable to a delay in treatment). On the other hand, in centers with the infrastructure for immediate embolectomy, surgery offers the fastest means of deobliterating the pulmonary arteries and should thus be considered as a therapeutic option in all patients with massive or even submassive pulmonary embolism.

Key Words: Massive pulmonary embolism; embolectomy; cardiopulmonary bypass.

From: *Contemporary Cardiology: Management of Acute Pulmonary Embolism*
Edited by: S. Konstantinides © Humana Press Inc., Totowa, NJ

HISTORY

Early Era

Surgical pulmonary embolectomy is one of the oldest cardiac operations and was introduced by Friedrich Trendelenburg, a German professor of surgery, in the early 20th century *(1)*. In his operation, performed 50 yr prior to the introduction of cardiopulmonary bypass, he extracted the embolus by introducing a specially designed forceps into the left pulmonary artery via a small arteriotomy. The extraction was blind, risking avulsion of the pulmonary artery wall with massive fatal hemorrhage. He reported three such attempts at extracting pulmonary emboli (PE), but all had a fatal outcome. The first successful embolectomy is reported to have occurred in 1924 and was performed by Martin Kirschner, a student of Trendelenburg, on a patient who developed acute PE after a hernia repair. In the subsequent decade, more than 300 embolectomies were performed, but, like the initial Trendelenburg operations, most attempts at surgical embolectomy were unsuccessful. In fact, a report in 1958 identified only 12 patients in the literature who had survived a pulmonary embolectomy *(2)*. The operation fast fell into disrepute, and in an address to the American Surgical Association in 1944, Alton Ochsner, a renowned surgeon and one of the pioneers in cardiovascular surgery, stated, "I hope we will not have any more papers on the removal of pulmonary emboli before this organization, an operation which should be of historical interest only" *(3)*. At that time, however, surgery was the only available treatment for PE; heparin had only just been discovered and its introduction into clinical practice was slow.

Introduction of Cardiopulmonary Bypass

The modern era of surgical embolectomy started with the introduction of cardiopulmonary bypass in the 1950s. Indeed, it was the desire to provide a safe means of treating PE that prompted the development of cardiopulmonary bypass. John Gibbon, who performed the first series of heart operations using cardiopulmonary bypass, had witnessed a patient die during a surgical embolectomy in 1930 and surmised that the patient might have been saved if there had been a mechanism to temporarily take over her circulation and cardiorespiratory function while the embolism was removed *(3)*. This event prompted Gibbon to spend the next 23 yr working on the development of an extracorporeal circulation device.

Gibbon himself never performed surgical embolectomy. Denton Cooley is credited with the first pulmonary embolectomy using extracorporeal circulation in 1961 *(3)*. Cooley's patient did not survive. The first successful embolectomy on cardiopulmonary bypass was reported in the literature by Sharpe 1 yr later *(4)*. With the use of cardiopulmonary bypass, it was now possible to open the pulmonary artery and extract the clot under direct vision, unlike the Trendelenburg operation in which the clot was extracted blindly with forceps. With this approach, the success rate for surgical embolectomy approached 50%, a great achievement for an otherwise fatal condition.

In the 1960s and 1970s, surgeons continued to perform the original Trendelenburg operation for embolectomies in patients collapsing at the bedside or in the community, and in patients having PE in hospitals where cardiopulmonary bypass was not available. As nonsurgical treatment for PE, intensive care, and respiratory support had not been sufficiently developed to cope with massive PE, this was a reasonable approach at that time and was occasionally life-saving *(5)*. Gradually, the classic Trendelenburg operation was abandoned and embolectomy using cardiopulmonary bypass became the surgical standard, as most patients can be stabilized for a few hours to allow transfer to a suitably equipped cardiac center.

A modification of the classic Trendelenburg operation that allows clot extraction under vision without use of cardiopulmonary bypass was introduced in the 1970s *(6)*. In this technique, the surgeon briefly occludes cardiac inflow by snaring the venae cavae, rapidly opens the pulmonary artery, extracts the clot under vision, then rapidly closes or clamps the pulmonary artery and unobstructs the cava allowing resumption of cardiac output. The caval occlusion period must be less than 3 min to prevent anoxic brain injury. This approach is occasionally still used by some surgeons *(7)*.

The principles of the standard surgical embolectomy procedure have remained largely unchanged over the last 40 yr—cardiopulmonary bypass, pulmonary arteriotomy, complete evacuation of emboli under direct vision, and consideration for caval interruption.

APPLICATION AND SURGICAL RESULTS

Incidence

With the advent of nonsurgical, particularly thrombolytic, treatment, only a small minority of patients with PE undergo surgery, and thus the experience of individual surgeons is generally very limited. The success of nonsurgical treatment combined with lack of enthusiasm by many surgeons and also lack of experience in dealing with this condition further reduced the interest in surgical embolectomy, such that many patients who could have potentially benefited from surgery are never referred to the surgeon, and embolectomy is now only occasionally performed. For example, in 2003 only 11 surgical embolectomies were reported in the United Kingdom by the 37 centers contributing to their national registry *(8)*. We recently reviewed 22 surgical series on pulmonary embolectomy published between 1970 and 1990 with a combined total of 837 patients *(9)* (Table 1). Probably the most startling feature was the rarity of surgical embolectomy in the current era, with an average of 2.9 embolectomies per year performed by contributing centers. This is a very low rate indeed, especially considering that published series usually represent the higher end of the volume spectrum and the some series date back to the 1970s, when embolectomy was more frequently applied. Unfortunately, the rarity of surgeons who perform this operation may limit access to surgical embolectomy in those patients for whom there is a clear indication for surgery.

Surgical Results

HISTORICAL SERIES

Pulmonary embolectomy is widely perceived as being an operation that carries a prohibitive mortality risk, and many physicians quote the 40% mortality rate seen in early series. In our review of the published literature *(9)* (Table 1), we found an overall mortality rate of 31% with nearly all centers reporting mortality rates between 20% and 40%. However, certain factors were found to predispose to higher mortality (Fig. 1), such as surgery before 1990, operations without cardiopulmonary bypass, and prior cardiac arrest. Preoperative cardiac arrest was in fact the strongest predictor of outcome, being associated with 59% mortality *(9)* (Fig. 1B). In contrast, patients who did not have prior cardiac arrest and underwent cardiopulmonary bypass had only 10% operative mortality. Patients with prior cardiopulmonary disease were also identified to be at greater risk of death, as they

Table 1
Surgical Series of Pulmonary Embolectomy

Lead author	Country	Publication date	Years covered	Number of years	Number of patients	Cases per year	Operative deaths	Operative mortality
Aklog (51)	United States	2001	1999–2001	2	29	14.5	3	10%
Doerge (13,15)	Germany	1999	1979–1998	19	41	2.2	12	29%
Ullman (14)	Germany	1999	1989–1997	8	40	5.0	14	35%
Jakob (16)	Germany	1995	1988–1994	7	25	3.6	6	24%
Gulba (46)	Germany	1994	1988–1993	5	13	2.6	3	23%
Stulz (12)	Switzerland	1994	1968–1992	26	50	1.9	23	46%
Laas, Schmid (17,20)	Germany	1993	1975–1992	17	34	2.0	15	44%
Meyns (18)	Belgium	1992	1973–1991	18	30	1.7	6	20%
Bauer (19)	Switzerland	1991	1978–1990	12	44	3.7	9	20%
Kieny (10)	France	1991	1970–1989	19	134	7.1	21	16%
Meyer (21)	France	1991	1968–1988	20	96	4.8	36	38%
Morshuis (22)	Netherlands	1990	1975–1988	13	16	1.2	6	38%
Gray (23)	England	1988	1964–1986	22	71	3.2	21	30%
Clarke (11)	England	1986	1960–1985	25	55	2.2	24	44%
Jaumin (47)	Belgium	1986	1969–1984	15	23	1.5	7	30%
Stalpaert (48)	Belgium	1986	1970–1984	14	29	2.1	10	34%
Mattox (27)	United States	1982	1961–1981	20	35	1.8	17	49%
Soyer (32)	France	1982	1977–1980	14	17	1.2	4	24%
Glassford (24)	United States	1981	1969–1979	10	20	2.0	8	40%
Tschirkov (25)	Germany	1978	1972–1976	4	24	6.0	7	29%
De Weese (26)	United States	1976	1961–1975	14	11	0.8	7	64%
Berger (49)	United States	1973			17		4	24%
Heimbecker (50)	Canada	1973			12		1	8%
Overall					837	2.9	261	31%

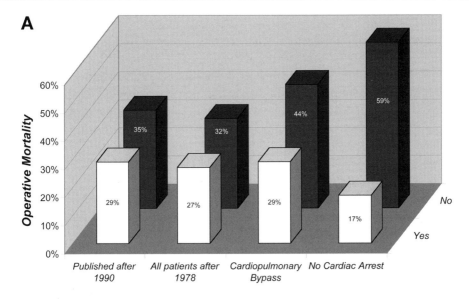

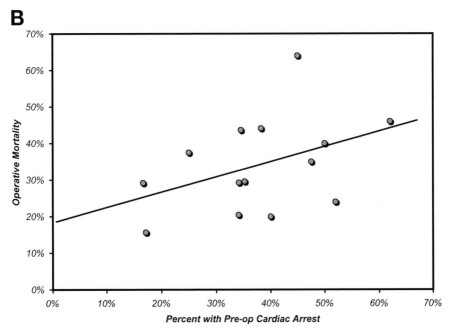

Fig. 1. (A) Mortality after pulmonary embolectomy. Mortality is lower in recent series, particularly those in which cardiopulmonary bypass was used and there was no prior cardiac arrest. **(B)** Relationship between operative mortality and preoperative cardiac arrest. (From ref. 9, with permission.)

have less cardiopulmonary reserve to tolerate even relatively low embolic loads. Of note, however, most of the literature on pulmonary embolectomy originates from series of operations performed in the 1970s and 1980s, which had higher mortality compared to recent series. These studies are largely of historical interest, as the indications, patient selection, and cardiac surgical management have changed over the past decade.

RECENT EXPERIENCE

The role of surgical embolectomy was recently revisited by some centers in the late 1990s, the most notable of which was the Brigham and Womens Hospital *(10)*. A team lead by Dr. Samuel Goldhaber and one of the authors (LA) decided to liberally apply surgical embolectomy to patients who had anatomically extensive PEs and moderate to severe right ventricular dysfunction, without ongoing hemodynamic compromise. Patients with preserved hemodynamics but impaired right ventricular function are known to have higher early mortality and higher incidence of recurrent PE compared to patients with preserved right ventricular function *(11,12)* (*see* Chapter 4). The Brigham strategy included rapid diagnosis by computed tomographic (CT) angiography, immediate assessment of right ventricular function by echocardiography, and prompt transfer to the operating room (without attempt at alternative nonsurgical treatment) when the criteria were met. We reported on the initial results in 2002 *(10)*, a series of 29 patients operated on between 1999 and 2001 with only 3 (10%) operative deaths (Table 1). These results represent a marked improvement in survival compared to the existing literature (most previously published series reported mortality between 20 and 40% *[9]*) and led to a renaissance of the interest in surgical embolectomy. A more recent report from the same group includes 47 patients with no further deaths (6% operative mortality) and documented an actuarial survival of 83% at 3 yr *(13)*.

Other recent series that also reported improved outcomes include that of Dauphine and colleagues *(14)*, who included 11 patients from 1998 through 2004 with 3 deaths among the patients with prior cardiac arrest ($n = 4$) and no deaths in the 7 patients without prior cardiac arrest. Yalamanchili et al. reported on 13 patients operated on between 2000 and 2002 with only 1 death *(15)*.

These recent series show that with rapid diagnosis, better patient selection, early surgical intervention, and modern surgical management, surgical embolectomy can be performed with a relatively low mortality (below 10%). It is relevant to note that surgical embolectomy is itself a relatively simple procedure carrying little risk inherent to the procedure itself, and that most deaths are due to right heart failure, multiorgan failure, and neurological injury (Fig. 2A). These fatal events are largely consequences of the patient's preoperative condition or a delayed intervention rather than direct complications of surgery *(9)*. In addition, the causes of late death are primarily related to underlying conditions (e.g., cancer) rather than recurrent thromboembolic disease (Fig. 2B). Thus, if patients are operated on at an earlier stage, before the onset of irreversible right ventricular dysfunction and protracted cardiogenic shock, then the mortality risk should be expected to be low.

INDICATIONS FOR SURGERY

With the advent of effective thrombolysis in the 1990s, surgery was generally regarded as a last resort when all other measures had failed or were unavailable. Reserving surgery for only such cases will predictably lead to poor outcomes. Surgery should be regarded as part of the armamentarium for treating PEs and should be applied early in suitable cases. In our opinion, surgery should be considered as an *alternative* to anticoagulation and thrombolysis, rather than as a bailout when medical treatment fails. The indications for surgery are not absolute and treatment strategy may vary from patient to patient. For some patients, surgery will be the most effective primary intervention, whereas for others medical therapy may be more appropriate. For this reason, a multidisciplinary approach, which includes

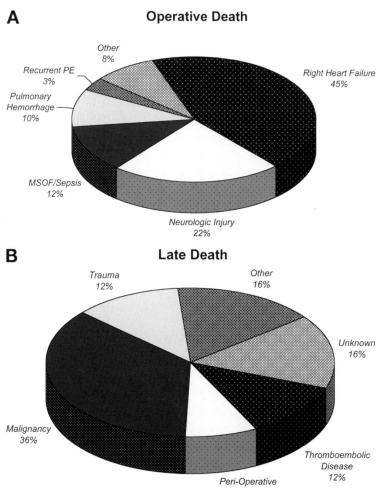

Fig. 2. Mortality following pulmonary embolectomy. (**A**) Causes of early mortality are related to the patient's preoperative condition and/or to delayed intervention. Right heart failure is the most frequent cause of early death. (**B**) Late mortality primarily depends on the patient's underlying condition(s), particularly cancer. (From 9, with permission.)

surgeons, should be applied to determine the appropriate management on an individual patient basis. Situations in which surgery should be considered are listed below and summarized in Table 2.

Lesion Amenable to Surgical Intervention

Surgery should be considered only in patients in whom most of the embolic burden can indeed be surgically extracted. The emboli have to be central in location (involving the main pulmonary trunk, or the left or right main pulmonary artery) and anatomically extensive, such that their extraction will most likely result in normalization of pulmonary artery pressures and right ventricular function. Thus, central clots that extend peripherally are most suitable for surgical treatment. On the other hand, if clots are limited to the periphery (i.e., lobar or sublobar branches), complete embolectomy cannot be performed without significant, blind instrumentation of the pulmonary arteries, and therefore such patients are not appropriate surgical candidates. Importantly, the history and radiological findings

Table 2
Factors to Consider in the Decision to Proceed With Surgical Pulmonary Embolectomy

Possible Indications for Embolectomy	Contraindications to Thrombolysis	
	Absolute	Relative
Embolus in the central pulmonary arteries	Active internal bleeding	Age greater than 75 years
More than 50% obstruction of pulmonary vasculature	Intracranial neoplasm, vascular malformation, or aneurysm	Recent (less than 10 days) major surgery, puncture of noncompressible puncture, or organ biopsy
Refractory cardiogenic shock	Neurosurgical procedure or stroke within the past 2 months	Pregnancy or early postpartum
Right atrial or ventricular thrombus	Severe uncontrolled hypertension	Recent trauma, including chest compressions
Severe right ventricular dysfunction	Known bleeding diathesis	Recent gastrointestinal bleeding or active ulcer disease (less than 10 days)
Elevated cardiac troponin T or I	Known allergy to thrombolytic agents	Known coagulation defects, including anticoagulant therapy and significant liver dysfunction
Moderate hemodynamic compromise or right ventricular dysfunction with contraindication to thrombolysis		High likelihood of left heart thrombus (e.g., mitral stenosis with atrial fibrillation)

should be consistent with *acute* PE without evidence for organized thromboembolic disease (chronic thromboembolic pulmonary hypertension; discussed in Chapter 19).

Hemodynamic Compromise

For patients with moderate or severe hemodynamic compromise resulting from massive PE, surgery offers the most rapid and effective method of relieving the obstruction. Although thrombolysis is often administered in this setting, and surgery has generally been reserved for patients in whom thrombolysis has failed or is contraindicated, there is no direct evidence that thrombolysis is superior to surgery. In institutions where rapid embolectomy can be undertaken with low mortality, this may be the preferred approach for this patient group.

For patients with cardiac arrest after massive embolism, surgery may, as an alternative to thrombolysis (*see* Chapter 11), offer a realistic chance of survival. However, pulmonary embolectomy in this setting carries very high mortality. When a patient with clinical suspicion of acute PE is successfully resuscitated after cardiac arrest, prompt transfer to the operating room and embolectomy should be considered even in the absence of preoperative radiological diagnosis. The diagnosis can usually be confirmed in the operating room by transesophageal echocardiography. On the other hand, emergency embolectomy under cardiopulmonary resuscitation (CPR) is rarely successful, probably because the pulmonary vascular obstruction and ventilatory dead space prevent effective forward flow during CPR. Although there are reports of successful emergency bedside peripheral cardiopulmonary bypass followed by transfer to the operating room for embolectomy *(16)*, the role of emergency cardiopulmonary bypass in this setting is not yet established.

Right-Ventricular Dysfunction

Moderate to severe right ventricular dysfunction, regardless of hemodynamic status, is associated with poorer survival after nonsurgical treatment; pulmonary embolectomy may offer better survival in this patient group compared to heparinization or thrombolysis *(12)*. For this reason, diagnosis of central PE should immediately be followed by an assessment of right ventricular function (*see* Chapter 4). Echocardiography is the method of choice for evaluating right ventricular function, although modern CT scanning may yield comparable diagnostic (and prognostic) information (*see* Chapter 2). If right ventricular function is compromised, discussion of the therapeutic strategy should, in our opinion, include the option of immediate embolectomy.

Failure of Medical Treatment

If cardiorespiratory compromise persists or worsens despite thrombolysis (Chapter 10) or catheter intervention (Chapter 13), then surgery is indicated. Many of these patients appear critically ill and are in a state of prolonged cardiogenic shock at this stage, but others may have less dramatic clinical presentation and preserved arterial blood pressure. Published series have repeatedly demonstrated that results are better when surgery is undertaken before the advent of severe hemodynamic compromise. Delaying surgery could therefore convert what might have been a low-risk procedure with a mortality risk of less than 10% into a high-risk procedure with 50% mortality. Because of this, we would advocate that surgeons be involved in the management of all patients with large central emboli and, if there is clinical deterioration or evidence of progressive right ventricular failure, immediate surgery should strongly be considered.

Other Indications

Other indications for surgery include the presence of right atrial or right ventricular thrombi in transit, as further embolism of even a small thrombus to an already obstructed pulmonary arterial system could be fatal. Some regard the presence of patent foramen ovale (*see* Chapter 6) as an indication for surgery, especially when paradoxical embolization has taken place.

Contraindications to Thrombolysis

Patients with stroke, intracranial tumors, recent surgery, recent trauma, bleeding diathesis, or active bleeding, are not ideal candidates for thrombolysis. Surgery is the treatment of choice for such patients, provided there is central clot amenable to surgical extraction. Advanced age alone is not a contraindication to surgery. Finally, surgery may also be the treatment of choice for massive PE in pregnancy.

SURGICAL MANAGEMENT AND TECHNIQUES

Little preoperative workup is required for surgical embolectomy, as the priority is immediate transfer to the operating room. Once the indication for surgery has been established, surgery should be undertaken. If surgery is available on site, and an operating room is available, then patients should be transferred directly from the radiology to the operating suite. Otherwise, the patient is transferred to an intensive care unit and arrangements are made for immediate transfer to a suitable facility. Resuscitation and stabilization should be continued en route to the operating room and should not delay surgery.

Anesthesia

Patients risk hemodynamic collapse on induction of anesthesia, as the right ventricle is preload-dependent and systemic blood pressure is maintained by an increased peripheral vascular tone. Venous and arterial dilatation on induction of anesthesia can therefore result in loss of these compensatory mechanisms. For this reason, the surgical and perfusion team must be ready to immediately perform sternotomy and proceed to cardiopulmonary bypass. Minimal monitoring lines are required and intracardiac catheters are avoided. Transesophageal echocardiography is a useful adjunct and helps identify the presence of clot in the right atrium and ventricle.

Surgical Technique

Median sternotomy and pericardiotomy are performed, the patient is heparinized, and the ascending aorta and right atrium are cannulated. If there is thrombus in the right atrium, care is taken to not to dislodge it during cannulation. Cardiopulmonary bypass is instituted. Some surgeons employ mild hypothermia. Cardioplegic arrest is not required and, in fact, avoidance of acute ischemia-reperfusion injury to the failing right ventricle is important in preventing postoperative right ventricular dysfunction. If echocardiography demonstrates thrombi in the right atrium or ventricle, these cavities are explored and the clot extracted. The patent foramen ovale, if present, is closed at this stage.

Pulmonary Arteriotomy and Embolectomy

An incision is made over the main pulmonary artery and the clot visualized (Fig. 3). Using gallbladder stone forceps, or any other suitable atraumatic forceps, the clot is extracted with every attempt made to extract it en bloc. Positioning the cardiotomy suction

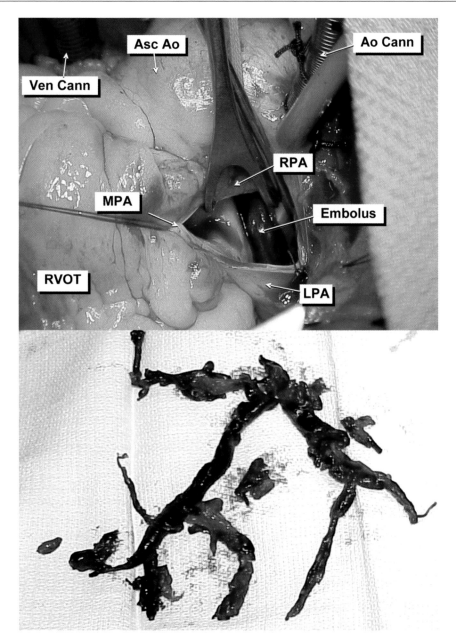

Fig. 3. Emergency pulmonary embolectomy for saddle embolus. Upper panel: operative view of an embolus straddling the bifurcation of the main pulmonary artery and resected specimen. Lower panel: note the cast of the lobar and sublobar branches in the resected specimen. Asc Ao, ascending aorta; Ao Cann, aortic cannula; LPA, left pulmonary artery; MPA, main pulmonary artery; RPA, right pulmonary artery; RVOT, right ventricular outflow tract; Ven Cann, cannula in appendage of the right atrium.

distal to the embolus can help with visualization and exposure of the emboli. Once all visible clot is removed, the pulmonary artery is repaired. There is no need to attempt to extract distal clot, as leaving small clots behind is preferable to the risks associated with blind extraction, namely pulmonary hemorrhage, which is usually fatal. Such distal clots will usually dissolve overtime and have no major hemodynamic or respiratory consequences.

Blind extraction of clot (such as by passing the forceps blindly into the distal arterial tree and grasping for clot) is dangerous and should be discouraged. Blind passage of instruments or blind grasping of clot can lead to fatal injury to the pulmonary arteries, one of the reasons for failures with the original Trendelenburg operation. Similarly, passage of balloon catheters distally to extract clots is a hazardous maneuver, as uncontrolled inflation of the balloon can lead to pulmonary artery rupture and catastrophic hemorrhage.

WEANING OFF CARDIOPULMONARY BYPASS

If embolectomy has been of brief duration and there is severe right ventricular dysfunction, it may be preferable to "rest" the heart on bypass for a period before attempting a wean. At this stage, a pulmonary artery catheter may be inserted for monitoring of right atrial and pulmonary artery pressures. Transesophageal echocardiography is used to assess ventricular function and to exclude residual thrombus in the right atrium, right ventricle, or pulmonary artery. Optimal preload for the right atrium is determined by volume loading and inotropic support used to assist right ventricular function. Other adjunctive measures such as nitric oxide may be helpful, but persistently elevated pulmonary artery pressures should raise the possibility of residual pulmonary artery obstruction.

INFERIOR VENA CAVAL (IVC) FILTERS

An IVC filter is inserted intraoperatively or in the immediate postoperative phase to prevent early recurrent embolization, which carries a high mortality. Caval filters will also help prevent late recurrent emboli. Filters can easily be inserted in the operating room under fluoroscopic guidance and directly through the right atrial pursestring. If the embolus is secondary to superior vena caval or right atrial thrombus, an IVC filter is not required.

Postoperative Care

Optimizing right heart function is the priority in the early postoperative phase, as heart failure is the most common cause of early postoperative death *(9)*. Invasive monitoring of central venous pressure is obligatory. A pulmonary artery catheter is usually placed for measurement of right atrial and pulmonary artery pressures, cardiac output, and mixed venous oxygen saturation. The optimal preload (central venous pressure) should be determined individually for each patient. Many patients require inotropic support pending recovery of right ventricular function; in some patients inotropic support may be required for days. Pulmonary vasoconstriction should be avoided at all cost by maintaining adequate ventilation and oxygenation and by avoidance of drugs that constrict the pulmonary arteries. Inotropes like milrinone, which dilate pulmonary arteries, may be preferable to catecholamines. Postoperative heparinization is instituted on the first postoperative day if there is no postoperative bleeding. An echocardiogram and ventilation-perfusion scan (or CT scan) should be obtained prior to hospital discharge.

SUMMARIZED ESSENTIALS
OF SURGICAL MANAGEMENT OF ACUTE PE

In surgical management of PE, a number of important aspects need to be kept in mind and are emphasized here, because they may determine the patient's outcome:

1. Appropriate patient selection—patients who have had cardiac arrest will rarely survive if spontaneous heart rate is not restored preoperatively.
2. Rapid transfer to the operating room—longer delays predispose to prolonged right ventricular failure and cardiogenic shock, both of which have adverse prognostic implications.
3. Placement of caval filters in the early postoperative period prevents early recurrent embolization.
4. Avoidance of aortic clamping prevents ischemia-reperfusion injury to the already compromised right ventricle.
5. Complete avoidance of blind techniques of extraction reduces likelihood of trauma to the pulmonary artery.

CONCLUSION

Pulmonary embolectomy can be undertaken with low mortality and morbidity when applied early before cardiorespiratory collapse. The poor results in historical series arose mainly because of its use as a salvage procedure. There is no longer a role for bedside embolectomy, and except under extreme circumstances, embolectomy without cardiopulmonary bypass should not be undertaken. In hospitals without bypass facility, thrombolysis is likely safer and outcomes more predictable than attempts at embolectomy without bypass. On the other hand, when the infrastructure for immediate surgical embolectomy is available, surgery may offer the fastest means of deobliterating the pulmonary arteries and may indeed offer superior long-term results. Surgery should, therefore, be one of the therapeutic options to consider in patients with massive or, perhaps, even submassive embolism. Because of the low case load, there is an argument for concentrating this surgery to few centers, or alternatively to designated surgeons within a center, thus allowing surgeons to consolidate experience. Further studies are required to compare the contemporary results of surgery with those of nonsurgical treatments.

REFERENCES

1. Trendelenburg F. Über die operative Behandlung der Embolite der Lungarterie. Arch Klin Chir 1908; 86:686–700.
2. Steenburg RW, Warren R, Wilson RE, Rudolf LE. A new look at pulmonary embolectomy. Surg Gynecol Obstet 1958;107(2):214–220.
3. Westaby S. The foundations of cardiac surgery. In: Westaby S, ed. Landmarks in Cardiac Surgery. Isis Medical Media, Oxford, 1997, pp. 1–47.
4. Sharp EH. Pulmonary embolectomy: successful removal of a massive pulmonary embolus with the support of cardiopulmonary bypass. Case report. Ann Surg 1962;156:1–4.
5. Bennett JG. Pulmonary embolectomy after "death". Cardiovasc Dis 1976;3(3):334–339.
6. Clarke DB, Abrams LD. Pulmonary embolectomy with venous inflow-occlusion. Lancet 1972;1(7754): 767–769.
7. Stulz P, Schlapfer R, Feer R, Habicht J, Gradel E. Decision making in the surgical treatment of massive pulmonary embolism. Eur J Cardiothorac Surg 1994;8(4):188–193.
8. Keogh BE, Kinsman R. Fifth National Adult Cardiac Surgical Database Report 2003. Henley-on-Thames, Dendrite, 2004.
9. Aklog L. Emergency surgical pulmonary embolectomy. Semin Vasc Med 2001;1(2):235–246.
10. Aklog L, Williams CS, Byrne JG, Goldhaber SZ. Acute pulmonary embolectomy: a contemporary approach. Circulation 2002;105(12):1416–1419.
11. Grifoni S, Olivotto I, Cecchini P, et al. Short-term clinical outcome of patients with acute pulmonary embolism, normal blood pressure, and echocardiographic right ventricular dysfunction. Circulation 2000; 101(24):2817–2822.
12. Sukhija R, Aronow WS, Lee J, et al. Association of right ventricular dysfunction with in-hospital mortality in patients with acute pulmonary embolism and reduction in mortality in patients with right ventricular dysfunction by pulmonary embolectomy. Am J Cardiol 2005;95(5):695–696.

13. Leacche M, Unic D, Goldhaber SZ, et al. Modern surgical treatment of massive pulmonary embolism: results in 47 consecutive patients after rapid diagnosis and aggressive surgical approach. J Thorac Cardiovasc Surg 2005;129(5):1018–1023.

14. Dauphine C, Omari B. Pulmonary embolectomy for acute massive pulmonary embolism. Ann Thorac Surg 2005;79(4):1240–1244.

15. Yalamanchili K, Fleisher AG, Lehrman SG, et al. Open pulmonary embolectomy for treatment of major pulmonary embolism. Ann Thorac Surg 2004;77(3):819–823.

16. Ohteki H, Norita H, Sakai M, Narita Y. Emergency pulmonary embolectomy with percutaneous cardiopulmonary bypass. Ann Thorac Surg 1997;63(6):1584–1586.

13

Interventional Approaches to the Treatment of Acute Massive Pulmonary Embolism

Nils Kucher, MD

CONTENTS

INTRODUCTION
PULMONARY ANGIOGRAPHY
INDICATIONS FOR CATHETER INTERVENTION IN PE
PERCUTANEOUS CATHETER DEVICES
CATHETER-DIRECTED THROMBOLYIS
COMPLICATIONS OF CATHETER INTERVENTIONS
REFERENCES

SUMMARY

Approximately one-third of the patients with acute massive pulmonary embolism (PE) and cardiogenic shock are not eligible for potentially life-saving systemic fibrinolysis because of major contraindications. Moreover, large-scale registries have shown that surgical embolectomy is carried out in only 1% of patients with massive PE and cardiogenic shock. Therefore, catheter-based thrombectomy or thrombus aspiration, as described in the present chapter, is a promising alternative if contraindications to fibrinolysis are present, or if surgical embolectomy is not readily available or feasible.

Key Words: Pulmonary embolism; fibrinolysis; catheter thrombectomy; cardiogenic shock; risk stratification.

INTRODUCTION

Right heart catheterization was first described in 1929 *(1)* and angiographic opacification of the pulmonary arteries was not performed until 1938 *(2)*. Selective pulmonary arteriography on serial cut films was first reported by Sasahara in 1964 *(3)*. Only a few years later, the first reports on percutaneous catheter interventions for massive pulmonary embolism (PE) were published. Currently, although noninvasive imaging modalities such as multidetector-row chest computed tomography (CT) are increasingly used to diagnose or exclude PE (Chapter 2), advanced knowledge of pulmonary angiography remains crucial for safely performing catheter interventions in acute massive PE. This chapter describes the basics of pulmonary angiography and focuses on percutaneous catheter interventions for treating patients with massive PE.

From: *Contemporary Cardiology: Management of Acute Pulmonary Embolism*
Edited by: S. Konstantinides © Humana Press Inc., Totowa, NJ

Table 1
Hemodynamic Parameters in the Pulmonary Circulation (Normal Range)

Right atrial pressure, mmHg	Mean	8–10
	A wave	2–10
	V wave	2–10
RV pressure, mmHg	Systolic	15–30
	End-diastolic	0–8
Pulmonary artery pressure, mmHg	Mean	10–20
	Systolic	15–30
	Diastolic	3–12
Cardiac output, L/min		4.0–8.0
Cardiac index, L/(min/m^2)		2.6–4.6
Pulmonary vascular resistance[a], Wood units		0.7–1.1

[a]Defined as (mean pulmonary artery pressure – pulmonary capillary wedge pressure)
/cardiac output.

PULMONARY ANGIOGRAPHY

Hemodynamic Measurements

Patients who undergo pulmonary angiography or catheter thrombectomy require continuous hemodynamic and electrocardiographic monitoring (Table 1). Complete heart block during right heart catheterization is likely to occur in patients with underlying left bundle branch block and may necessitate temporary pacing. Transient tachyarrhythmias are common during catheter advancement through the right heart chambers, particularly the right-ventricular (RV) outflow tract.

Continuous monitoring of the pressure wave form during catheter manipulation is mandatory. The catheter should not be advanced in the absence of an appropriate pressure wave form. Damping of the pressure in the main pulmonary artery may indicate massive PE with the catheter holes embedded in the embolus.

In patients with acute massive PE, RV systolic pressure rarely exceeds 50–60 mmHg. Acute increase in RV afterload with a systolic pressure greater than 60 mmHg will result in acute RV dilation and systolic failure. In contrast, patients with recurrent PE or pre-existing cardiopulmonary disorders may tolerate higher RV systolic pressures prior to the development of failure. In patients with cardiogenic shock and RV failure, the RV end-diastolic pressure often exceeds 20 mmHg and typically shows a prominent dip followed by a rapid rise (Fig. 1A). Right atrial pressure is elevated with a prominent A-wave and a steep X descent (Fig. 1B).

Catheterization Techniques

Most catheters used for diagnostic pulmonary angiography have a size of 5 to 7 F. Catheters of this size are necessary to provide a lumen that will accommodate flow rates of 20–25 mL/s. The presence of an inferior vena caval filter, such as the Greenfield, Bird's Nest, or Gunter Tulip filter, does not necessarily preclude a transfemoral approach.

There are two basic designs of pulmonary angiographic catheters. The standard Grollman pulmonary artery catheter (Cook Inc., Bloomington, IN) is a 6.7-F polyethylene catheter with a 90° reversed secondary curve 3 cm proximal to the pigtail. The distal loop of the angled pulmonary pigtail catheter is less than 1 cm, permitting use of the same catheter for subselective injections. In contrast, balloon-tipped catheters, such as the 7-F

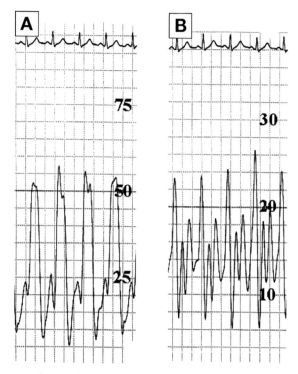

Fig. 1. Typical pressure tracings in a patient with massive PE and cardiogenic shock. (**A**) Right-ventricular (RV) pressure tracing. The RV systolic pressure rarely exceeds 60 mmHg in patients without preexisting cardiopulmonary disease. If the end-diastolic pressure exceeds 20 mmHg, the patient likely has RV failure. (**B**) Right atrial pressure tracing, with a prominent A wave and a steep X descent.

Berman balloon catheter (Critikon Inc., Tampa, FL), are passively carried by blood flow through the right-heart chambers and into the pulmonary arteries. Side-holes in the catheter shaft then allow power injection into the main branches, and an end-hole makes balloon occlusion angiography possible with the same catheter.

All pigtail catheters should be removed from the pulmonary arteries only after straightening with a floppy tip guide wire under fluoroscopic observation. An easy and atraumatic approach to probe the right or left pulmonary arteries is to use a coronary diagnostic catheter, such as a left Judkins 4 catheter, which may be used in combination with a 0.035-inch exchange-length J-tipped wire.

The contrast injection rate is determined by the catheter used for angiography, the volume and rate of flow in the selected vessel, the pulmonary artery pressure, and imaging modes. For digital subtraction angiography, less contrast is necessary to obtain adequate opacification of segmental and subsegmental arteries (Table 2). As smaller vessels are selected, the rate and volume are decreased. Contrast injection should be performed using an automated injector system if adequate opacification of segmental and subsegmental vessels is to be obtained. For balloon occlusion angiography of segmental vessels, a hand injection of 5 to 10 mL is used. In the presence of pulmonary hypertension, the amount of contrast should be reduced (4).

A minimum of two radiographic series for each lung is usually required. The two validated standard views are the frontal and 45° ipsilateral posterior oblique view. If available, biplane filming is preferred over monoplane filming.

Table 2
Suggested Contrast Injection Rates

Site of contrast injection	Cine angiography	DSA
Right atrium/main pulmonary artery	20–25 (40–50)	15–20 (30–40)
Right/left main pulmonary artery	15–20 (30–40)	10–15 (20–30)
Lobar pulmonary arteries	10–15 (20–30)	5–10 (10–20)

Numbers are contrast injection rates in mL per second, and the total amount of contrast in mL is given in parentheses. DSA, digital subtraction angiography.

Interpretation and Validity of Pulmonary Angiograms

Several studies have validated the angiographic criteria for acute PE (5–7). The primary angiographic criterion is a persistent central or marginal intraluminal radiolucency, the trailing edge of which causes a varying degree of obstruction to contrast flow. Complete obstruction showing abrupt vessel cut-off with a concave border of the contrast column is also considered as a primary sign of acute PE. Secondary signs include oligomeric or avascular regions, a focal prolonged arterial phase, abruptly tapered peripheral vessels, or focally diminished venous flow.

In PIOPED (8), interobserver agreement for cut-film pulmonary angiography decreased with diminishing pulmonary artery caliber. For example, it was 98% for lobar PE and 90% for segmental PE, but only 66% for subsegmental PE. The diagnostic sensitivity and specificity of pulmonary angiography were 98% and 95–98%, respectively. The validity of pulmonary angiography also was assessed by clinical follow-up of patients with negative angiograms, in whom anticoagulation was withheld. In 5 studies, 840 patients had a follow-up of at least 3 mo duration (9–13). Recurrent venous thromboembolism was documented in 1.9% of these patients.

INDICATIONS FOR CATHETER INTERVENTION IN PE

In patients with massive PE, systemic thrombolysis (14) or surgical embolectomy (15) are, in addition to anticoagulation, established and potentially life-saving treatment options, facilitating rapid reversal of RV failure and cardiogenic shock. However, thrombolysis for PE is accompanied by a particularly high risk of bleeding complications, and approx one-third of the patients with massive PE are not eligible for thrombolysis because of major contraindications such as recent surgery, trauma, stroke, or advanced cancer (16). Among 304 patients from the International Cooperative Pulmonary Embolism registry (ICOPER) who received PE thrombolysis, 66 (21.7%) suffered major bleeding and 9 (3.0%) had intracranial bleeding (17). On the other hand, few tertiary care centers offer emergency surgical embolectomy with round-the-clock availability for patients with massive PE and contraindications to thrombolysis (15). This operation mandates a median sternotomy, incision of the main pulmonary artery, and circulatory arrest with cardiopulmonary bypass (see Chapter 12 for details). In the two largest PE registries, surgical embolectomy was used in only 1% of patients with massive PE and cardiogenic shock (16,17).

The only alternative to thrombolysis or surgical embolectomy for reversing PE-related right heart failure and cardiogenic shock is percutaneous catheter thrombectomy (18). Catheter thrombectomy may be particularly useful if contraindications to thrombolysis are present or if surgical embolectomy is not feasible or available.

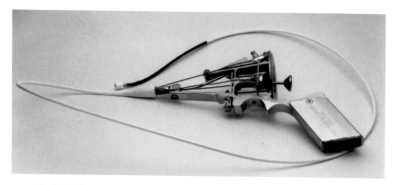

Fig. 2. The steerable 10-F Greenfield pulmonary embolectomy catheter (*see* text). Figure kindly provided by Lazar Greenfield, MD, Professor of Surgery and Chair Emeritus, University of Michigan, MI.

The author proposes that all of the following criteria should be fulfilled to consider catheter thrombectomy in a patient with acute PE:

1. Acute PE with cardiogenic shock, defined as systolic arterial pressure no greater than 90 mmHg, a drop in systolic arterial pressure of at least 40 mmHg for at least 15 min, or ongoing adminsitration of catecholamines for systemic arterial hypotension *(16)*.
2. Subtotal or total filling defect in the left and/or right main pulmonary artery by chest CT or by conventional pulmonary angiography *(19)*.
3. RV dysfunction, defined as RV systolic hypokinesis and/or RV dilation on echocardiography *(20)*, or RV enlargement on reconstructed CT four-chamber view *(21,22)*, or positive cardiac troponin test *(23–25)*.
4. Presence of at least one of the following contraindications to PE thrombolysis *(14)*:
   a. Active bleeding;
   b. History of intracranial bleeding, head injury, ischemic stroke, brain tumor, or neurosurgery;
   c. Surgery, delivery, organ biopsy, or puncture of a noncompressible vessel within the past 10 d;
   d. Gastrointestinal bleeding within the past 15 d;
   e. Major trauma within the past 15 d;
   f. Active cancer with known hemorrhagic risk;
   g. Platelet count less than 50,000/μL, or international normalized ratio greater than 2.0;
   h. Pregnancy.

PERCUTANEOUS CATHETER DEVICES

Greenfield Embolectomy Catheter

The Greenfield embolectomy device (Boston Scientific/Meditech, Watertown, MA) is a 10-F steerable catheter with a 5- or 7-mm plastic suction cup at the tip (Fig. 2). This device was the first catheter designed for the treatment of massive PE and has been available for more than three decades. Its major disadvantage is that it has to be inserted through a venotomy via the femoral or jugular vein, and that there is no guide wire to advance the bulky device into the pulmonary circulation. The device removes the centrally located fresh embolus by manual suction with a large syringe, and requires retrieval of the device and the thrombus as a unit through the venotomy. In the hands of Dr. Greenfield, the device was successful in extracting pulmonary thrombus in 76% of the patients, with

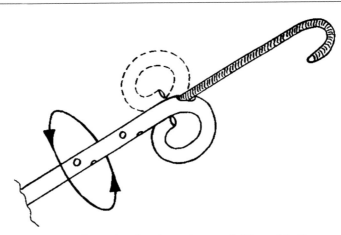

Fig. 3. The tip of the 5-F pigtail rotational catheter (*see* text). Figure kindly provided by Thomas Schmitz-Rode, MD, Professor of Radiology, University Hospital Aachen, Germany.

significant improvement in hemodynamics *(26,27)*. The 30-d mortality rate was 30%. The device was less useful in chronic PE, and it was not adopted by many other interventional cardiologists or radiologists for the treatment of patients with massive PE. Another major limitation of the device is the risk of fracture of the entrapped thrombus while removing the device from the pulmonary circulation, which may result in massive reembolization and hemodynamic deterioration.

Balloon Angioplasty and Stents

Balloon angioplasty of obstructing emboli has been used for many years in an attempt to restore pulmonary blood flow and improve hemodynamics *(28,29)*. Balloon angioplasty using balloon sizes of 6 to 16 mm results in compression of the embolus to the vessel wall but also to partial fragmentation of the thrombus with distal embolization. Most of the patients who have been treated with balloon angioplasty also received local thrombolysis, with a decrease in pulmonary artery pressure over time. Therefore, it is unknown whether balloon angioplasty without concomitant thrombolysis is effective. Self-expanding wallstents *(30)* and self-expandable Gianturco Z stents *(31)* were used in patients with massive PE and failed thrombolysis or failed thrombus fragmentation.

Pigtail Rotational Catheter

The rotatable pigtail catheter (Cook Europe, The Netherlands) is a modified 115-cm 5-F pigtail catheter with a radiopaque tip and 10 side holes for contrast material injection. A jugular version of the catheter is 105 cm long. An oval side hole in the outer (convex) surface of the pigtail loop allows direct passage of a 0.035-inch guide wire through the hole to act as a central axis around which the catheter rotates (Fig. 3). The catheter is rotated bimanually to break apart large fresh clots. The pigtail tip of the catheter disrupts the clot in multiple smaller fragments, which embolize distally in the pulmonary circulation. A smaller version of the pigtail catheter has also been used in segmental arteries. In 20 patients with massive PE, catheter intervention with the pigtail rotational catheter showed a 33% recanalization rate by fragmentation alone, but the catheter was more effective with adjuvant thrombolytic therapy with recombinant tissue plasminogen reactivor *(32,33)*.Mortality in this series was 20%. One disadvantage with this catheter device is the risk of macroembolization *(34)*. Macroembolization may cause further deterioration of hemodynamics when a large centrally located nonobstructive thrombus breaks and embolizes into a previously nonobstructed lobar branch.

Amplatz Thrombectomy Device

The Amplatz Thrombectomy Device (ATD) (Bard-Microvena, White Bear Lake, MN) is a 120-cm long, 7-F polyurethane catheter with a distal metal can, housing an impeller mounted on a drive shaft. The high speed of the impeller creates a vortex of circulating blood, pulling the clots toward the impeller, which pulverizes fresh thrombus. The metal can has side ports behind the impeller used as exit for macerated thrombus particles and blood. The system is propelled by an air turbine that can generate 150,000 rpm. Infusion of saline through the catheter lubricates and cools the system. The ATD cannot be used in combination with a guide wire. Therefore, a 10-F-long guiding catheter is advanced close to the PE and the ATD is introduced through the catheter. Then, the device can be activated and gently moved back-and-forth. The device should not be advanced into segmental branches because of the risk of perforation.

Initial experience with the ATD device showed clinical improvement in a limited number of patients, with improvement in symptoms and systemic arterial pressure *(35)*. There is a risk of severe hemoptysis with the ATD, and it is unclear whether hemoptysis is the result of perforation, dissection, or reperfusion injury. Because of recirculation of macerated blood and thrombus, the ATD always causes some degree of transient mechanical hemolysis.

Hydrodynamic Thrombectomy Catheter Devices

None of the currently available hydrodynamic catheter devices were designed for the treatment of the large-size pulmonary arteries, but they have been successfully used in small case series of patients with massive PE.

The Hydrolyser (Cordis, Warren, NJ) is a 7-F, 80-cm over-the-wire catheter, with a large side hole near the distal tip. The larger catheter lumen is used for aspiration of the fragmented clots and blood, and the smaller one is the injection channel with a metallic tubing looped at 180° to enable reversal of flow. High-velocity injection through the small lumen creates lower pressure dynamics in the larger lumen and a vortex, causing fragmentation and aspiration of the clots by the pressure gradient *(36,37)*. The Hydrolyser is effective in vessels up to 9 mm in diameter. When used in larger vessels, it tends to create a tract within the clot. The device can be used only via the jugular approach and is advanced over a 0.025-inch guide wire into the pulmonary artery. The rigidity of the catheter causes some difficulty in advancing into the pulmonary artery. In addition, the Hydrolyser may often be ineffective for removal of large, centrally located thrombi.

The Oasis catheter (Boston Scientific/Medi-Tech, Watertown, MA) also uses the Venturi effect. It creates a vortex that causes fragmentation and aspiration of the clots, with modest efficacy in larger vessels *(38,39)*.

The AngioJet Xpeedior (Possis, Minneapolis, MN) is a 6-F, 120-cm over-the-wire catheter and is probably the most efficacious catheter among the hydrodynamic devices (Table 3) (Figs. 4 and 5). However, because AngioJet was not designed to treat larger vessels greater than 12 mm in diameter, it is also of limited effectiveness in the therapy of massive PE *(41–43)*. Nervertheless, even minor improvement in pulmonary perfusion is often sufficient to improve hemodynamics and clinical outcome in these patients (Fig. 6).

Table 3
Effectiveness of Catheter Devices for Thrombus Removal

Catheter device	Company	French	Guide wire compatible	Embolectomy	Time and completeness of thrombus removal[a]
Aspirex	Straub Medical, Switzerland	11	Yes	Yes	69 s, ≈100% complete
Amplatz thrombectomy device	BARD-Microvena, USA	7	No	No	83 s, 66% complete
Hydrolyser	Cordis Europe, The Netherlands	6	Yes	Yes	124 s, 32% complete
Oasis	Medi-Tech/Boston Scientific, USA	6	Yes	Yes	185 s, 43% complete
Angiojet Xpeedior	Possis Medical, USA	6	Yes	Yes	118 s, 67% complete

[a]Measurements obtained from flow models using 16.3–16.5 g of ex vivo generated thrombus in test tubes with an internal diameter of 14 mm without stenosis (Aspirex) (44); and in test tubes with 20-mm internal diameter and 66% stenosis (Amplatz thrombectomy device, Angiojet Xpeedior, Hydrolyser, and Oasis) (40).

For the use in larger vessels, the company will launch in 2006 a modified 6-F AngioJet DVX catheter with improved aspiration capacity.

Aspirex PE Catheter

The Aspirex catheter thrombectomy device (Straub Medical, Wangs, Switzerland) was specifically designed and developed for percutaneous interventional treatment of PE in pulmonary arteries ranging from 6 to 14 mm in caliber. The central part of the catheter system is a high-speed rotational coil within the catheter body, which: (1) creates negative pressure through an L-shaped aspiration port at the catheter tip; (2) macerates aspirated thrombus; and (3) removes macerated thrombus (Fig. 7). The catheter is easily connected to a motor via an electromagnetic clutch. A small control unit ensures steady motor speed at 40,000 rpm.

The aspiration capacity of the Aspirex device was adjusted to remove thrombus from obstructed major pulmonary arteries and to minimize the risk of vascular collapse and vessel wall engagement. This was achieved by adjusting the caliber of the device, the pitch of the rotational coil, motor speed, and size and configuration of the aspiration port at the catheter tip. Aspirated blood cools off and lubricates the catheter system. The design of the Aspirex catheter does not allow recirculation of aspirated blood. In static in-vitro tests using human blood samples, aspiration with the Aspirex device was not associated with an increase in plasma-free hemoglobin (44).

A 12-F sheath is mandatory to introduce the device into the internal jugular or femoral vein. The Aspirex device is then advanced over the wire. An 80-cm long instead of the standard-length 12-F sheath may be used to provide more support to introduce the Aspirex device into the pulmonary arteries, monitor RV or pulmonary artery pressures, and inject contrast agent for pulmonary angiography. The distal part of the catheter shaft has enhanced

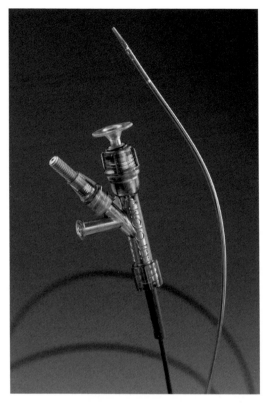

Fig. 4. The 6-F AngioJet Xpeedior catheter. The inflow channel, the pumpset channel, and the outflow channel are shown. Figure kindly provided by the manufacturer, Possis.

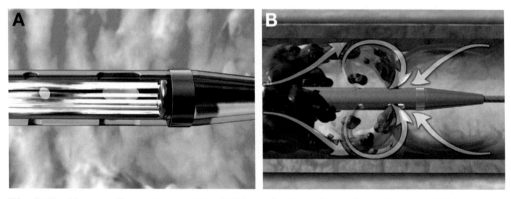

Fig. 5. The Venturi effect at the tip of the 6-F AngioJet Xpeedior catheter. Reversed high pressure saline jets within the catheter (**A**) cause cross-stream blood flow (**B, arrows**), resulting in fragmentation and aspiration of thrombus into the suction ports of the catheter. Figures kindly provided by the manufacturer, Possis.

flexibility, facilitating right heart passage and selective advancement into proximal pulmonary arteries. The Aspirex device is introduced and activated using a hydrophilic 0.035-inch J-tipped wire, such as the Terumo wire. The device should be gently moved back and forth to achieve an optimal thrombectomy result. Aspirex should be used in the

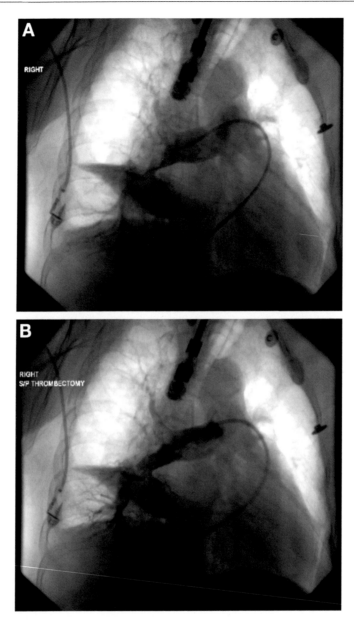

Fig. 6. Digital pulmonary cine angiogram of the right pulmonary artery using a left anterior oblique view (**A**) in a patient with massive PE and cardiogenic shock who had neurosurgery 2 d prior to the event. Although thrombectomy with the 6-F AngioJet Xpeedior catheter resulted only in modest angiographic improvement of blood flow into the lower lobe pulmonary artery, the patient had hemodynamic and rapid clinical improvement (**B**). The patient received a temporary Gunter Tulip filter after completion of the thrombectomy.

main and lobar but not in segmental pulmonary arteries. A large cohort study is currently being performed in Europe to investigate effectiviness and safety of the Aspirex device in patients with massive PE and contraindications to thrombolysis.

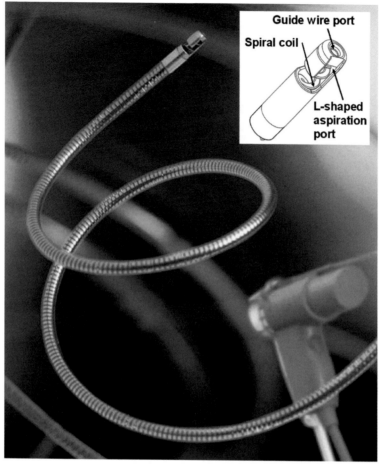

Fig. 7. The 11-F Aspirex PE catheter thrombectomy device (*see* text). Figure kindly provided by the manufacturer, Straub Medical.

CATHETER-DIRECTED THROMBOLYIS

Catheter-directed thrombolytic therapy with intrapulmonary administration of a fibrinolytic drug has been used by several authors *(45–48)*. It aims at accelerating clot lysis and achieving rapid reperfusion of the pulmonary arteries. The technique requires positioning of an infusion catheter within the embolus, with injection of a bolus of thrombolytic drug followed by a continuous infusion. The following intrapulmonary thrombolytic regimens have been used in combination with a therapeutic infusion of unfractionated heparin in patients with massive PE: Urokinase 250,000 IU/h over 2 h, followed by 100,000 IU/h of urokinase over 12–24 h; alteplase bolus of 10 mg followed by 20 mg/h over 2 h, or 100 mg over 7 h.

Another possibility is the administration of local thrombolysis via the AngioJet Xpeedior catheter using the power-pulse-spray technique (Fig. 8). Short-acting, newer-generation fibrinolytic drugs, such as alteplase (10–20 mg), reteplase (2.5–5 U), or tenecteplase (5–10 mg) may be used.

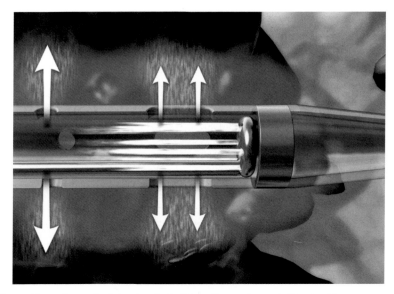

Fig. 8. If the outflow channel of the AngioJet Xpeedior catheter is blocked by a stop cock, thrombolytic drugs may be delivered locally into the thrombus (power-pulse-spray technique). Figure kindly provided by the manufacturer of the device, Possis.

In the author's opinion, catheter-directed thrombolysis is of limited value. If thrombolysis is being considered, it should rather be given systemically, and an invasive catheter approach may not be necessary.

COMPLICATIONS OF CATHETER INTERVENTIONS

Rare but serious complications of catheter thrombectomy for PE include pericardial tamponade, pulmonary hemorrhage, and hemothorax. The most serious complication is the perforation or dissection of a major pulmonary arterial branch, which may cause massive pulmonary hemorrhage and immediate death. The myocardium of the right ventricle, particularly the RV outflow tract, is thin and fragile, and caution is warranted when advancing any device into the pulmonary arteries. The interventionalist must be able to perform an emergency pericardiocentesis in case of a perforation and should be familiar with measures to achieve rapid reversal of anticoagulation. To minimize the risk of perforation or dissection, thrombectomy should be performed only in the main and lobar but not in the segmental pulmonary arteries. The procedure should be terminated as soon as hemodynamic improvement is achieved, regardless of the angiographic result.

Device-related complications also include blood loss and mechanical hemolysis, or arrhythmia from catheter passage through the right heart. Other complications include bleeding from heparin anticoagulation, contrast-induced nephropathy, anaphylactic reaction to iodine contrast, and vascular access complications, such as hematoma, pseudoaneurysm, or arteriovenous fistula.

REFERENCES

1. Ludwig JW. Heart and coronaries—the pioneering age. In: Rosenbusch G, Oudkerk M, Amman E, eds. Radiology in medical diagnostics—evolution of X-ray applications 1895–1995. Blackwell Science, Oxford, 1995, pp. 213–224.

2. Robb GP, Steinberg I. A practical method of visualization of the chambers of the heart, the pulmonary circulation, and the great blood vessels in man. J Clin Invest 1938;17:507.
3. Sasahara AA, Stein M, Simon M, Littmann D. Pulmonary angiography in the diagnosis of thromboembolic disease. N Engl J Med 1964;270:1075–1081.
4. Oudkerk M, van Beek EJR, Reekers JA. Pulmonary angiography: technique, indications and interpretation. In: Oudkerk M, van Beek EJR, ten Cate JW, eds. Pulmonary embolism. Blackwell Science, Berlin, 1999, pp. 135–159.
5. Stein PD, Athanasoulis C, Alavi A, et al. Complications and validity of pulmonary angiography in acute pulmonary embolism. Circulation 1992;85:462–468.
6. Dalen JE, Brooks HL, Johnson LW, et al. Pulmonary angiography in acute pulmonary embolism: indications, techniques, and results in 367 patients. Am Heart J 1971;81:175–185.
7. Hull RD, Hirsh J, Carter CJ, et al. Pulmonary angiography, ventilation lung scanning, and venography for clinically suspected pulmonary embolism with abnormal perfusion lung scan. Ann Intern Med 1983; 98:891–899.
8. PIOPED Investigators. Value of the ventilation/perfusion scan in acute pulmonary embolism. Results of the Prospective Investigation of Pulmonary Embolism Diagnosis (PIOPED). JAMA 1990;263:2753–2759.
9. Cheely R, McCartney WH, Perry JR, et al. The role of noninvasive tests versus pulmonary angiography in the diagnosis of pulmonary embolism. Am J Med 1998;70:17–22.
10. Van Beek EJ, Reekers JA, Batchelor DA, Brandjes DP, Buller HR. Feasibility, safety and clinical utility of angiography in patients with suspected pulmonary embolism. Eur Radiol 1996;6:415–419.
11. Bookstein JJ. Segmental arteriography by pulmonary embolism. Radiology 1969;93:1007–1012.
12. Novelline RA, Baltarowich OH, Athanasoulis CA, et al. The clinical course of patients with suspected pulmonary embolism and a negative pulmonary arteriogram. Radiology 1978;126:561–567.
13. Henry JW, Relyea B, Stein PD. Continuing risk of thromboemboli among patients with normal pulmonary angiograms. Chest 1995;107:1375–1378.
14. Guidelines on diagnosis and management of acute pulmonary embolism. Task Force on Pulmonary Embolism, European Society of Cardiology. Eur Heart J 2000;21:1301–1336.
15. Aklog L, Williams CS, Byrne JG, et al. Acute pulmonary embolectomy: a contemporary approach. Circulation 2002;105:1416–1419.
16. Kasper W, Konstantinides S, Geibel A, et al. Management strategies and determinants of outcome in acute major pulmonary embolism: results of a multicenter registry. J Am Coll Cardiol 1997;30:1165–1171.
17. Goldhaber SZ, Visani L, De Rosa M. Acute pulmonary embolism: clinical outcomes in the International Cooperative Pulmonary Embolism Registry (ICOPER). Lancet 1999;353:1386–1389.
18. Uflacker R. Interventional therapy for pulmonary embolism. J Vasc Interv Radiol 2001;12:147–164.
19. Kucher N, Luder CM, Dornhofer T, et al. Novel management strategy for patients with suspected pulmonary embolism. Eur Heart J 2003;24:366–376.
20. Goldhaber SZ. Echocardiography in the management of pulmonary embolism. Arch Intern Med 2002; 136:691–700.
21. Quiroz R, Kucher N, Kipfmueller F, et al. Right ventricular enlargement on chest computed tomography: prognostic role in acute pulmonary embolism. Circulation 2004;109:2401–2404.
22. Schoepf UJ, Kucher N, Kipfmueller F, et al. Right ventricular enlargement on chest CT: a predictor of early death in acute pulmonary embolism. Circulation 2004;110:3276–3280.
23. Kucher N, Goldhaber SZ. Cardiac biomarkers for risk stratification of patients with acute pulmonary embolism. Circulation 2003;108:2191–2194.
24. Meier T, Binder L, Hruska N, et al. Cardiac troponin I elevation in acute pulmonary embolism is associated with right ventricular dysfunction. J Am Coll Cardiol 2000;36:1632–1636.
25. Giannitsis E, Müller-Bardorf M, Kurowski V, et al. Independent prognostic value of cardiac troponin T in patients with confirmed pulmonary embolism. Circulation 2000;102:211–217.
26. Greenfield LJ, Proctor MC, Williams DM, Wakefield TW. Long-term experience with transvenous catheter pulmonary embolectomy. J Vasc Surg 1993;18:450–458.
27. Greenfield LJ, Kimmell GO, McCurdy WC III. Transvenous removal of pulmonary emboli by vacuum-cup catheter technique. J Surg Res 1969;9:347–352.
28. Handa K, Sasaki Y, Kiyonaga A, et al. Acute pulmonary thromboembolism treated successfully by balloon angioplasty: a case report. Angiology 1988;8:775–778.
29. Fava M, Loyola S, Flores P, Huete I. Mechanical fragmentation and pharmacologic thrombolysis in massive pulmonary embolism. J Vasc Interv Radiol 1997;8:261–266.

30. Haskal ZJ, Soulen MC, Huetti EA, Palevsky HI, Cope C. Life-threatening pulmonary emboli and cor pulmonale: treatment with percutaneous pulmonary artery stent placement. Radiology 1994;191:473–475.
31. Koizumi J, Kusano S, Akima T, et al. Emergent Z stent placement for treatment of cor pulmonale due to pulmonary emboli after failed lytic treatment: technical considerations. Cardiovasc Intervent Radiol 1998;21:254–255.
32. Schmitz-Rode T, Janssens U, Duda SH, et al. Massive pulmonary embolism: percutaneous emergency treatment by pigtail rotation catheter. J Am Coll Cardiol 2000;36:375–380.
33. Schmitz-Rode T, Janssens U, Schild HH, et al. Fragmentation of massive pulmonary embolism using a pigtail rotation catheter. Chest 1998;114:1427–1436.
34. Schmitz-Rode T, Janssens U, Hanrath P, et al. Fragmentation of massive pulmonary embolism by pigtail rotation catheter: possible complication. Eur Radiol 2001;11:2047–2049.
35. Uflacker R, Stange C, Vujic I. Massive pulmonary embolism: preliminary results of treatment with the Amplatz thrombectomy device. J Vasc Interv Radiol 1996;7:519–528.
36. Reekers J, Kromhout J, van der Wall K. Catheter for percutaneous thrombectomy: first clinical experience. Radiology 1993;188:871–874.
37. Fava M, Loyola S, Huete I. Massive pulmonary embolism: treatment with the hydrolyser thrombectomy catheter. J Vasc Interv Radiol 2000;11:1159–1164.
38. Sharafuddin MJA, Hicks ME. Current status of percutaneous mechanical thrombectomy. Part I: general principles. J Vasc Interv Radiol 1997;8:911–921.
39. Sharafuddin MIA, Hicks ME. Current status of percutaneous mechanical thrombectomy. Part II: devices and mechanisms of action. J Vasc Interv Radiol 1998;9:15–31.
40. Muller-Hulsbeck S, Grimm J, Leidt J, Heller M. In vitro effectiveness of mechanical thrombectomy devices for large vessel diameter and low-pressure fluid dynamic applications. J Vasc Interv Radiol 2002; 13:831–839.
41. Koning R, Cribier A, Gerber L, et al. A new treatment for severe pulmonary embolism. Circulation 1997; 96:2498–2500.
42. Voigtlander T, Rupprecht HJ, Nowak B, et al. Clinical application of a new rheolytic thrombectomy catheter system for massive pulmonary embolism. Cathet Cardiovasc Intervent 1999;47:91–96.
43. Zeni PT Jr, Blank BG, Peeler DW. Use of rheolytic thrombectomy in treatment of acute massive pulmonary embolism. J Vasc Interv Radiol 2003;14:1511–1515.
44. Kucher N, Windecker S, Banz Y, et al. Percutaneous catheter thrombectomy device for acute pulmonary embolism. Radiology 2005;236:852–858.
45. Molina HE, Hunter DW, Yedlick JW, et al. Thrombolytic therapy for post operative pulmonary embolism. Am J Surg 1992;163:375–381.
46. Gonzales-Juanatey JR, Valdes L, Amaro A, et al. Treatment of massive pulmonary thromboembolism with low intrapulmonary dosages of urokinase: short term angiographic and hemodynamic evolution. Chest 1992;102:341–346.
47. Vujic I, Young JWR, Gobien RP, et al. Massive pulmonary embolism treatment with full heparinization and topical low-dose streptokinase. Radiology 1983;148:671–675.
48. Verstraete M, Miller GAH, Bounameaux H, et al. Intravenous and intrapulmonary recombinant tissue-type plasminogen activator in the treatment of acute massive pulmonary embolism. Circulation 1988;77: 353–360.

14

Vitamin K Antagonists and Novel Oral Anticoagulants

Giancarlo Agnelli, MD
and Cecilia Becattini, MD

CONTENTS

SUMMARY

Vitamin K antagonists (VKAs) are the agents of choice for long-term treatment and secondary prophylaxis of pulmonary embolism (PE), as they were shown to be effective in preventing recurrence of the disease. At present, VKAs are the only available anticoagulants allowing oral administration, an essential feature in agents intended for long-term use. The currently recommended duration of anticoagulant treatment for PE is related to the features of the thromboembolic event, ranging from a minimum of 3 mo to life-long treatment. Patients presenting with idiopathic or unprovoked PE generally require longer treatment than patients with an event associated with temporary risk factors. On the other hand, the need for laboratory monitoring and dose adjustment, and the risk for bleeding complications, are the main pitfalls of treatment with VKAs and limit their use for long-term anticoagulation. Therefore, new oral anticoagulants are currently under development. To be of clinical value, these agents should be at least as effective as VKAs, possibly safer and easier to administer, and they should not require routine laboratory monitoring.

Key Words: Anticoagulation; pulmonary embolism; recurrence; vitamin K antagonists.

From: *Contemporary Cardiology: Management of Acute Pulmonary Embolism*
Edited by: S. Konstantinides © Humana Press Inc., Totowa, NJ

INTRODUCTION

In the large majority of patients, therapy of pulmonary embolism (PE) begins with a brief period of parenteral anticoagulation using unfractionated heparin (UFH) or low-molecular-weight heparin (LMWH) followed by long-term treatment with oral vitamin K antagonists (VKAs) *(1)*. Thrombolysis in the acute phase (*see* Chapter 10), or LMWH for long-term treatment, are reserved for only a few of the patients with PE. The aim of long-term treatment with oral anticoagulants after venous thromboembolism (VTE) is the secondary prevention of recurrences and deaths due to PE. VKAs are effective in preventing recurrence of VTE, although more recently, LMWHs were shown to be more effective than VKAs in the prevention of recurrence in cancer patients *(2–9)*.

Only a few studies on the long-term clinical outcome of VTE focused on patients with PE *(2,10–13)*, whereas most of the studies included patients with deep venous thrombosis (DVT) *(5–7,9,14–16)*. However, as it is widely accepted that DVT and PE are two manifestations of the same disease, VTE, information obtained in patients with DVT is usually extrapolated to patients with PE.

In this chapter, we will review the long-term clinical course of PE, the risk factors for recurrence, the treatment options available at present, and the new oral anticoagulants currently under development.

LONG-TERM CLINICAL COURSE AND PROGNOSIS AFTER PE

Patients with PE are at risk for recurrent VTE and death during long-term follow-up. A population-based study showed that VTE recurs frequently, especially within the first 6 to 12 mo, and continues to recur for at least 10 yr after the initial episode *(17)*. The reported rates of recurrent VTE vary widely, ranging from 0.6 to 5% at 90 d, and from 13 to 25% at 5 yr *(4,16,18–20)*. Recent trials showed that patients with PE are at higher risk of having a second, potentially fatal PE episode than are patients with DVT *(21–22)*. In particular, the risk of being readmitted to the hospital because of acute PE is 4.2-fold elevated in patients with previous PE compared to patients with previous DVT *(17)*. Nevertheless, currently available data do not suffice for recommending longer duration of anticoagulant treatment for patients with PE.

In a study focusing on 399 patients with objectively confirmed acute PE, 33 clinically apparent recurrences of PE (8.3%) and 95 deaths (23.8%) were observed during 1-yr follow-up after the initial thromboembolic event *(10)*. The most frequent causes of death were PE itself during the in-hospital phase and cancer during the follow-up period.

More recently, a high incidence of arterial complications such as acute myocardial infarction (1.0% of patients per year), stroke (0.5% of patients per year), and sudden otherwise unexplained death (0.3% of patients per year) was observed in the first 2–3 yr after a first PE episode *(11)*. The incidence was particularly high in patients with idiopathic PE as opposed to those with PE associated with temporary risk factors.

RISK FACTORS FOR RECURRENCE OF VTE

Patients with permanent (or persistent) risk factors for VTE (cancer, known thrombophilia), idiopathic DVT, or a history of previous VTE have a higher incidence of recurrent VTE in comparison with patients with VTE associated with temporary risk factors *(3–5)*. This concept is supported by the results of a prospective cohort study that included 355 consecutive patients who received anticoagulant treatment for 3 mo after a first episode of VTE *(16)*. In this study, the cumulative incidence of recurrent VTE was 17.5% at 2 yr, 25% at 5 yr, and 30% at 8 yr. The presence of cancer was associated with an increased risk of recurrent VTE (hazard ratio, 1.7), as was the presence of molecular thrombophilic abnormalities like deficiency of antithrombin, protein C, or protein S, or the presence of lupus-like anticoagulant (hazard ratio, 1.4).

On the other hand, patients with VTE associated with transient risk factors (e.g., surgery or recent trauma) have a low risk of recurrent thromboembolism. For example, in a study of patients with a first episode of PE, the incidence of recurrence was 12.2% in patients with idiopathic PE compared to 7.6% in those with PE associated with transient risk factors *(2)*. In another study of patients with VTE, recurrence occurred during 2-yr follow-up in 6.7% of patients with VTE associated with transient risk factors compared to 18.1% of patients with VTE associated with a permanent risk factor or idiopathic VTE *(4)*. Thus, based on the available data, three risk groups with regard to recurrence of thromboembolism can be identified within the population of patients who have suffered an episode of VTE: (1) patients with VTE associated with temporary risk factors; (2) patients with VTE associated with persistent risk factors; and (3) patients with idiopathic VTE.

Idiopathic or "unprovoked" VTE deserves further analysis and risk stratification. The term "idiopathic" stands for an episode of VTE occurring in the absence of any identifiable temporary or persistent risk factors for thrombosis. In order to identify patients at particularly high risk for recurrent VTE within the group of patients with idiopathic PE, potential risk factors have been proposed *(23–30)*. Of note, however, is that most of these data were derived from retrospective studies and in only a few cases were confirmed by prospective studies. At present, identification of patients at high risk for recurrence of VTE is based on screening for thrombophilic abnormalities, the D-dimer assay, and the assessment of residual thrombosis.

A large variety of thrombophilic abnormalities have been identified (*see also* Chapter 15). Although the increase in the risk for VTE (either for the first episode or for a recurrent event) has been well documented for some of them, the importance of other thrombophilias needs to be further investigated. In addition, high D-dimer levels measured 1 mo after discontinuation of oral anticoagulants have been reported to be associated with an increased risk of recurrence in patients with a first idiopathic episode of VTE *(29)*. Finally, persistence of residual DVT detected by compression ultrasonography after adequate treatment with oral anticoagulants has been reported to translate into an increased risk of recurrent VTE *(30)*. However, whether these conditions (possibly) associated with high risk for recurrence require different treatment strategies remains unclear. Nevertheless, based on all the available data regarding risk assessment in patients with idiopathic PE, the overall number of risk groups with regard to recurrence can increase from three (as described previously) to five, namely:

1. First episode of VTE secondary to a temporary risk factor;
2. First episode of VTE in patients with active cancer;
3. First episode of unprovoked VTE;
4. First episode of VTE associated with a prothrombotic genotype (deficiency of antithrombin III, protein C, or protein S; prothrombotic gene mutation [factor V Leiden or prothrombin 20210]; high levels of antiphospholipid antibodies, homocysteinemia, or factor VIII), or with a prognostic marker indicating increased risk of recurrence (persistent residual thrombosis on repeated compression ultrasonography); and
5. Patients with recurrent VTE (two or more episodes).

We recommend that these patient groups, which represent an escalating risk of recurrence, be taken into account when deciding on the duration of oral anticoagulant treatment.

VKAs

Coumarins, the only VKAs currently available in most countries, exert their anticoagulant effect by interfering with the vitamin K-mediated γ-carboxylation of the coagulation factors II, VII, IX, and X (31–32). After oral administration, coumarins are rapidly absorbed and have a high bioavailability (33). The relationship between the dose of these agents and the anticoagulant response is influenced by genetic and environmental factors. These factors include the absorption of coumarins, their pharmacokinetics and pharmacodynamics as well their metabolism. The wide interindividual variation in the dose-effect relation of VKAs is also linked to interactions with other drugs and nutrition. The use of VKAs is further complicated by their narrow therapeutic window. All these features make laboratory monitoring and dose adjustment necessary in order to maintain the anticoagulant effect within the therapeutic range and thus ensure efficacy and reduce the risk of bleeding complications. Prothrombin time is currently used to monitor the anticoagulant effect of VKAs, and the results are usually reported as the international normalized ratio (INR). The currently recommended intensity of oral anticoagulant for treatment of VTE is to target an INR between 2.0 and 3.0 (1). This value has been established by the results of randomized trials that included patients with DVT and PE (8,34–36).

The superiority of oral anticoagulants over long-term use of UFH was shown in a randomized trial evaluating subcutaneous low-dose UFH (5000 U bid) as an alternative to oral anticoagulation for long-term treatment of patients with DVT (18). In this trial, the low-dose UFH regimen was shown to be ineffective and resulted in a high rate (47%) of recurrent VTE.

OPTIMAL DURATION OF TREATMENT WITH VKAs FOR PE

The currently recommended duration of oral anticoagulant treatment for PE is a balance between the risks and inconvenience of treatment itself on one side and the risk of recurrent VTE once treatment is discontinued on the other.

Several clinical trials focusing on the optimal duration of oral anticoagulant treatment randomized patients affected by DVT with or without concomitant PE to different time periods of oral anticoagulant treatment (3–9). The earliest among these studies showed a higher incidence of recurrent VTE during the 6 mo to 1 yr after treatment discontinuation in patients randomized to shorter courses (4 to 6 wk) of oral anticoagulant treatment, as opposed to those randomized to longer treatment periods (3 to 6 mo) (3–5).

Further studies evaluated the risk-benefit ratio of extended anticoagulant therapy (1 to 2 yr) in comparison to the standard treatment (3 to 6 mo) in patients with idiopathic DVT (2,6–8). These studies showed that extended treatment with VKAs was highly effective in reducing the incidence of recurrent VTE, the recurrence rate on anticoagulant treatment being as low as 1%. However, the second important finding obtained from these randomized studies is that the clinical benefit achieved during extended oral anticoagulant treatment is not maintained after its discontinuation. In fact, the incidence of recurrent VTE after treatment discontinuation is approx 5% per year in patients with a first idiopathic VTE, regardless of prolongation of treatment beyond the first 3 mo. Thus, prolonging anticoagulant treatment only delays recurrences until anticoagulant is stopped rather than reducing the risk of recurrence.

In conclusion, the risk of recurrent VTE is high after a first episode of idiopathic vVTE, but the benefit of extended treatment is partially offset by the risk of bleeding (particularly major bleeding episodes), and the benefit is lost when treatment is withdrawn. At present, oral anticoagulant treatment for at least 6 mo to 1 yr is generally recommended after a first episode of idiopathic PE. However, physicians should also consider that some high-risk patients (as defined previously) may be candidates for indefinite anticoagulation (1).

The issue of the optimal duration of anticoagulant treatment specifically for patients with PE was addressed by a recent trial that evaluated the clinical benefit of extending oral anticoagulant treatment beyond 3 mo in patients with a first episode of symptomatic, objectively confirmed PE (2). This study also showed that extending VKA treatment to 12 mo (as opposed to 3 mo) in patients with idiopathic PE only delayed the time to recurrence but did not reduce the incidence of recurrences after discontinuation of treatment. On the other hand, in patients with PE associated with temporary risk factors, this study showed a trend towards reduction in the risk for recurrence after 6 mo of oral anticoagulation compared with the 3-mo treatment regimen.

OPTIMAL INTENSITY OF TREATMENT WITH VKAs FOR PE

As some patients with VTE may require indefinite oral anticoagulation, it has been proposed that the initial period of conventional oral anticoagulant treatment (INR 2.0 to 3.0) be followed by low-intensity warfarin treatment (8,35). This strategy might be expected to reduce the incidence of bleeding complications and the frequency of monitoring. The efficacy and safety of low-intensity warfarin therapy (target INR below 2.0 and above 1.5) has been evaluated in two trials of long-term treatment of patients with idiopathic VTE. In one of these studies, after at least 3 mo of standard-intensity warfarin therapy, patients were randomized in a double-blind fashion to receive low-intensity warfarin therapy (target INR, 1.5 to 1.9) or standard-intensity warfarin therapy (INR, 2.0 to 3.0) (35). During an average follow-up of 2.3 yr, recurrence rate of VTE was 1.9% per year among the 370 patients in the low-intensity group compared to 0.6% per year in the 369 patients of the standard-intensity group (hazard ratio, 3.3; 95% confidence interval [CI], 1.2 to 9.1). The incidence of major bleeding was similar in the two treatment groups. In the other study, patients with idiopathic VTE who had received full-dose anticoagulant therapy for a median of 6.5 mo were randomly assigned to placebo or low-intensity warfarin (target INR, 1.5 to 2.0) (8). The incidence of recurrent VTE was 7.2 and 2.6% per year in patients assigned to placebo and low-intensity warfarin, respectively (hazard ratio, 0.36; 95% CI, 0.19 to 0.67; $p < 0.001$). Risk reduction was similar in all subgroups, including those with and those without inherited thrombophilia. The incidence of bleeding complications also was similar in patients receiving standard-intensity and low-intensity warfarin therapy. Taken together, these results may be interpreted as indicating that although low-intensity warfarin therapy is more effective than placebo, it is less effective than standard-intensity therapy (INR, 2.0 to 3.0) and does not reduce the incidence of bleeding complications.

Patients persistently positive for antiphospholipid antibodies and a history of thromboembolism (venous or arterial) were randomized to standard-intensity warfarin therapy (INR, 2.0 to 3.0) or high-intensity warfarin therapy (INR, 3.1 to 4.0) for the prevention of recurrent thromboembolism (36). Recurrent thromboembolism occurred in 3.4% of patients receiving standard-intensity therapy compared with 10.7% of patients receiving high-intensity therapy (hazard ratio, 3.1; 95% CI, 0.6 to 15) during an average follow-up of 2.7 yr. Thus, high-intensity warfarin therapy did not provide additional antithrombotic protection. Furthermore, in a number of randomized trials, this regimen has been shown to be associated with a high risk (20%) of clinically important bleeding in patients with DVT.

BLEEDING COMPLICATIONS WITH VKAs

The risk of bleeding complications is one of the major limitations of long-term anticoagulant treatment. A meta-analysis of 33 prospective studies assessed the incidence of fatal bleeding during VKA therapy (target INR, 2.0 to 3.0) for treatment of VTE (37). Overall, 275 major bleeding events were observed. The overall case fatality was 13%. Case fatality was 46% for intracranial bleedings and 10% for major extracranial bleedings. This meta-analysis showed that the risk of bleeding in patients receiving oral anticoagulants is higher during the first 3 mo of treatment and then decreases, whereas the case fatality of bleeding events is constant and does not decrease with time.

A 3.0% incidence of major bleeding has been observed during the first month of outpatient warfarin therapy. The incidence decreased to 0.8% per month during the rest of the first year of therapy, and to 0.3% per month thereafter (38). Age over 75 is associated with a particularly high risk for bleeding (5.1% per year) compared to younger age (1% per year), and this is particularly the case for the risk of intracranial bleeding (39). The incidence of total bleeding and major bleeding in patients receiving oral anticoagulant treatment for VTE also has been shown to be consistently associated with the use of higher-intensity regimens (INR, 2.6 to 4.4) (40–42). The intensity of anticoagulation is probably the most important risk factor for intracranial hemorrhage, with the risk increasing dramatically at an INR of 4.0 to 5.0 (43–45). In a case–control study, the risk of intracerebral hemorrhage doubled for each increase of the INR by approx 1.0 (45). On the other hand, and as mentioned previously, a recent study showed that lower-intensity coumarin treatment (INR, 1.5 to 1.9) does not reduce the risk of bleeding complications compared to standard regimens (targeted INR, 2.0 to 3.0) (35). Finally, recent trials on the treatment of VTE (initial treatment with UFH or LMWH followed by oral anticoagulants) showed that the incidence of major bleeding complications was slightly higher in cancer patients than in the general population (2–9).

LMWH FOR LONG-TERM TREATMENT OF VTE

Recently, a randomized, controlled study in cancer patients showed that long-term administration of LMWH may be a better treatment option for this group of patients (46). In that study, patients were randomized to receive initial treatment with once-daily dalteparin (200 IU/kg), followed by either dalteparin or warfarin. The results of the study demonstrated a significant reduction in recurrence of VTE in patients who received dalteparin in comparison to those who received heparin and warfarin. Importantly, this benefit was obtained without an increase in the risk of bleeding.

Idraparinux, a long-half-life derivative of the synthetic pentasaccharide, fondaparinux, is currently under evaluation in two large clinical trials in patients with DVT and PE, respectively.

NOVEL ORAL ANTICOAGULANTS FOR TREATMENT OF VTE

An oral antithrombin agent, ximelagatran, has been evaluated in two phase III trials on treatment of VTE. The oral anti-Xa agent Bay 59-7939 is currently under evaluation in two phase II studies.

Ximelagatran is the prodrug of the active site-directed thrombin inhibitor, melagatran. After oral administration, ximelagatran is absorbed in the small intestine. Neither nutrition nor drugs seem to influence its absorption. After absorption, ximelagatran rapidly undergoes biotransformation to melagatran via intermediate metabolites *(47)*. The plasma half-life of ximelagatran is 3 to 4 h. Melagatran, the active agent, is eliminated via the kidneys *(47)*.

Ximelagatran does not need laboratory monitoring of coagulation. The drug has been evaluated for prophylaxis of VTE in high-risk orthopedic patients, for the treatment of VTE, for the prevention of cardioembolic events in patients with nonvalvular atrial fibrillation, and for the prevention of recurrent ischemia in patients who have recently experienced acute myocardial infarction.

The efficacy of monotherapy with ximelagatran in the treatment of VTE was first evaluated in a phase II, dose-ranging study. In this study, 350 patients with DVT were randomized to receive ximelagatran (dose ranging from 24 to 60 mg twice daily) or subcutaneous dalteparin followed by warfarin for 2 wk *(48)*. The primary end point was the rate of thrombus regression as assessed by venography. The incidence of thrombus regression plus improvement of clinical symptoms was similar in patients receiving ximelagatran and in those receiving dalteparin plus warfarin. There was a trend towards more thrombus progression with ximelagatran than with dalteparin, but this difference was not statistically significant. The bleeding rate was similar in the two treatment groups. In a further phase III study, ximelagatran (36 mg twice daily) was compared with enoxaparin (1 mg/kg subcutaneously twice daily) followed by warfarin (target INR 2.0 to 3.0); both treatment regimens were continued for 6 mo *(49)*. Overall, 2489 patients with VTE (approx 35% of them with PE) were included in the study. Recurrent VTE occurred in 2.1 and 2.0% and major bleeding in 1.3 and 2.2% of the patients randomized to ximelagatran or enoxaparin/warfarin, respectively. These differences were not statistically significant. All-cause mortality occurred in 2.3 and 3.4% of patients randomized to ximelagatran and enoxaparin/warfarin, respectively.

A second randomized trial evaluated the long-term efficacy and safety of treatment with fixed-dose oral ximelagatran initiated after 6 mo of standard anticoagulant therapy for VTE *(50)*. In this trial, 1233 patients who had completed 6 mo of anticoagulant therapy were randomized to receive ximelagatran (24 mg twice daily) or placebo for an additional 18 mo. Recurrent VTE occurred in 12 and 71 patients who had been randomized to ximelagatran or placebo, respectively (hazard ratio, 0.16; $p = 0.001$). Major bleeding occurred in six and five patients, respectively. No fatal or intracranial bleeding was observed.

Approximately 4 to 10% of patients randomized to receive long-term treatment with ximelagatran in clinical trials developed an increase in alanine aminotransferase levels. This event typically occurred after 6 wk to 4 mo of treatment and usually was asymptomatic and reversible. Although the increase in transaminase levels with ximelagatran therapy is benign in most cases, it is a reason for concern. Whether patients receiving long-term ximelagatran treatment will need to monitor liver enzymes levels during the initial period of therapy is unclear.

CONCLUSIONS

PE frequently recurs, especially within the first year, and continues to have a high risk of recurrence for at least 10 yr after the initial event. Patients with a first episode of PE are at risk for recurrent episodes of VTE, which often present (again) as PE. Currently available oral anticoagulants such as the VKAs are effective for the treatment of PE, and recurrence is a rare event while on anticoagulant treatment. Long-term treatment with LMWH is reserved for cancer patients with thromboembolic complications. However, the need for anticoagulation monitoring and dose adjustment, as well as the risk of bleeding complications, are major limitations of VKAs. Thus, new oral anticoagulants that are easier to use in clinical practice are currently under investigation. The efficacy and safety of these new drugs need further confirmation in randomized clinical trials.

REFERENCES

1. Buller HR, Agnelli G, Hull RD, et al. Antithrombotic therapy for venous thromboembolic disease. Chest 2004;126:401S–428S.
2. Agnelli G, Prandoni P, Becattini C, et al. Extended oral anticoagulant therapy after a first episode of pulmonary embolism. Ann Intern Med 2003;139:19–25.
3. Research Committee of the British Thoracic Society. Optimum duration of anticoagulation for deep-vein thrombosis and pulmonary embolism. Lancet 1992;340:873–876.
4. Schulman S, Rhedin AS, Lindmarker P, et al. A comparison of six weeks with six months of oral anticoagulant therapy after a first episode of venous thromboembolism. Duration of Anticoagulation Trial Study Group. N Engl J Med 1995;332:1661–1665.
5. Levine MN, Hirsh J, Gent M, et al. Optimal duration of oral anticoagulant therapy: a randomized trial comparing four weeks with three months of warfarin in patients with proximal deep vein thrombosis. Thromb Haemost 1995;74:606–611.
6. Kearon C, Gent M, Hirsh J, et al. A comparison of three months of anticoagulation with extended anticoagulation for a first episode of idiopathic venous thromboembolism. N Engl J Med 1999;340:901–907.
7. Agnelli G, Prandoni P, Santamaria MG, et al. Three months versus one year of oral anticoagulant therapy for idiopathic deep venous thrombosis. N Engl J Med 2001;345:165–169.
8. Ridker PM, Goldhaber SZ, Danielson E, et al. Long-term, low-intensity warfarin therapy for the prevention of recurrent venous thromboembolism. N Engl J Med 2003;348:1425–1434.
9. Pinede L, Ninet J, Duhaut P, et al. Comparison of 3 and 6 months of oral anticoagulant therapy after a first episode of proximal deep vein thrombosis or pulmonary embolism and comparison of 6 and 12 weeks of therapy after isolated calf deep vein thrombosis. Circulation 2001;103:2453–2460.
10. Carson JL, Kelley MA, Duff A, et al. The clinical course of pulmonary embolism. N Engl J Med 1992;326:1240–1245.
11. Becattini C, Agnelli G, Prandoni P, et al. A prospective study on cardiovascular events after acute pulmonary embolism. Eur Heart J 2005;26:77–83.
12. Eichinger S, Weltermann A, Minar E, et al. Symptomatic pulmonary embolism and the risk of recurrent venous thromboembolism. Arch Intern Med 2004;164:92–96.
13. Meneveau N, Ming LP, Seronde MF, et al. In-hospital and long-term outcome after sub-massive and massive pulmonary embolism submitted to thrombolytic therapy. Eur Heart J 2003;24:1447–1454.
14. Beyth RJ, Cohen AM, Landefeld S. Long-term outcomes of deep-vein thrombosis. Arch Intern Med 1995;155:1031–1037.
15. Lindner DJ, Edwards JM, Phinney ES, et al. Longterm hemodynamic and clinical sequelae of lower extremity deep vein thrombosis. J Vasc Surg 1986;4:436–442.
16. Prandoni P, Lensing AW, Cogo A, et al. The long-term clinical course of acute deep venous thrombosis. Ann Intern Med 1996;125:1–7.
17. Heit JA, Silverstein MD, Mohr DN, et al. Predictors of survival after deep vein thrombosis and pulmonary embolism: a population-based, cohort study. Arch Intern Med 1999;159:445–453.
18. Hull R, Delmore T, Genton E, et al. Warfarin sodium versus low-dose heparin in the long-term treatment of venous thrombosis. N Engl J Med 1979;301:855–858.
19. Brandjes DP, Heijboer H, Büller H, et al. Acenocoumarol and heparin compared with acenocoumarol alone in the initial treatment of proximal vein thrombosis. N Engl J Med 1992;327:1485–1489.
20. Hirsh J. Duration of anticoagulant therapy after first episode of venous thrombosis in patients with inherited thrombophilia. Arch Intern Med 1997;157:2174–2177.
21. Douketis JD, Kearon C, Bates S, et al. Risk of fatal pulmonary embolism in patients with treated venous thromboembolism. JAMA 1998; 279:458–462.

22. Murin S, Romano PS, White RH. Comparison of outcomes after hospitalization for deep venous thrombosis or pulmonary embolism. Thromb Haemost 2002;88:407–414.
23. van Den Belt AG, Sanson BJ, Simioni P, et al. Recurrence of venous thromboembolism in patients with familial thrombophilia. Arch Intern Med 1997;157:2227–2232.
24. Simioni P, Prandoni P, Lensing AW, et al. The risk of recurrent venous thromboembolism in patients with an Arg506→Gln mutation in the gene for factor V (factor V Leiden). N Engl J Med 1997;336:399–403.
25. De Stefano V, Martinelli I, Mannucci PM, et al. The risk of recurrent deep venous thrombosis among heterozygous carriers of both factor V Leiden and the G20210A prothrombin mutation. N Engl J Med 1999;341:801–806.
26. Kyrle PA, Minar E, Hirschl M, et al. High plasma levels of factor VIII and the risk of recurrent venous thromboembolism. N Engl J Med 2000;343:457–462.
27. Schulman S, Svenungsson E, Granqvist S. Anticardiolipin antibodies predict early recurrence of thromboembolism and death among patients with venous thromboembolism following anticoagulant therapy. Duration of Anticoagulation Study Group. Am J Med 1998;104:332–338.
28. Khamashta MA, Cuadrado MJ, Mujic F, et al. The management of thrombosis in the antiphospholipid-antibody syndrome. N Engl J Med 1995;332:993–997.
29. Palareti G, Legnani C, Cosmi B, et al. Risk of venous thromboembolic recurrence: high negative predictive value of D-dimer performed after oral anticoagulation is stopped. Thromb Haemost 2002;87:7–12.
30. Prandoni P, Lensing AW, Prins MH, et al. Residual venous thrombosis as a predictive factor of recurrent venous thromboembolism. Ann Intern Med 2002;137:955–960.
31. Friedman PA, Rosenberg RD, Hauschka PV, et al. A spectrum of partially carboxylated prothrombins in the plasmas of coumarin treated patients. Biochim Biophys Acta 1977;494:271–276.
32. Malhotra OP, Nesheim ME, Mann KG. The kinetics of activation of normal and gamma carboxy glutamic acid deficient prothrombins. J Biol Chem 1985;260:279–287.
33. Breckenridge AM. Oral anticoagulant drugs: pharmacokinetic aspects. Semin Hematol 1978;15:19–26.
34. Hull R, Hirsh J, Jay R, et al. Different intensities of oral anticoagulant therapy in the treatment of proximal-vein thrombosis. N Engl J Med 1982;307:1676–1681.
35. Kearon C, Ginsberg JS, Kovacs MJ, et al. Comparison of low-intensity warfarin therapy with conventional-intensity warfarin therapy for long-term prevention of recurrent venous thromboembolism. N Engl J Med 2003;349:631–639.
36. Crowther MA, Ginsberg JS, Julian J, et al. A comparison of two intensities of warfarin for the prevention of recurrent thrombosis in patients with the antiphospholipid antibody syndrome. N Engl J Med 2003;349:1133–1138.
37. Linkins L, Choi PT, Douketis JD. Clinical impact of bleeding in patients taking oral anticoagulant therapy for with venous thromboembolism: a meta-analysis. Ann Intern Med 2003;139:893–900.
38. Landefeld S, Goldman L. Major bleeding in outpatients treated with warfarin: incidence and prediction by factors known at the start of outpatient therapy. Am J Med 1989;87:144–152.
39. Altman R, Rouvier J, Gurfinkel E, et al. Comparison of two levels of anticoagulant therapy in patients with substitute heart valves. J Thorac Cardiovasc Surg 1991;101:427–431.
40. Hull R, Hirsh J, Jay R, et al. Different intensities of oral anticoagulant therapy in the treatment of proximal-vein thrombosis. N Engl J Med 1982;307:1671–1681.
41. Turpie AGG, Gunstensen J, Hirsh J, et al. Randomized comparison of two intensities of oral anticoagulant therapy after tissue heart valve replacement. Lancet 1988;1:1242–1245.
42. Saour JN, Sieck JO, Mamo LAR, et al. Trial of different intensities of anticoagulation in patients with prosthetic heart valves. N Engl J Med 1990;322:428–432.
43. Cannegieter SC, Rosendaal FR, Wintzen AR, et al. Optimal oral anticoagulant therapy in patients with mechanical heart valves. N Engl J Med 1995;333:11–17.
44. Hylek EM, Singer DE. Risk factors for intracranial hemorrhage in outpatients taking warfarin. Ann Intern Med 1994;120:897–902.
45. Algra A, Franke CL, Koehler PJJ, et al. A randomized trial of anticoagulants versus aspirin after cerebral ischemia of presumed arterial origin. Ann Neurol 1997;42:857–865.
46. Lee AYY, Levine MN, Baker RI, et al. Low-molecular weight heparin versus a coumarin for the prevention of recurrent venous thromboembolism in patients with cancer. N Engl J Med 2003;349:146–153.
47. Gustafsson D, Nystrom JE, Carlsson S, et al. The direct thrombin inhibitor melagatran and its oral prodrug H 376/95: intestinal absorption properties, biochemical and pharmacodynamic effects. Thromb Res 2001;101:171–181.

48. Eriksson H, Wahlander K, Gustafsson D, et al. A randomized, controlled, dose-guiding study of the oral direct thrombin inhibitor ximelagatran compared with standard therapy for the treatment of acute deep vein thrombosis: THRIVE I. J Thromb Haemost 2003;1:41–47.

49. Fiessinger JN, Huisman MV, Davidson BL; the THRIVE Investigators. Ximelagatran vs low-molecular-weight heparin and warfarin for the treatment of deep vein thrombosis a randomized trial. JAMA 2005;293:681–689.

50. Schulman S, Wahlander K, Lundstrom T, et al. Secondary prevention of venous thromboembolism with the oral direct thrombin inhibitor ximelagatran. N Engl J Med 2003;349:1713–1721.

III SPECIFIC ASPECTS

15 Hereditary and Acquired Thrombophilia

Hanno Riess, MD

Contents

Summary

Acquired and hereditary disorders predisposing to venous thromboembolism (VTE) may coexist in an individual and result in latent or overt thrombophilia. Hereditary risk factors are detectable in approx 50% of patients with VTE events and a positive family history. Deficiencies of antithrombin, protein C, and its cofactor protein S, were the first disorders found to increase the risk of recurrent thrombotic events among carriers. Among Caucasians, resistance against activated protein C caused by factor V Leiden (factor V R506Q), and the mutation in the prothrombin promoter region (G20210A), are the most common hereditary prothrombotic defects, with a prevalence of 3 to 5% in the general population. In addition, several other rare defects have been reported. In heterozygous carriers, these disorders increase the risk of suffering a thromboembolic event between 2- and 10-fold. The risk is clearly higher in homozygous individuals, and in those with combined defects. To result in acute VTE, however, inherited deficiencies of hemostasis usually have to interact with acquired transient or permanent risk factors, such as perioperative bedrest, intake of oral contraceptives, or malignancy. Laboratory methods for the diagnosis of the most relevant hereditary defects, and for some acquired thrombophilic disorders such as the antiphospholipid syndrome, have been established and are available at present. Preliminary studies suggest that the laboratory detection of thrombophilic risk factors may not only help explain the cause of VTE in an individual but also affect the management strategy for these patients. This is particularly true for the recommended duration of secondary prophylaxis with vitamin K antagonists after a first thromboembolic event, which needs to take into account the overall risk of recurrence vs that of anticoagulation-related hemorrhage.

From: *Contemporary Cardiology: Management of Acute Pulmonary Embolism*
Edited by: S. Konstantinides © Humana Press Inc., Totowa, NJ

Key Words: Thrombophilia; venous thromboembolism; laboratory diagnosis; anti-coagulation therapy.

INTRODUCTION

Thrombophilia is generally defined as an increased risk for developing thrombosis that may be caused by hereditary or acquired disorders (Tables 1 and 2). It may affect the arterial side, the venous side, or both, but the term thrombophilia is commonly (and in this chapter) used in association with *venous* thromboembolism (VTE). Accordingly, acquired risk factors for thrombophilia include diseases, conditions, or laboratory abnormalities that predispose to the development of venous thrombosis and pulmonary embolism (PE). On the other hand, inherited thrombophilia is a genetically fixed tendency to develop VTE, usually characterized by (recurrent) thromboembolic episodes within several members of a given family.

When considering the issue of thrombophilia, it needs to be mentioned that the risk of developing recurrent thromboembolism is usually determined by an interaction of both permanent and temporary risk factors. To make the issue even more complicated, both prothrombotic and prohemorrhagic, hereditary and acquired risk factors may exist in an individual or kindred. These factors interact with each other and define the overall balance of hemostasis.

Anticoagulants are highly effective for primary prevention of PE in high-risk situations (e.g., perioperatively), for treatment in the acute phase of thromboembolic events (to prevent further thrombus extension or embolization), and for secondary long-term prevention. An increase in the intensity of anticoagulation does decrease the risk of recurrent thromboembolism (*see* Chapter 14) but may cause minor, severe, or even life-threatening bleeding *(1–3)*. A treatment plan must therefore not only consider the underlying provoking condition and the possible existence of a thrombophilic disorder, but also take into account the treatment-associated bleeding risk, which may vary widely depending on the predisposition and the clinical condition of the individual patient.

HEREDITARY THROMBOPHILIA

The main causes of hereditary thrombophilia *(4–9)* may be classified into: (1) loss of function of inhibitors of hemostasis; and (2) gain of function of procoagulants. In addition, very rare hereditary defects resulting in disturbance of the fibrinolytic system or in enhanced platelet aggregation have been described. Hereditary risk factors are detectable in a relative high percentage (40 to 60%) of patients with VTE events and a positive family history. Typical clinical features include a first thromboembolic event at an early age (<50 yr) and positive family history of thrombosis or recurrent thromboembolism.

Deficiencies of Specific Coagulation Inhibitors

DEFICIENCY OF ANTITHROMBIN, PROTEIN C, AND ITS COFACTOR, PROTEIN S

These were the first hereditary disorders found to increase the risk of recurrent thrombotic events among carriers as opposed to noncarriers *(5,7,10,11)*. Overall, these deficiencies are rare, being found in less than 1% of the population (Table 1), and a very small proportion of patients with VTE carry one of these defects. Thus, most of the data currently available in the literature have been obtained in family studies. These findings must be interpreted with caution, however, because thrombophilic patients may harbor more

Table 1
Hereditary Risk Factors for VTE

Deficiency	Prevalence (among Caucasians)	Incidence (in patients with positive family history)	Relative risk
Antithrombin <0.1%	<5%[a]	8–12	
Protein C	<0.5%[a]	<5%	5–10
Protein S	<0.5%[a]	<5%	2–8
Factor V Leiden (G1691A)	approx 5%[a]	<50%	2–8
Factor V Leiden (G1691A)	<0.02%[b]	<2%	30–80
Prothrombin (G20210A)	<3%[a]	<20%	2–5
Prothrombin (G20210A)	<0.01%[b]	<1%	10–20
MTHFR[c] (C677T)	<5%[b]	<20%	1.5–3

[a]Heterozygous mutation.
[b]Homozygous mutation.
[c]Methylene tetrahydrofolate reductase (resulting in hyperhomocysteinemia).

Table 2
Acquired Risk Factors for VTE

Acquired factors	Acquired and/or hereditary factors
Age	Hyperhomocysteinemia
Antiphospholipid syndrome	High level of factor VIII
Essential thrombocytosis	High level of factor IX
Hormonal contraceptives	High level of factor XI
Hospitalization	High level of TAFI
Immobilization	
Malignancy	
Paroxysmal nocturnal hemoglobinuria	
Polycythaemia vera	
Puerperium	
Postmenopausal hormonal replacement therapy	
Pregnancy	
Previous thrombosis	
Surgery	

TAFI, thrombin-activatable fibrinolysis inhibitor.

than one defect, including unknown defects. These "confounding" factors may, at least in some studies, have resulted in an increased risk among members of a given thrombophilic family who did not carry the specific defect under investigation (11,12). Therefore, it remains questionable whether the risk estimates derived from these studies can be extrapolated to other individuals with the same abnormalities.

Overall, deficiencies of the previously mentioned coagulation inhibitors appear to increase the risk of VTE approx 10-fold in heterozygotes. It is believed that antithrombin deficiency, especially type I, carries a higher risk than protein C or protein S deficiencies (5,11). On the other hand, homozygous deficiency of natural anticoagulants is extremely rare and results in a marked thrombotic tendency (presenting, among others, as purpura fulminans) that occurs shortly after birth or may already become lethal during fetal development (11).

Activated Protein C (APC) Resistance—Factor V Leiden

Among Caucasians, APC resistance caused by factor V Leiden (factor V R506Q) is the most common hereditary prothrombotic defect, with an overall prevalence of approx 5% in the population *(13–16)*. However, because of other confounding factors, the population-based prevalence varies widely between different regions. In general, this mutation is found in up to 20% of unselected patients with VTE, and in up to 50% of those with the first event before the age of 50 and a positive family history. Factor V Leiden is the result of a mutation in one of the cleavage sites in factor V, where APC inactivates factor Va. As a result, it produces a phenotype of resistance to APC (thus termed APC resistance). Heterozygous Factor V Leiden mutation is a rather weak thrombophilic disorder, believed to increase the risk of VTE only three- to fivefold. In homozygous carriers, representing approx 1 individual per 5000 population, the risk is reported to increase 50- to 80-fold.

G20210A-Prothrombin Mutation

This mutation in the prothrombin promoter region is found in approx 3% of Caucasians with wide regional variations *(17,18)*. Among patients with VTE, the mutation has a prevalence of approx 6%. The defect is reported to increase the risk of thrombosis approx three-fold because of elevated prothrombin levels. Thus, the mutation results in a rather weak prothrombotic disorder.

Other Hereditary Thrombophilic Factors

Hyperhomocysteinemia results in an increased risk of VTE. A variation in the gene for methylene-tetrahydro-folate reductase (MTHFR 677C), which plays a role in homocysteine metabolism, is an established weak thrombophilic risk factor, at least in homozygote carriers *(19,20)*. More often, however, hyperhomocysteinemia is an acquired disorder, usually resulting from low intake of folate or vitamins B6 or B12.

As compared to blood group 0, carriers of the blood groups A, B, or AB do have a two- to fourfold increased risk of VTE, most likely associated with higher von Willebrand factor and factor VIII levels.

Elevated levels of prothrombin (*see* previous section), factor VIII, factor IX, or factor XI, as well as of the thrombin-activatable fibrinolysis inhibitor (TAFI), all are associated with a slightly increased risk of VTE. Little is known about the reason for the (constantly) elevated levels of these factors in some individuals, but familial clustering has been reported, suggesting, at least in part, genetic causes. Finally, elevated levels of lipoprotein (a), a recognized risk factor for cardiovascular disease, have been shown to be an independent risk factor for VTE as well.

A number of further hereditary disorders including polymorphisms in coagulation-related factors and inhibitors may also increase the risk of VTE, but their exact role is currently under discussion.

ACQUIRED RISK FACTORS

Numerous acquired risk factors predispose to VTE *(4,20,21)* (Table 2). These may either be permanent or transient in nature. Despite the availability of effective anticoagulant prophylaxis, acquired risk factors are still responsible for a large number of thrombotic events. Some of these factors are briefly reviewed here.

There is an increased risk of VTE with *increasing age*, resulting in a 1000-fold difference in risk between the very young and the very old. Therefore estimation of the thromboembolic risk of an individual always needs to be adjusted for this person's age.

The presence of *cancer* is one of the most important factors associated with VTE *(22, 23)* (*see* Chapter 16). There is a complex relation between cancer and hemostasis, which may further be aggravated by anticancer therapies. In this context, it is important to realize that, among unselected patients with a first episode of VTE, approx 10 to 20% present with known preexisting malignancy, 5 to 10% have undiagnosed but readily detectable malignancy, and in another 5 to 10% of the patients, more intensive screening procedures may be necessary to detect an underlying, early-stage, (hopefully) curable malignancy.

Without thromboprophylaxis, *surgery* leads to thrombosis in a high percentage of patients depending on the extent and the site of the operation *(24)*. For example, in orthopedic surgery of the hip or the knee, the risk of thrombosis without thromboprophylaxis reaches 50–70%. Major *nonsurgical trauma* is also an important risk factor for VTE. Taken together, surgery and trauma are still associated with a high risk of thrombosis despite the routine use of anticoagulant prophylaxis, resulting in an overall 10–20% risk of VTE episodes confirmed by imaging procedures. This number translates into an approx 5% risk of clinically overt VTE and/or PE. Besides surgery and trauma, other situations associated with prolonged *immobilization* such as bedrest, plaster clasts, paralysis (e.g., stroke), and prolonged travel (*see* Chapter 18) increase the risk of VTE.

Oral contraceptives and hormonal replacement therapy (25). Most oral contraceptives contain an estrogen and progesterone. Shortly after the introduction of these drugs, it became apparent that they may increase the risk of thrombosis as much as fourfold. Until now, there is no convincing evidence that modifying the content or kind of hormones abolishes this risk. Hormone replacement therapy using oral, transdermal, or subcutaneous applications also is associated with a two- to fourfold increased risk of VTE.

Pregnancy and puerperium (26). Pregnancy (*see* Chapter 17) increases the risk of VTE about 10-fold compared to age-matched nonpregnant women. This means that approx 0.05% of women will develop VTE during pregnancy. The risk may even be higher during the first 6 to 8 wk after delivery.

Lupus anticoagulant—antiphospholipid antibodies. The so-called antiphospholipid syndrome is clinically characterized by recurrent venous and arterial thromboembolism and fetal loss *(27,28)*. Antiphospholipid antibodies and/or lupus anticoagulant are detectable in the circulation. Approximately one-half of the patients with this syndrome have concomitant or underlying diseases such as autoimmune disorders (e.g., lupus erythematosus), malignancies (especially lymphatic neoplasias) or infections (e.g., HIV). The clinical presentation and the risk of thrombosis vary widely in patients with the antiphospholipid syndrome, but, overall, the risk of VTE is increased approx 10-fold, with a high percentage of patients suffering recurrence after the end of anticoagulation.

INTERACTIONS OF THROMBOPHILIC DISORDERS

Many of the risk factors for VTE mentioned previously are frequently present in the general population, at least temporarily. Therefore, the coexistence of genetic and/or acquired risk factors in the same individual is likely in several cases of VTE. It is indeed possible that, for the development of clinically overt VTE, the combination and interactions of several thrombophilic factors may be required. In fact, the risk of patients with two coexisting

Table 3
Interactions of Hereditary Risk Factors for VTE
(Estimated Relative Risk)

Deficiencies (heterozygous)	Relative risk
Factor V Leiden	5
Prothrombin mutation	3
Protein C deficiency	10
Factor V Leiden + prothrombin mutation	30
Protein C + factor V Leiden	50

Data from refs. *29–40.*

Table 4
Interaction of Acquired and Hereditary Risk Factors for VTE
(Estimated Relative Risk)

Hereditary heterozygous deficiency	Oral contraceptives	Pregnancy
None	4	6
Factor V Leiden (1691A)	34	60
Prothrombin mutation (G20210A)	27	40
Factor V Leiden + prothrombin mutation	240	400

Data from refs. *25,26,29,41–45,61,62.*

hereditary risk factors is supra-additively elevated (Table 3), and the same has been demonstrated for the interaction of hereditary and acquired risk factors (Table 4). The existence and importance of such supra-additive interactions needs to be considered when advising and treating individual patients.

LABORATORY TESTS FOR THE DETECTION OF THROMBOPHILIA

The search for thrombophilia remains a controversial issue in clinical practice *(4,6,8, 9,46–48).* In particular, there is ongoing discussion about the value of routinely screening patients with VTE and their family members for thrombophilia. Thus, at present, no general recommendations can be given, and decisions should be met on an individual basis.

First of all, the clinical situation and the family history should be considered. An underlying hereditary thrombophilia is much more likely in younger patients, in patients with an unprovoked, idiopathic, or recurrent thrombotic event, and in those with a positive family history. If the clinical evaluation of the patient favors screening, testing should be comprehensive and include all clinically relevant parameters in order to help clinicians make an "optimal" therapeutic decision.

Testing of the phenotype can be performed using an initial blood sample taken before starting anticoagulation therapy. To avoid misleading results due to the acute thrombotic process itself or the effects of anticoagulant therapy, some investigators recommend testing at least 6 mo after the acute thrombotic event and, specifically for protein C and protein S, at least 2 wk after oral anticoagulation is discontinued. Personally, I do prefer taking the blood sample for thrombophilia testing *before* oral anticoagulation is initiated in order to include the screening result in the initial management of the patient (discussed later).

After all, genetic defects are not expected to be influenced by an acute ongoing thrombotic process or anticoagulation. A "normal" phenotype (within the reference range) with regard to natural coagulation inhibitors definitely rules out deficiencies in patients with acute thromboembolism. If, on the other hand, phenotype testing yields an abnormal result, confirmation using another blood sample taken several weeks apart (also considering interfering conditions, such as acute phase reaction for factor VIII elevation or low protein S levels, or vitamin K deficiency for low protein C or S levels) is required. Especially with regard to decreased protein S activity or elevated levels of coagulation factors such as factor VIII, it is a challenging task to rule out reactive changes, such as those that occur, for example, in patients with chronic inflammatory diseases.

MANAGEMENT OF VTE IN THROMBOPHILIA

The presence of a known inherited or acquired thrombophilic disorder may alter the recommendations given to an individual with regard to prophylactic use of anticoagulants, the type and intensity of therapy of acute VTE, and the duration of secondary prophylaxis after a venous thrombotic event.

Prevention of VTE

The in-hospital use of anticoagulant drugs to prevent VTE is based on the fact that most hospitalized patients have one or more thrombophilic risk factors. In this setting, it is widely accepted that patients can be classified into different risk categories, but it is, of course, not possible to predict which individual will develop a thromboembolic event in a given situation. Focusing on early detection of symptoms or signs of (beginning) thrombosis is definitely an unreliable strategy to prevent clinically important thromboembolic events. Massive (fulminant) PE often occurs without warning, and the chances of successfully resuscitating such patients are usually very low (*see* Chapter 11). In approx three-quarters of patients who die of PE in the hospital, this diagnosis has not even been considered prior to death. Thus, as routine screening of patients for asymptomatic thrombosis is difficult and probably also not cost-effective, routine thromboprophylaxis remains the appropriate strategy to reduce the risk of overt thromboembolism.

Based on prospective data, a classification system has been developed categorizing patients into three to four risk levels with regard to the likelihood of developing VTE. This has successfully been implemented in everyday care, especially in surgical patients, and also is increasingly being used in medical patients. Patients with underlying thrombophilia due to recognized hereditary or acquired risk factors such as antithrombin deficiency, antiphospholipid antibodies, malignancy, or prior VTE are categorized as the group at highest risk. In these patients, prolonged prophylaxis is recommended following established regimens, such as those recommended by the American College of Chest Physicians guidelines *(48)*. For example, thromboembolism can be effectively prevented using fondaparinux, some preparations of low-molecular-weight heparin (LMWH), or combinations of mechanical methods of thromboprophylaxis together with anticoagulant drugs *(48)*.

Therapy of Acute VTE Disease

The presence of a known inherited or acquired thrombophilic risk factor will not alter the intensity of anticoagulant therapy in the acute phase, except if treatment with heparins or fondaparinux is met with heparin resistance in the presence of antithrombin deficiency

(50). In this latter case, an increased dose of the anticoagulant agent may be required to obtain therapeutic anticoagulation levels. When unfractionated heparin is used, laboratory monitoring of the activated partial thromboblastin time is, as in all other patients, mandatory for dose adjustment (*see* Chapter 9). However, if antithrombin deficiency is known, it may be preferable to control the intensity of heparin anticoagulation based on anti Xa-activity, as is occasionally done in patients treated with LMWHs or fondaparinux. Substitution therapy with antithrombin concentrates is rarely necessary *(50,51)*, but may be indicated during peripartum in women with VTE.

Heparin-induced thrombocytopenia (HIT) is a rare but clinically important complication of heparin treatment resulting in an additional thrombogenic stimulus. This syndrome is attributed to activation of the platelets and the endothelium by heparin-induced antibodies directed against complexes of platelet factor 4 and heparin, resulting in enhanced thrombin generation. In historical controls, the onset of thrombocytopenia was followed by acute (recurrent) VTE in 25–50% of affected patients even after heparin was discontinued. HIT is less likely to complicate LMWH therapy and has not been reported for fondaparinux. Anticoagulant therapy in patients with HIT, or history thereof, should be based on noncrossreacting alternatives to heparin such as lepirudin (recombinant hirudin), danaparoid (a mixture of heparan sulfate, dermatan sulfate, and chondroitin sulfate), and argatroban (a small molecular size thrombin inhibitor) *(63)*. These drugs are used to treat patients with acute or subacute HIT. In patients with a previous history of HIT, these drugs, and possibly fondaparinux as well, are effective and safe for prevention of thromboembolism. Of note, the previously mentioned drugs vary with regard to the anticoagulant mechanism, biological half-life, and route of elimination. Therefore, drug-specific recommendations must be followed.

Deficiency in protein C or protein S is associated with an increased risk of developing skin necrosis during the early days of treatment with vitamin K antagonists (VKAs; also termed *warfarin-induced skin necrosis*) *(52)*. Taking the standard precaution of a several day overlap with the heparin anticoagulant may reduce this complication, which also can be minimized by avoiding high loading doses of VKAs. Moreover, and importantly, VKAs should not be started during the acute or subacute phase of HIT, i.e., not until the platelet count has returned to normal. Otherwise, VKAs may contribute to venous limb gangrene.

Duration of Anticoagulation in Patients With Thrombophilia

VTE can be considered a chronic disorder, as the cumulative risk of recurrence during long-term follow-up after a first episode of VTE reaches more than 20% after 5 yr and is higher in patients with thrombophilia *(53–58)*. Recurrence rates after acute VTE are determined by the initial "trigger" (idiopathic/permanent vs transient), an ongoing predisposition to thrombosis (e.g., known hereditary thrombophilia, active malignancy), the extent and location of the event (PE, proximal vs distal vein thrombosis), and a history of previous thromboembolism. Recurrence is effectively suppressed by prolonged oral anticoagulant therapy with a target international normalized ratio (INR) of 2.0–3.0, resulting in less than 1% of patients experiencing recurrences per year (*see* Chapter 14).

Detection of congenital thrombophilia or the chronic presence of acquired thrombophilic risk factors implies that prolonged duration of secondary prophylaxis will be needed. On the other hand, prolonged oral anticoagulation is limited by the cumulative anticoagulation-related risk of hemorrhage. It is estimated that 1–2% of patients suffer severe bleeding episodes per year of treatment, including the complications with a lethal outcome (<0.8% per year). Factors increasing the risk of hemorrhage include age greater than 65 yr, previous stroke or gastrointestinal bleeding, comorbidities such as previous myocardial infarction, diabetes mellitus, anemia, or decreased renal function, and intake of antiplatelet drugs. Reducing the intensity of oral anticoagulant therapy to an INR of 1.5 to 2.0 appears to decrease the efficacy of secondary prevention without clearly reducing the risk of hemorrhage (64), and, therefore, prolonged reduced-intensity anticoagulation cannot be recommended at present. Furthermore, wide fluctuations of the INR below and above the therapeutic range decrease efficacy and increase the risk of oral anticoagulation, respectively.

When deciding on the optimal duration of anticoagulation, it needs be considered that patients who have suffered PE are more likely to present again with PE recurrence than with (recurrent) symptomatic deep venous thrombosis, and they may thus be at higher risk of death when compared to patients with recurrence of leg vein thrombosis "alone" (59). Therefore, the optimal duration of anticoagulation needs to be individualized. In general, however, the higher the thrombosis risk and the lower the bleeding risk, the longer the optimal treatment duration. Accordingly, patients with deficiency of natural coagulant inhibitors (particularly antithrombin deficiency, followed in severity by protein C and protein S deficiency), those with homozygote factor V Leiden or prothrombin mutation, and double heterozygotes for factor V Leiden and the prothrombin mutation, are considered to be candidates for long-term anticoagulation when the bleeding risk is not elevated (65). The same is true for patients with antiphospholipid antibodies or lupus anticoagulant after a first episode of thromboembolism (60,65).

Following identification of an acquired "reversible" condition provoking the development of VTE, the patient should be instructed to avoid further predisposing factors (e.g., use of oral contraceptives) and to start anticoagulant prophylaxis in high-risk situations (Table 2). This may also be the case for patients with congenital thrombophilia. Finally, VTE complicated by active malignancy or the antiphospholipid syndrome needs special consideration (22,23,27,28) (Chapter 16). For example, recent clinical trials demonstrated that prolonged use of LMWHs may have a better risk/benefit ratio than use of VKAs in patients with cancer (61,65), and this is possibly also the case for patients with the antiphospholipid syndrome.

CONCLUSION

Appropriate testing for an inherited or acquired predisposition to VTE has clinical utility. Results may help not only explain the onset of thrombosis and select patients for prolonged anticoagulant therapy, but also provide optimal thromboprophylaxis in relatives affected by inborn thrombophilia. On the other hand, overestimation of the utility of thrombophilia testing and inappropriate counseling about the risks and remedies may confuse patients and have unintended consequences. Today, there are still only few answers and many unanswered questions in this rapidly developing field of research and clinical practice.

REFERENCES

1. Ridker PM, Goldhaber SZ, Danielson E, et al. Long-term, low-intensity Warfarin for the prevention of recurrent venous thromboembolism. N Engl J Med 2003;348:1425–1434.
2. Van den Belt AG, Hutten BA, Prins MH, Bossuyt PMM. Duration of oral anticoagulant treatment in patients with venous thromboembolism and a deficiency of antithrombin, protein C or protein S—a decision analysis. Thromb Haemost 2000;84:758–763.

3. Hutten BA, Prins MH, Gent M, et al. The incidence of recurrent thromboembolic and bleeding complications among patients with venous thromboembolism in relation to both malignancy and achieved INR. A retrospective analysis. J Clin Oncol 2000;18:3078–3083.

4. Bauer KA. The thrombophilias: well-defined factors with uncertain therapeutic implications. Ann Intern Med 2001;135:367–373.

5. De Stefano V, Leone G, Mastrangelo S, et al. Clinical manifestations and management of inherited thrombophilia: retrospective analysis and follw-up after diagnosis of 238 patients with congenital deficiency of antithrombin II, proten C, and protein S. Thromb Haemost 1994;72:352–358.

6. Greaves M, Baglin T. Laboratory testing for heritable thormbophilia: impact on clinical management of thrombotic disease. Br J Haematol 2000;109:699–703.

7. Heijboer H, Brandjes DPM, Büller HR, et al. Deficiencies of coagulation-inhibiting and fibrinolytic proteins in outpatients with deep venous thrombosis. N Engl J Med 1990;323:1512–1516.

8. Loew A, Völler H, Riess H. Thrombophilia—Diagnostic steps and therapeutic consequences after deep vein thrombosis. Dtsch Med Wochenschr 2002;127:273–278.

9. Walker ID, Geaves M, Preston FE. Investigation and management of heritable thrombophilia. Br J Haematol 2001;1145:512–528.

10. Finazzi G, Caccia R, Barbui T. Different prevalence of thromboembolism in the subtypes of congenital antithrombin III deficiency: review of 404 cases. Thromb Haemost 1987;58:1094.

11. Sanson BJ, Simioni P, Tormene D, et al. The incidence of venous thromboembolism in asymptomatic carriers of a deficiency of antithrombin, protein C, or protein S: a prospective cohort study. Blood 1999; 94:3702–3706.

12. Langlois NJ, Wells PS. Risk of venous thromboembolism in realatives of symptomatic probands with thrombophilia: a systematic review. Thromb Haemost 2003;90:17–26.

13. Dahlbäck B, Carlosson M, Svensson PJ. Familial thrombophilia due to a previously unrecognised mechanism characterized by poor anticoagulant response to activated protein C: prediction of a cofactor to activated protein C. Proc Natl Acad Sci USA 1993;9:1004–1008.

14. De Vissser MCH, Rosendaal FR, Bertina RM. A reduced sensitivity for activated protein C in the absence of factor V Leiden increased the risk of venous thrombosis. Blood 1997;93:1271–1276.

15. Hille ET, Westendorp RG, Vandenbroucke JP, Rosendaal FR. Mortality and causes of death in families with the factor V Leiden mutation (resistance to activated protein C). Blodd 1997;89:1963–1967.

16. Loew A, Jacob D, Neuhaus P, Riess H. Resistance to activated protein C caused by factor V Leiden mutation and orthotopic liver transplantation. Transplantation 2005;79:1422–1427.

17. Nguyen A. Prothrombin G20210A polymorphism and thrombophilia. Mayo Clin Proc 2000;75:595–504.

18. Poort SR, Rosendaal FR, Reitsma PH, Bertina RM. A common genetic variation of the 3'-untranslated region of the porthrombin levels and increase in venous thrombosis. Blood 1996;88:3698–3703.

19. Cattaneo M. Hyperhomocysteinemia, atherosclerosis and thrombosis. Thromb Haemost 1999;81:165–176.

20. Van Cott EM, Laposata M, Prins MH. Laboratory evaluation of hypercoagulability with venous or arterial thrombosis: venous thromboembolism, myocardial infarction, stroke, and other conditions. Arch Pathol Lab Med 2002;126:1281–1295.

21. Riess H. Acquired blood coagulation disorders. Haemostaseologie 2004;27:506–511.

22. Falang A. Thrombosis and malignancy: an underestimated problem. Haematologica 2003;88:607–610.

23. Prandoni P, Falanga A, Piccioli A. Cancer and venous thromboembolism. Lancet Oncol 2005;6:401–410.

24. Wu O, Clark P, Lowe GDO, et al. Thrombophilia and venous thromboembolsim after total hip or knee rerplacement surgerey: a stematic review. Int Soc Thromb Heamost 2005;3:811–813.

25. Martinelli I, Taioli E, Bucciarelli P, et al. Interaction between the G2010A mutation of the prothrombin gene and oral contraceptive use in deep vein thrombosis. Arterioscler Thormb Vasc Biol 1999;19:700–703.

26. Grandone E, Margaglione M, Colaizzo D, et al. Genetic susceptibility to pregnancy-related venous thromboembolism: roles of factor V Leiden, prothrombin G20210A, and methylenetetrahydrofolate reductase C677T mutations. Am J Obstet Gynecol 1998;179:1324–1328.

27. Levine JS, Branch DW. The antiphospholipid syndrome. N Engl J Med 2002;346:752–763.

28. Baglin T, Luddington R, Brown K, Baglin C. Incidence of recurrent venous thromboembolism in relation to clinical and thrombophilic risk factors: prospective cohort study. Lancet 2003;362:523–526.

29. De Stefano V, Martinelli I, Mannucci PM, et al. The risk of recurrent deep venous thrombosis among heterozygous carriers of both factor V Leiden and the G20210A prothrombin mutation. N Engl J Med 1999;341:801–806.

30. Eichinger S, Pabinger I, Schneider B, et al. The risk of reccurence of venous thromboembolsim in patients with and without factor V Leiden. Thromb Haemost 1997;77:624–628.

31. Eichinger S, Minar E, Hirschl M, et al. The risk of early recurrent venous thromboembolism after oral anticoagulant therapy in patients with the G20210A transition in the prothrombin gene. Thromb Haemost 1999;81:14–17.

32 Emmerich J, Rosendaal FR, Cattaneo M, et al. Combined effect of factor V Leiden and prothrombin 20210A on the risk of venous thromboembolism: polled analysis of 8 case-control studies including 2310 cases and 3204 controls. Thromb Haemost 2001;86:809–816.

33. Koeleman BPC, Reitsma PH, Allaart CF, Bertina RM. Activated protein C resistance as an additional risk factor for thrombosis in protein C-deficient families. Blood 1994;84:1031–1035.

34. Lindmarker P, Schulman S, Sten-Linder M, et al. The risk of recurrent venous thromboembolsim in carriers and non-carriers oft the G1691A allele in the coagulation factor V gene and the G20210A allele in the prothrombin gene. Thromb Haemost 1999;81:684–690.

35. Margaglione M, D'Andrea G, Colaizzo D, et al. Coexistence of factor V Leiden and factor II A20210 mutations and recurrent venous thromboembolism. Thromb Haemost 1999;82:1583–1587.

36. Martinelli I, Bucciarelli P, Margaglione M, et al. The risk of venous thromboembolism in family members with mutations in the genes of factor V or prothormbin or both. Br J Haematol 2000;111:1223–1229.

37. Simioni P, Prandoni P, Lensing AWA, et al. The risk of recurrernt venous thromboembolism in patients with an Arg^{506}φGln mutation in the gene factor V (factor V Leiden). N Engl J Med 1997;336:399–403.

38. Simioni P, Prandoni P, Lensing AWA, et al. Risk for subsequent venous thromboembolic complications in carriers of the prothrombin or the factor V gene mutation with a first episode of deep vein thrombosis. Blood 2000;96:3329–3333.

39. Wahlander K, Larson G, Lindahl TL, et al. Factor V Leiden (G1691A) and prothrombin gene 20210A mutations as potential risk factors for venous thromboembolism after total hip or total knee replacement surgery. Thromb Haemost 2002;87:580–585.

40. Baglin C, Brown K, Luddington R, Baglin T. Risk of recurrent venous thromboembolism in patient with the factor V Leiden (FVR506Q) mutation: effect of warfarin and prediction by precipitating factors. East Anglian Thrombophilia Study Group. Br J Haematol 1998;100:764–768.

41. Heit JA, Mohr DN, Silverstein MD, Petterson TM, O'Falloon WM, Melton LJ. Predictors of recurrence after deep vein thrombosis and pulmonary embolism: a population-based cohort study. Arch Intern Med 2000;160:761–768.

42. Lowe GD, Haverjate F, Thompson SG, et al. Prediction of deep vein thrombosis after elective hip replacement surgery by preoperative clinical and haemostatic variables: the ECAT DVT Study. European Concerted Action on Thrombosis. Thromb Haemost 1999;81:879–886.

43. Martinelli I, Taaioli E, Battaglioli T, et al. Risk of venous thromboembolism after air travel: interaction with thrombophilia and oral contraceptives. Ach Intern Med 2003;163:2771–2774.

44. Vossen CY, Conrad J, Fontcuberta J, et al. Risk of a first venous thrombotic event in carriers of a familial thrombophilic defect. The European Prospective Cohort on Thrombophilia (EPCOT). J Thromb Haemost 2005;3:459–464.

45. Green D. Genetic hypercoaguability: screening should be an informed choice. Blood 2001;98:20.

46. Mannucci PM. Genetic hypercoagulability: prevention suggests testing family members. Blood 2001;98: 21–22.

47. Tripodi A. A review of the clinical and diagnostic utility of laboratory tests for the detection of congenital thrombophilia. Semin Thromb Hemost 2005;31:11–16.

48. Geerts WH, Pineo GF, Heit JA, et al. Prevention of venous thromboembolism: the Seventh ACCP Conference on Antithrombotic and Thrombolytic Therapy. Chest 2004;126:338S–400S.

49. Kearon C, Gent M, Hirsh J, et al. A comparison of three months of anticoagulation with extended anticoagulation for a first episode of idiopathic venous thromboembolism. N Engl J Med 1999;340:901–907.

50. Lemmer JH Jr, Desposits GJ. Antithrombin III concentrate to treat heparin resistance in patients undergoing cardiac surgery. J Thorac Cardiovasc Surg 2002;123:213–217.

51. Riess H. Antithrombin: mechansim of action and clinical useage. Blood Coagul Fibrinolysis 1998;9: S23–S34.

52. Chan YC, Valenti D, Mansfield AO, Stansby G. Warfarin induced skin necrosis. Br J Surg 2000;87: 266–272.

53. Agnelli G, Prandoni P, Santamaria MG, et al. The duration of oral anticoagulant therapy after a second episode of venous thromboembolism. N Engl J Med 1997;333:393–398.

54. Agnelli G, Prandoni P, Santamaria MG, et al. Three months versus one year of oral anticoagulant therapy for idiopathic deep venous thrombosis. N Engl J Med 2001;345:165–169.

55. Sarasin FP, Bounameaux H. Decision analysis model of prolonged oral anticoagulant treatment in factor V Leiden carriers with first episode of deep vein thrombosis. BMJ 1998:316:95–99.

56. Schulman S, Granqvist S, Halmström M, et al. The duration of oral anticoagulant therapy after a second episode of venous thromboembolism. N Engl J Med 1997;336:393–398.

57. van den Belt AG, Sanson BJ, Simioni P, et al. Recurrence of venous thromboembolsim in patients with familial thrombophilia. Arch Intern Med 1997;157:2227–2232.

58. Prandoni P, Lensing AWA, Cogo A, et al. The long-term clinical course of acute deep venous thrombosis. Ann Intern Med 1996;125:1–7.

59. Murin S, Romano PS, White RH. Comparisons of outcomes after hospitalisation for deep venous thrombosis or pulmonary embolism. Thromb Haemost 2002;88:407–414.

60. De Stefano V, Rossi E, Leone G. Inherited thrombophilia, pregnancy, and oral contraceptive use: clinical implications. Semin Vasc Med 2003;3:47–60.

61. Yilmazer M, Kurtay G, Sonmezer M, et al. Factor V Leiden and prothrombin 20210 G-A mutations in controls and in patients with thromboembolic events during pregnancy or the puerperium. Arch Gynecol Obstet 2003;8:304–308.

62. Hassell K. The management of patients with heparin-induced thrombocytopenia who require anticoagulant therapy. Chest 2005;127:1S–8S.

63. Lewis BE, Wallis BE, Berkowtz SD, et al. Argatroban anticoagulant therapy in patients with heparin-induced thrombocytopenia. Circulation 2001;103:1838–1856.

64. Kearon C, Ginsberg JS, Kovacs MJ, et al. Comparison of low-intensity warfarin therapy with conventional-intensity warfarin therapy for long-term prevention of recurrent venous thromboembolism. N Engl J Med 2003;349:631–639.

65. Buller HR, Agnelli G, Hull RD, et al. Antithrombotic therapy for venous thromboembolic disease. Chest 2004;126:401S–428S.

16 Venous Thromboembolism and Cancer

Paolo Prandoni, MD, Anna Falanga, MD, and Andrea Piccioli, MD

Contents

Summary

Venous thromboembolism (VTE) is a common occurrence in patients with cancer. The pathogenetic mechanisms of thrombosis in malignancy involve complex interactions between tumor cells and the hemostatic system. In addition, clinical risk factors for thromboembolism are frequently present in patients with cancer and include prolonged immobilization (especially during the hospital stay), surgery, and chemotherapy with or without adjuvant hormone therapy. Although prophylaxis and treatment of VTE in patients with cancer is based on the same agents as those used in patients free from malignancy, there are many unique issues in patients with cancer that often make the choice and duration of treatment more problematic. Low-molecular-weight heparins are the cornerstone of prophylaxis and treatment of VTE in patients with cancer. Furthermore, they have the potential to prolong survival, at least among patients with more favorable prognosis. Approximately 10% of patients with idiopathic VTE harbor an underlying malignancy that can be detected by an extensive diagnostic workup. However, whether screening for occult malignancies ultimately improves prognosis and prolongs patient survival remains to be demonstrated.

Key Words: Venous thromboembolism; cancer; anticoagulation; low-molecular-weight heparin; warfarin.

From: *Contemporary Cardiology: Management of Acute Pulmonary Embolism*
Edited by: S. Konstantinides © Humana Press Inc., Totowa, NJ

INTRODUCTION

Venous thromboembolism (VTE) in cancer is a well recognized challenge and a serious concern. Clinical manifestations vary from VTE and disseminated intravascular coagulation, which are more commonly observed in patients with hematological malignancies and those with widespread metastatic cancer, to arterial embolism, the latter being more common in patients undergoing chemotherapy and in those with nonbacterial thrombotic endocarditis. This overview will focus on the relationship between cancer and VTE.

PATHOGENESIS OF THROMBOSIS IN CANCER

A subclinical activation of blood coagulation, or hypercoagulable state, characterizes the development of malignant disease. Indeed, abnormalities in laboratory coagulation tests, demonstrating an ongoing process of fibrin formation and removal, are commonly present in patients with cancer even in the absence of clinical thrombosis. These features help explain the thrombophilic condition of these patients, but they are also involved in the progression of the malignant disease itself, as fibrin and other coagulation products participate in tumor growth and metastatic spread *(1)*. In fact, histopathological studies have repeatedly demonstrated the presence of fibrin and/or platelet plugs in and around many types of tumors, suggesting a local activation of blood coagulation and an involvement of clotting mechanisms in the growth of malignant tissues *(2)*.

Prothrombotic Mechanisms in Malignancy

The pathogenesis of clotting activation in cancer is complex and reflects the interaction of different mechanisms. General prothrombotic mechanisms are related to the host response to the tumor and include the acute phase reaction, paraprotein production, inflammation, necrosis, and hemodynamic disorders. Procoagulant effects are also exerted by anticancer therapies (i.e., chemo- or radiotherapy). However, a prominent role is also played by tumor-specific, clot-promoting mechanisms, as a result of the capacity of tumor cells to exhibit their own prothrombotic properties (Fig. 1). These properties are unique to malignancy and distinguish the pathogenesis of thrombosis associated with cancer from that of other thrombophilic conditions.

The principal mechanisms by which malignant cells are able to activate blood coagulation can be classified into the following categories:

1. procoagulant, fibrinolytic, and proaggregatory activity;
2. release of proinflammatory and proangiogenic cytokines; and
3. direct adhesion to host vascular and blood cells by means of adhesion molecules.

Tumor cells produce *procoagulant factors*, among which the most studied are tissue factor (TF) and cancer procoagulant (CP) *(3)*. TF, the primary activator of normal blood coagulation, forms a complex with Factor VII to proteolytically activate Factors X and IX. In normal vascular cells, TF expression is tightly controlled, being induced by inflammatory stimuli such as the cytokines interleukin (IL)-1β, tumor necrosis factor (TNF)-α, and bacterial lipopolysaccharides *(4)*. In contrast, in malignant cells, TF is constitutively expressed. The other procoagulant, CP, is a cysteine proteinase that directly activates Factor X independently of FVII *(5)*. It has been found in tumor cells and in amnion-chorion tissues but not in normal differentiated cells.

Tumor cells express numerous *proteins regulating the fibrinolytic system*, including the urokinase-type and tissue-type plasminogen activators (u-PA and t-PA), PA inhibitors

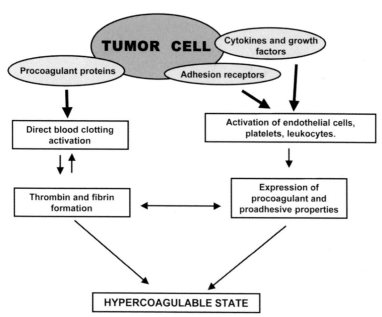

Fig. 1. Prothrombotic properties of tumor cells. Tumor cells can interfere with the hemostatic system through: (1) the expression of procoagulants; (2) the release of proinflammatory cytokines and proangiogenic factors; and (3) the expression of cell membrane adhesion receptors, which allow the direct interaction of tumor cells with the vascular cells. Overall, these tumor-specific characteristics lead to increased thrombin generation and fibrin formation, resulting in a hypercoagulable state.

(PAI-1 and PAI-2) *(6)*, and PA receptors (u-PAR) *(7)*. Moreover, tumor cells induce platelet activation and aggregation by a direct cell-to-cell contact or by releasing soluble factors such as adenosine diphosphate, thrombin, and other proteases *(8)*. Activated platelets have an increased capacity to interact through specific adhesive mechanisms with endothelial cells, leukocytes, and blood-borne tumor cells *(9)*.

Tumor cells produce and release various *cytokines*. Among them, TNF-α, IL-1β, and vascular endothelial growth factor (VEGF) may be involved in the onset of thrombotic disorders of cancer patients. The major targets of tumor-derived cytokines are the vascular endothelium and leukocytes. In the endothelium, TNF-α and IL-1β can induce the expression of TF and downregulate the expression of thrombomodulin *(10)*, thus leading to a prothrombotic state in the vascular wall *(11)*. The same cytokines stimulate the endothelium to produce the PAI-1 *(12)*. Tumor-derived VEGF can also induce the expression of TF by endothelial cells, a mechanism probably contributing to tumor neovascularization *(13)*. Similarly to endothelial cells, monocytes are activated by tumor cells and/or tumor cell products to express TF on their surface *(1)*. Furthermore, tumor-derived cytokines are able to attract and activate polymorphonuclear leukocytes, which release reactive oxygen species and intracellular proteases that possess several activities on endothelial cells, and platelets and may modify the hemostatic balance towards a prothrombotic state *(14,15)*.

Because of the expression of *cell-adhesion molecules*, tumor cells may directly interact with various host cells. In particular, cancer cells may activate platelets both directly and indirectly (i.e., by promoting fibrin deposition and thrombus formation). They may come in contact with endothelial cells in the process of adhesion and migration through the

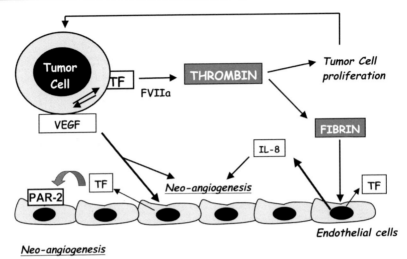

Fig. 2. Influence of tumor cell-derived tissue factor (TF) on tumor progression by coagulation-dependent and coagulation-independent mechanisms. The former mechanisms are represented by the proliferative and proangiogenic activities exerted by thrombin and fibrin on tumor and endothelial cells. The latter consist in the capacity of TF to stimulate endothelial cell angiogenesis through the interaction with the endothelial protease activated receptor (PAR)-2, and indirectly by increasing the expression of the proangiogenic factor VEGF by tumor cells. In turn, VEGF as well as β-FGF, TNF-α, and fibrin, upregulate TF expression by endothelial cells.

vessel wall and may be assisted by granulocytes in their interaction with endothelial cells. The tumor cell capacity to adhere to both resting and cytokine-stimulated endothelium is well described, and adhesion molecule pathways specific to different tumor cell types have been identified *(16)*.

Role of Thrombosis in Cancer Progression

Most of the tumor-specific prothrombotic properties discussed previously can also be involved in tumor growth and dissemination. These effects are mediated both by coagulation-dependent and coagulation-independent mechanisms.

The *coagulation-dependent mechanisms* mainly rely on the formation of thrombin and fibrin, the final products of clotting activation. Thrombin is a potent proliferative factor for tumor cells *(17)*. Furthermore, it binds to and activates the endothelial protease activated receptors (PARs), which mediate new vessel formation *(18)*. Fibrin also plays important roles in tumor metastasis and neoangiogenesis *(19)*. Fibrin deposits on potentially metastatic blood-born malignant cells mediate the attachment of these cells to the vascular endothelium, a process that preceeds extravasation and migration to distant organs. The deposition of fibrin(ogen), along with other adhesive glycoproteins, in the extracellular matrix serves as a scaffold to support binding of growth factors and promote cellular responses of adhesion, proliferation, migration, and neoangiogenesis. On the other hand, fibrinolysis is also a key component in tumor progression, as it is essential for releasing tumor cells from their primary site, promoting neoangiogenesis and favoring cell mobility and motility *(20)*.

The *coagulation-independent mechanisms* of tumor progression involve the noncoagulant activities of TF and other clotting components *(1,3)* (Fig. 2). Overexpression of TF by tumor cells markedly increases the production of VEGF, and the two proteins co-localize at sites of angiogenesis. The production of VEGF by malignant cells plays an important role in tumor-induced angiogenesis. Regulation of VEGF by TF in malignant and normal vascular cells provides an important link between activation of coagulation, inflammation, thrombosis, and tumor progression and metastasis.

EPIDEMIOLOGY AND RISK FACTORS OF VTE IN PATIENTS WITH CANCER

It was nearly 140 yr ago when Armand Trousseau first described migratory thrombophlebitis in patients with cancer. Since then, numerous studies have addressed the relationship between cancer and VTE. VTE is a well-established and frequent complication in patients with cancer. Importantly, it sometimes acts as an epiphenomenon of occult cancer, thus offering opportunities for early cancer diagnosis and treatment (21). Approximately 15% of patients with cancer have relevant thrombosis, which is seen in virtually all cancer types (albeit at different rates), and is the second leading cause of death in patients with malignant disease (21). According to the Medicare Provider Analysis and Review Record, a database that records the diagnosis at discharge in the US, the rate of initial or recurrent thromboembolism in patients with cancer exceeds by far that recorded in those without malignancy (22). The majority of thrombotic episodes occur spontaneously, i.e., in the absence of triggering factors commonly accounting for thromboembolic complications in subjects without cancer. Patients with cancer have a highly increased risk of VTE in the first few months after diagnosis, and also in the presence of distant metastases (23). This risk is further enhanced in the presence of inherited thrombophilic abnormalities (23). The most common situations that make patients with cancer at higher risk of VTE include immobilization, surgery, chemotherapy with or without hormone therapy, and the insertion of central venous catheters (CVCs) (21).

One of the most important triggering factors for VTE is *prolonged immobilization*, especially during hospital stay. This pattern was clearly confirmed by Shen and Pollack, who reported that as many as 14% of patients with cancer admitted to hospital died of autopsy-confirmed PE, compared with 8% of those who were free from cancer (24).

Patients with cancer are at a markedly high risk of developing deep vein thrombosis (DVT) when they undergo *surgical procedures*. In the absence of adequate prophylaxis, the overall incidence of postoperative DVT in patients with cancer is approximately twice as high as that in patients free from malignancy (21). If thromboprophylaxis is not prolonged beyond the hospital stay, patients with cancer remain at risk of developing late VTE complications (25).

Cancer patients also face a particularly high risk of developing both venous and arterial thrombosis when they receive *chemotherapy (26)*. Most data on the incidence of chemotherapy-associated VTE comes from studies in women with breast cancer. Patients with breast cancer are at a markedly high risk for developing both venous and arterial thrombosis when receiving chemotherapy. For example, the incidence of chemotherapy-induced thromboembolic complications in women with stage II breast cancer undergoing chemotherapy was found to be 7% on average (26). Hormone therapy in combination with chemotherapy further enhances the incidence of thromboembolic complications in women with breast cancer (27). Tamoxifen, either as adjuvant therapy or for prevention of breast cancer in women at high risk, slightly increased the rate of VTE (28). In comparison to tamoxifen, third-generation oral aromatase inhibitors, such as the irreversible steroidal inactivator, exemestane, may be associated with a lower rate of thromboembolic events (29).

Long-term *CVCs* have considerably improved the management of many patients with cancer, who usually have a long-term CVC inserted for chemotherapy. However, their use has been associated with the occurrence of upper-limb DVT, especially in those patients who require the administration of chemotherapy *(30)*.

PREVENTION OF VTE IN CANCER

Prevention of VTE in patients with cancer represents an important challenge, because patients with cancer experiencing a thrombotic episode have a poor outcome with greater probability of death. Although patients with active cancer often develop thrombotic complications spontaneously, i.e., in the absence of additional risk factors, there is probably little rationale behind providing thromboprophylaxis to all patients with cancer who are not receiving surgical or medical therapy. However, a history of thromboembolism places cancer patients at such a high risk of recurrence that the systematic use of either mechanical or pharmacological prophylaxis may be considered even in the absence of the common risk factors for thrombosis.

Surgical Interventions

According to widely accepted guidelines, low-molecular-weight heparin (LMWH) in low doses, low-dose unfractionated heparin (UFH), or physical measures should be adopted in patients with cancer who require prolonged immobilization or undergo low-risk surgical procedures *(31)*. Extensive surgery places patients with cancer at a remarkably high risk of postoperative VTE. Accordingly, these patients require more intensive prophylactic regimens such as higher doses of LMWHs (on average, twice as high as those suggested for low-risk procedures), adjusted-dose heparin, or oral anticoagulants *(31)*.

Once-daily injections of LMWH are at least as effective and safe as multiple injections of UFH for prevention of postoperative VTE in cancer patients *(32,33)*. Of interest, a recent trial suggested that prolonging the administration of LMWH until the completion of the first month after surgical intervention provides an additional thromboprophylactic effect without increasing the hemorrhagic risk *(25)*.

Chemotherapy and Radiotherapy

In the only available study, fixed low-dose warfarin (1 mg/d) for 6 wk, followed by doses that maintained the international normalized ratio (INR) at 1.3 to 1.9 was an effective and safe method for prevention of chemotherapy-induced thromboembolism in women with metastatic breast cancer *(34)*. Whether this strategy or strategies that involve LMWHs are effective and safe in other oncologic patterns as well remains to be demonstrated.

Unfortunately, no proper study has been performed as yet to assess the preventive value of antithrombotic strategies in patients undergoing radiotherapy.

CVCs

The role of antithrombotic prophylaxis in the prevention of CVC-related thrombosis is controversial. Two randomized, controlled studies documented the benefit of fixed low-dose warfarin in decreasing the incidence of arm vein thrombosis related to in-dwelling CVC *(35,36)*. The subcutaneous administration of dalteparin (2500 IU once-daily) for 90 d also was shown to be beneficial in this setting *(37)*. However, four recent clinical trials failed to show a benefit from a 1-mg daily dose of warfarin *(38,39)*, dalteparin (5000 IU o.i.d.) *(40)*, and enoxaparin *(41)*, respectively, compared to no prophylaxis. Thus, neither "mini-dose" warfarin nor prophylactic LMWH can be recommended on a routine basis as prophylaxis for patients with cancer with in-dwelling central venous lines *(31)*.

TREATMENT AND SECONDARY PREVENTION OF VTE

Initial Treatment

Except for selected patients requiring aggressive treatment, the large majority of patients with cancer should receive the subcutaneous injection of therapeutic doses (adjusted to body weight) of a LMWH by once- or twice-daily injection. Alternatively, a proper course of full-dose UFH, i.e., a heparin regimen that prolongs the activated partial thromboplastin time (APTT) up to 1.5 to 3.0 times the control value can be employed *(42)* (*see* Chapter 9). Whenever possible, LMWH should be administered as soon as there is a reasonable suspicion that venous thrombosis exists *(42)*. LMWHs make the treatment of selected patients with cancer feasible on an ambulatory basis or directly at home *(43)*. Thrombolytic drugs are rarely indicated. The limited cases in which thrombolysis may be considered include massive pulmonary embolism (PE), extension of venous thrombosis despite extensive anticoagulation, and upper-extremity thrombosis in patients who have an in-dwelling CVC, which must be kept patent *(42)*. Finally, the insertion of an inferior vena caval filter should be considered whenever a full-dose anticoagulation is contraindicated or unsuccessful.

Long-Term Anticoagulation

What are the main questions clinicians deal with when facing patients with cancer with an episode of venous thrombosis? The main controversies deal with the most appropriate duration and intensity of anticoagulation, the risk of extension and/or recurrence of VTE during anticoagulation, and the potential for an increased risk of bleeding during the course of proper anticoagulant therapy.

According to the results of recent prospective cohort and population-based studies *(44, 45)*, after discontinuation of warfarin, patients with cancer and venous thrombosis exhibit a risk for recurrence that is almost twice as high as that observed in patients free from malignancy. In view of the persistently high risk of recurrent thrombotic events, prolongation of warfarin should be considered for as long as the malignant disorder is active, provided that it is not contraindicated. The suggested policy is to administer warfarin to maintain the INR between 2.0 and 3.0.

Of interest, patients with cancer have a three- to fourfold higher risk of recurrent VTE than cancer free patients while on anticoagulation *(46–48)*. This risk correlates with the extent of cancer. Accordingly, more aggressive initial or long-term treatment has the potential to reduce the risk of recurrent thrombosis. However, a complicating factor in intensifying anticoagulant therapy in patients with cancer is the occurrence of excess bleeding in combination with excess recurrent thromboembolism. Although some improvement can be expected from optimizing laboratory monitoring of anticoagulant therapy, most bleeding and thrombotic complications occur in patients with anticoagulant parameters within the therapeutic range. Possibilities for improvement using the current paradigms of anticoagulation seem, therefore, limited.

According to the results of recent randomized clinical trials, full-dose dalteparin for the first month followed by three-fourths of the initial regimen has the potential to provide a more effective antithrombotic regimen in patients with cancer and venous thrombosis than conventional treatment, and is not associated with an increased hemorrhagic risk

(49,50). Although LMWHs are more expensive than oral anticoagulants, they are easier to administer, more convenient and flexible, and not influenced by nutrition or liver function. Thus, long-term administration of subtherapeutic doses of LMWH can now be considered as the treatment of choice in patients with aggressive disease and in those with conditions limiting the use of oral anticoagulants *(42)*.

The anticoagulation strategy for the treatment of patients with *recurrent VTE* during oral anticoagulation is not rigidly standardized. A patient who develops recurrent VTE while the INR is subtherapeutic can be retreated with UFH or LMWH for a few days, and oral anticoagulant therapy can be continued with the INR kept between 2.0 and 3.0. For those who experience warfarin failure and develop a recurrence while the INR is therapeutic, the long-term management is less clear. Three options are acceptable after initial retreatment with UFH or LMWH: (1) continue with oral anticoagulant therapy aiming for a higher target INR of 3.0 to 3.5; (2) switch to adjusted-dose twice-daily subcutaneous standard heparin to maintain a therapeutic APTT; (3) or use once-daily weight-based therapeutic doses of LMWH. For patients with a high risk of PE, or who are hemodynamically unstable, an inferior vena caval filter can be inserted in addition to one of the previously described options.

IMPACT OF ANTITHROMBOTIC DRUGS ON CANCER PROGRESSION

Anticoagulant treatment of cancer patients, particularly those with lung cancer, has been reported to improve survival *(51)*. These interesting, albeit preliminary, results of controlled trials provide some support to the argument discussed previously, namely that activation of blood coagulation plays a role in the natural history of tumor growth.

Numerous studies have been performed in recent years to address the value of LMWH in comparison with standard heparin in the treatment of VTE, and an updated meta-analysis of the most adequate reports was published in 2000 *(52)*. In eight of the nine studies reporting on long-term follow-up, analysis of total mortality exhibited a surprising trend in favor of LMWH. In the five studies that provided subgroup analysis, this effect was entirely attributable to the differences in the subgroup of patients with cancer.

The evidence for reduction of cancer-related mortality in patients on LMWH has stimulated renewed interest in these agents as antineoplastic drugs. Four randomized studies have recently compared the long-term survival of patients with cancer receiving conventional treatment with that of patients receiving a supplementary dose of LMWH in therapeutic or prophylactic doses *(53–56)*. All four studies showed a favorable impact of the tested heparin on patients' survival. This result was particularly evident in patients with a better prognosis. However, further, larger studies are needed before LMWH can be recommended for routine treatment of patients with cancer.

Of interest, in a recent trial addressing the value of different periods of warfarin treatment for prevention of recurrent thromboembolism in patients with the first episode of VTE, the development of late malignancies was recorded much more frequently in patients allocated to 6 wk than in those allocated to 6 mo of anticoagulation *(57)*. These results suggest that cancer and thrombosis share common mechanisms, and that antithrombotic drugs may interfere with cancer progression.

RISK OF CANCER IN PATIENTS WITH VTE

In patients presenting with VTE, the prevalence of *concomitant* cancer, defined as cancer not known before VTE and discovered by routine investigation (history taking, physical examination, urinalysis, routine blood tests, and chest-X-ray) varied considerably between the studies. Overall, the risk of concomitant cancer was increased among patients with idiopathic VTE by a factor of 3–19 *(58)*. According to the results of a recent study, particularly high D-dimer concentrations in patients with DVT seem to suggest an increased probability of overt or occult cancer *(59)*.

The risk of developing *subsequent* overt malignancy also was found to be consistently higher (four to five times) in patients with idiopathic VTE than in those with secondary thrombosis *(21)*. Newly discovered malignancies, whose incidence in patients with idiopathic VTE consistently amounted to 10% in various studies, involve virtually all body systems. The risk of cancer is even higher in patients with recurrent thromboembolism *(60)* and in those with bilateral VTE *(61)*.

These findings were confirmed by those of three large, population-based studies conducted in Denmark, Sweden, and Scotland *(62–64)*. By examining data from both cancer and thromboembolic disease national registries, the authors of all three studies found a significantly increased risk for developing cancer among patients discharged with the diagnosis of VTE. The risk was highest during the first year after hospitalization. Of interest, in two of these studies, risk elevation persisted for up to 10 yr, suggesting that either a malignant disorder can induce hypercoagulability many years prior to its overt clinical development or, more likely, cancer and thrombosis may share common pathogenetic mechanisms *(62,63)*.

By assessing the survival rate in patients with cancer diagnosed in the first year following the thrombotic episode in comparison with that of matched cancer patients without thrombosis, Sorensen and coworkers found increased mortality in the former group *(65)*. The same was true of cancer diagnosed at the time of hospitalization for VTE. From these data, it appears that whenever cancer is preceded by a clinical manifestation of thrombosis, its prognosis is far worse. However, because of the retrospective nature of the study design, it is possible that the large majority of identified tumors were already symptomatic at the time of detection.

Monreal and colleagues published the results of a prospective cohort follow-up study in consecutive patients with acute VTE *(66)*. All patients underwent routine clinical evaluation for malignancy, which, if negative, was followed by a limited diagnostic work-up consisting of abdominal and pelvic ultrasound and laboratory markers for malignancy. The routine clinical evaluation was performed in 864 patients and revealed malignancy in 34 (3.9%) of them. Among the remaining 830 patients, the limited diagnostic work-up revealed 13 further malignancies. During follow-up, cancer became symptomatic in 14 patients who were negative for cancer at screening (sensitivity of limited diagnostic work-up, 48%). Malignancies that were identified by the limited diagnostic work-up were early-stage in 61% of cases. Most patients with occult cancer had idiopathic VTE and were older than 70 yr. According to these study results, a limited diagnostic work-up for occult cancer in patients with VTE has the capacity to identify approximately one-half of the malignancies, predominantly in an early stage.

We recently conducted a multicenter randomized clinical trial (the SOMIT study) patients who were apparently cancer-free but had acute idiopathic VTE or PE *(67)*. Of 201 patients with a first episode of idiopathic VTE, 99 were randomized to undergo extensive screening after initial negative routine battery tests (Table 1), whereas 102 had no further testing for malignancy. All patients were followed until the completion of 2 yr of follow-up. Of the 14 malignancies that occurred in the extensive screening group, screening was able to

Table 1
Extensive Screening Procedure According to the SOMIT Study

Procedures:
- Ultrasound of abdomen/pelvis
- Computed tomographic scan of abdomen and pelvis
- Gastroscopy or double contrast barium swallowing
- Flexible sigmoidoscopy or rectoscopy followed by barium enema or colonoscopy
- Haemoccult, sputum cytology, tumor markers (CEA, αFP, CA125)
- Mammography and pap smear in women
- Transabdominal ultrasound of the prostate and PSA in men

PSA, prostate specific antigen.

detect 13 (mostly detected by CT scanning), resulting in a sensitivity of greater than 90%. The risk for occult cancer was higher among elderly patients and in those without thrombophilic abnormalities. In the follow-up of patients allocated to the control group, 10 malignancies developed. Overall, malignancies identified in the extensive screening group were at an earlier stage and the mean delay to diagnosis was reduced from 11 mo to 1 mo. The earlier discovery and subsequent treatment resulted in a slightly improved cancer-related mortality (2.0 vs 3.9%) and cancer-free survival (5.1 vs 7.9%) of the patients in the extensive screening group. Although these differences were not statistically significant, the reduction observed is in line with the hypothesis and would translate into a "number needed to screen" of only 50 patients to prevent one cancer-related death over a 2-yr period.

Thus, although the data from either study do not conclusively demonstrate that extensive screening for cancer in patients with VTE ultimately prolongs life, the observations taken together make such a beneficial effect likely. The earlier discovery of cancer may be of decisive importance for a (possibly) considerable number of patients, especially nowadays when continuous therapeutic innovations are providing growing chances of success in the cure of malignancies.

REFERENCES

1. Rickles FR, Falanga A. Molecular basis for the relationship between thrombosis and cancer. Thromb Res 2001;102:V215–224.
2. Falanga A, Donati MB. Pathogenesis of thrombosis in patients with malignancy. Int J Hematol 2001;73: 137–144.
3. Gale AJ, Gordon SG. Update on tumor cell procoagulant factors. Acta Haematol 2001;106:25–32.
4. Nemerson Y. The tissue factor pathway of blood coagulation. Sem Hematol 1992;29:170–176.
5. Falanga A, Gordon SG. Isolation and characterization of cancer procoagulant: a cysteine proteinase from malignant tissue. Biochemistry 1985;24:5558–5567.
6. Kwaan HC, Keer HN. Fibrinolysis and cancer. Semin Thromb Haemost 1990;16:230–235.
7. Hajjar KA. Cellular receptors in the regulation of plasmin generation. Thromb Haemost 1995;74:294–301.
8. Varon D, Brill A. Platelets cross-talk with tumor cells. Haemostasis 2001;31(Suppl 1):64–66.
9. Felding-Habermann B. Tumor cell-platelet interaction in metastatic disease. Haemostasis 2001;31(Suppl 1):55–58.
10. Cines DB, Pollak ES, Buck CA, et al. Endothelial cells in physiology and in the pathophysiology of vascular disorders. Blood 1998;91:3527–3561.
11. Falanga A, Marchetti M, Giovanelli S, Barbui T. All-trans-retinoic acid counteracts endothelial cell procoagulant activity induced by a human promyelocytic leukemia-derived cell line (NB4). Blood 1996;87: 613–617.

12. Van Hinsberg VWM, Bauer KA, Kooistra T, et al. Progress of fibrinolysis during tumor necrosis factor infusion in humans. Concomitant increase of tissue-type plasminogen activator, plasminogen activator inhibitor type-1, and fibrin(ogen) degradation products. Blood 1990;76:2284–2289.

13. Contrino J, Hair G, Kreutzer DL, Rickles FR. In situ detection of tissue factor in vascular endothelial cells: correlation with the malignant phenotype of human breast disease. Nature Med 1996;2:209–215.

14. Falanga A, Marchetti M, Evangelista V, et al. Neutrophil activation and hemostatic changes in healthy donors given granulocyte-colony stimulating factor. Blood 1999;93:2506–2514.

15. Falanga A, Marchetti M, Evangelista V, et al. Polymorphonuclear leukocyte activation and hemostasis in patients with Essential Thrombocythemia and Polycythemia Vera. Blood 2000;96:4261–4266.

16. Marchetti M, Falanga A, Giovanelli S, et al. All-trans-retinoic acid increases the adhesion to endothelium of the acute promyelocytic leukemia cell line NB4. Br J Haematol 1996;93:360–366.

17. Darmoul D, Gratio V, Devaud H, Lehy T, Laburthe M. Aberrant expression and activation of the thrombin receptor protease-activated receptor-1 induces cell proliferation and motility in human colon cancer cells. Am J Pathol 2003;162:1503–1513.

18. Costantini V, Zacharski LR. Fibrin and cancer. Thromb Haemost 1993;69:406–414.

19. Rickles FR, Shoji M, Abe K. The role of the hemostatic system in tumor growth, metastasis, and angiogenesis: tissue factor is a bifunctional molecule capable of inducing both fibrin deposition and angiogenesis in cancer. Int J Hematol 2001;73:145–150.

20. McMahon GA, Petitclerc E, Stefansson S, et al. Plasminogen activator inhibitor-1 regulates tumor growth and angiogenesis. J Biol Chem 2001;276:3964–3968.

21. Prandoni P, Piccioli A, Girolami A. Cancer and venous thromboembolism: an overview. Haematologica 1999;84:437–445.

22. Levitan N, Dowlati A, Remick SC, et al. Rates of initial and recurrent thromboembolic disease among patients with malignancy versus those without malignancy. Risk analysis using Medicare claims data. Medicine (Baltimore) 1999;78:285–291.

23. Blom JW, Doggen CJ, Osanto S, Rosendaal FR. Malignancies, prothrombotic mutations, and the risk of venous thrombosis. JAMA 2005;293:715–722.

24. Shen VS, Pollak EW. Fatal pulmonary embolism in cancer patients: is heparin prophylaxis justified? South Med J 1980;73:841–843.

25. Bergqvist D, Agnelli G, Cohen AT, et al. Duration of prophylaxis against venous thromboembolism with enoxaparin after surgery for cancer. N Engl J Med 2002;346:975–980.

26. Levine MN. Prevention of thrombotic disorders in cancer patients undergoing chemotherapy. Thromb Haemost 1997;78:133–136.

27. Tempelhoff GF, Dietrich M, Hommel G, Heilmann L. Blood coagulation during adjuvant epirubicin/cyclophosphamide chemotherapy in patients with primary operable breast cancer. J Clin Oncol 1996; 14:2560–2568.

28. Deitcher SR, Gomes MPV. The risk of venous thromboembolic disease associated with adjuvant hormone therapy for breast carcinoma. Cancer 2004;101:439–449.

29. Coombes RC, Hall E, Gibson LJ, et al. A randomized trial of exemestane after two to three years of tamoxifen therapy in postmenopausal women with primary breast cancer. N Engl J Med 2004;350:1081–1092.

30. Verso M, Agnelli G. Venous thromboembolism associated with long-term use of central venous catheters in cancer patients. J Clin Oncol 2003;21:3665–3675.

31. Geerts WH, Pineo GF, Heit JA, et al. Prevention of venous thromboembolism: the seventh ACCP conference on antithrombotic and thrombolytic therapy. Chest 2004;126:338S–400S.

32. Enoxacan Study group. Efficacy and safety of enoxaparin versus unfractionated heparin for prevention of deep vein thrombosis in elective cancer surgery: a double-blind randomized multicentre trial with venographic assessment. Br J Surg 1997;84:1099–103.

33. McLeod RS, Geerts WH, Sniderman KW, et al. Subcutaneous heparin versus low-molecular-weight heparin as thromboprophylaxis in patients undergoing colorectal DVT prophylaxis trial: a randomized, double-blind trial. Ann Surg 2001;233:438–444.

34. Levine MN, Hirsh J, Gent M, et al. Double-blind randomized trial of very-low-dose warfarin for prevention of thromboembolism in stage IV breast cancer. Lancet 1994;343:886–889.

35. Bern MM, Lokich JJ, Wallach SR, et al. Very low dose of warfarin can prevent thrombosis in central venous catheters. A prospective trial. Ann Intern Med 1990;112:423–428.

36. Bern MM, Bothe A Jr, Bistrian B, Champagne CD, Keane MS, Blackburn GL. Prophylaxis against central vein thrombosis with low-dose warfarin. Surgery 1986;99:216–221.

37. Monreal M, Alastrue A, Rull M, et al. Upper extremity deep venous thrombosis in cancer patients with venous access devices- prophylaxis with a low molecular weight heparin (fragmin). Thromb Haemost 1996;75:251–253.

38. Couban S, Goodyear M, Burnell M, et al. Randomized placebo-controlled study of low-dose warfarin for the prevention of central venous catheter-associated thrombosis in patients with cancer. J Clin Oncol 2005;23:4063–4069.

39. Heaton DC, Han DY, Inder A. Minidose warfarin as prophylaxis for central vein catheter thrombosis. Intern Med 2002;32:84–88.

40. Karthaus M, Kretzschmar A, Kroning H, et al. Dalteparin for prevention of catheter-related complications in cancer patients with central venous catheters: final results of a double-blind, placebo-controlled phase III trial. Ann Oncol 2006;17:289–296.

41. Verso M, Agnelli G, Bertoglio S, et al. Enoxaparin for the prevention of venous thromboembolism associated with central vein catheter: a double-blind, placebo-controlled, randomized study in cancer patients. J Clin Oncol 2005;23:4057–4062.

42. Büller HR, Agnelli G, Hull RD, Hyers TM, Prins MH, Raskob GE. Antithrombotic therapy for venous thromboembolic disease: the seventh ACCP conference on antithrombotic and thrombolytic therapy. Chest 2004;126:401S–428S.

43. Ageno W, Grimwood R, Limbiati S, Dentali F, Steidl L, Wells PS. Home-treatment of deep vein thrombosis in patients with cancer. Haematologica 2005;90:220–224.

44. Prandoni P, Lensing AWA, Cogo A, et al. The long-term clinical course of acute deep venous thrombosis. Ann Intern Med 1996;125:1–7.

45. Heit JA, Mohr DN, Silverstein MD, Petterson TM, O'Fallon WM, Melton LJ III. Predictors of recurrence after deep vein thrombosis and pulmonary embolism. A population-based cohort study. Arch Intern Med 2000;160:761–768.

46. Hutten B, Prins M, Gent M, Ginsberg J, Tijsen JGP, Buller HR. Incidence of recurrent thromboembolic and bleeding complications among patients with venous thromboembolism in relation to both malignancy and achieved international normalized ratio: a retrospective analysis. J Clin Oncol 2000;18:3078–3083.

47. Palareti G, Legnani C, Agnes L, et al. A comparison of the safety and efficacy of oral anticoagulation for the treatment of venous thromboembolic disease in patients with or without malignancy. Thromb Haemost 2000;84:805–810.

48. Prandoni P, Lensing AWA, Piccioli A, et al. Recurrent venous thromboembolism and bleeding complications during anticoagulant treatment in patients with cancer and venous thrombosis. Blood 2002;100: 3484–3488.

49. Lee AY, Levine MN, Baker RI, et al. Low-molecular-weight heparin versus a coumarin for the prevention of recurrent venous thromboembolism in patients with cancer. N Engl J Med 2003;349:146–153.

50. Meyer G, Marjanovic Z, Valcke J, et al. Comparison of low-molecular-weight heparin and warfarin for the secondary prevention of venous thromboembolism in patients with cancer. Arch Intern Med 2002; 162:1729–1735.

51. Zacharski LR, Henderson WG, Rickles FR, et al. Effect of warfarin anticoagulation on survival in carcinoma of the lung, colon, head and neck, and prostate. Cancer 1984;53:2046–2052.

52. Dolovich LR, Ginsberg JS, Douketis JD, Holbrook AM, Cheah G. A meta-analysis comparing low-molecular-weight heparins with unfractionated heparin in the treatment of venous thromboembolism. Arch Intern Med 2000;160:181–188.

53. Kakkar AK, Levine MN, Kadziola Z, et al. Low molecular weight heparin, therapy with dalteparin, and survival in advanced cancer: The Fragmin Advanced Malignancy Outcome Study. J Clin Oncol 2004;22: 1944–1948.

54. Klerk CPW, Smorenburg SM, Otten HYM, et al. The effect of low-molecular-weight heparin on survival in patients with advanced malignancy. J Clin Oncol 2005;23:2130–2135.

55. Lee AY, Rickles FR, Julian JA, et al. Randomized comparison of low molecular weight heparin and coumarin derivatives on the survival of patients with cancer and venous thromboembolism. J Clin Oncol 2005;23:2123–2129.

56. Altinbas M, Coskun HS, Er O, et al. A randomized clinical trial of combination chemotherapy with and without low-molecular-weight heparin in small cell lung cancer. J Thromb Haemost 2004;2:1266–1271.

57. Schulman S, Lindmarker P. Incidence of cancer after prophylaxis with warfarin against recurrent venous thromboembolism. N Engl J Med 2000;342:1953–1958.

58. Otten HM, Prins MH. Venous thromboembolism and occult malignancy. Tromb Res 2001;102:V187–V194.

59. Schutgens RE, Beckers MM, Haas FJ, Biesma DH. The predictive value of D-dimer measurement for cancer in patients with deep vein thrombosis. Haematologica 2005;90:214–219.
60. Prandoni P, Lensing AWA, Büller HR, et al. Deep-vein thrombosis and the incidence of subsequent symptomatic cancer. N Engl J Med 1992;327:1128–1133.
61. Bura A, Cailleux N, Bienvenu B, et al. Incidence and prognosis of cancer associated with bilateral venous thrombosis: a prospective study of 103 patients. J Thromb Haemost 2004;2:441–444.
62. Sorensen HT, Mellemkjaer L, Steffensen H, Olsen JH, Nielsen GL. The risk of a diagnosis of cancer after primary deep-venous thrombosis or pulmonary embolism. N Engl J Med 1998;338:1169–1173.
63. Baron JA, Gridley G, Weiderpass E, Nyren G, Linet M. Venous thromboembolism and cancer. Lancet 1998;351:1077–1080.
64. Murchison JT, Wylie L, Stockton DL. Excess risk of cancer in patients with primary venous thromboembolism: a national, population-based cohort study. Br J Cancer 2004;91:92–95.
65. Sorensen HT, Mellemkjaer L, Olsen JH, Baron JA. Prognosis of cancers associated with venous thromboembolism. N Engl J Med 2000;343:1846–1850.
66. Monreal M, Lensing AWA, Prins MH, et al. Screening for occult cancer in patients with acute deep vein thrombosis or pulmonary embolism. J Thromb Haemost 2004;2:876–881.
67. Piccioli A, Lensing AWA, Prins MH, et al. Estensive screening for occult malignant disease in idiopathic venous thromboembolism. J Thromb Haemost 2004;2:884–889.

17

Pulmonary Embolism in Pregnancy

Simon J. McRae, MBBS

and Shannon M. Bates MDCM, MSc

CONTENTS

SUMMARY

Pregnancy is associated with a 5- to 10-fold increase in the incidence of venous thromboembolism. Pulmonary embolism (PE) remains a leading cause of maternal mortality in developed countries. The diagnosis, treatment, and prevention of PE during pregnancy continue to present a challenge to healthcare professionals. Many commonly used diagnostic tests are less accurate in pregnant than in nonpregnant patients, and some radiological procedures expose the fetus to ionizing radiation. There are limited data regarding the efficacy of anticoagulant therapy in the treatment and prophylaxis of PE during pregnancy. The treatment of PE in pregnant women is also made more difficult because warfarin can cause embryopathy and other adverse fetal effects, and unfractionated heparin and low-molecular-weight heparins, the cornerstones of therapy in this patient population, may have maternal side effects. This chapter reviews areas of controversy and provides recommendations for the diagnostic workup and treatment of PE, as well as thromboprophylaxis, in pregnant women.

Key Words: Pregnancy; pulmonary embolism; anticoagulation; prophylaxis; diagnosis.

INTRODUCTION

It has been recognized for many years that pregnant women are at increased risk of developing venous thromboembolism (VTE), which may manifest as deep vein thrombosis

From: *Contemporary Cardiology: Management of Acute Pulmonary Embolism*
Edited by: S. Konstantinides © Humana Press Inc., Totowa, NJ

(DVT) or pulmonary embolism (PE). The fact that PE remains a leading cause of maternal mortality in developed countries emphasizes the importance of this association and provides an ongoing challenge to healthcare professionals involved in the care of pregnant women. The following chapter focuses on the diagnosis and treatment of PE during pregnancy, both of which are influenced by changes in maternal physiology and the potential impact of any intervention on fetal well-being.

EPIDEMIOLOGY

Incidence of Fatal Pregnancy-Related PE

Comprehensive data on the incidence of fatal pregnancy-related PE has been available in the United Kingdom since 1952, from the Confidential Enquiries into Maternal Deaths *(1)*. The rate of fatal PE during pregnancy has fallen progressively from approx 7 deaths in 100,000 maternities in the 1950s to 1.2 deaths per 100,000 maternities in the latest report covering the period from 2000 to 2002 *(2)*. Despite the reduction in incidence, PE remained the leading direct cause of maternal death in the most recent report, being responsible for 30% of all cases.

Although a mandatory reporting system for maternal deaths does not exist in the United States, data derived from death certification also have documented a fall in fatal PE in the past decades *(3–5)*. Thus, the Pregnancy Mortality Surveillance System (PMSS) reported fatal PE rates of 1.8 and 2.3 per 100,000 live deliveries for the periods 1987–1990 and 1991–1999, respectively *(5,6)*. In the latter period, PE was responsible for 21% of maternal fatalities. In the United States, the rate of fatal PE, like all-cause maternal mortality, has been consistently found to be two- to threefold higher in African American compared to Caucasian women, a ratio maintained despite reductions in the overall incidence of VTE *(3,6)*. Whether this relates to differences in severity of disease, diagnostic methods, or treatment remains unclear.

Incidence of Nonfatal Pregnancy-Associated PE

The incidence of nonfatal PE during pregnancy and the puerperium is less certain *(7)*. Studies designed to accurately determine the rate of asymptomatic DVT or PE during pregnancy have not been performed, as sensitive tests for asymptomatic VTE are often invasive and involve exposure to radiation. In nonpregnant women of childbearing age, the annual incidence of symptomatic VTE is approx 1 in 10,000 individuals *(8–10)*. Early studies *(11–13)*, in which the diagnosis of acute thrombosis was made entirely on clinical grounds, are likely to have overestimated the incidence of VTE, as the majority of individuals with clinically suspected DVT or PE during pregnancy do not have the diagnosis confirmed by objective testing *(14,15)*. Results from more recent studies (Table 1), in which the majority or all patients underwent accurate diagnostic testing, are therefore more likely to reflect true disease incidence. These retrospective studies used national *(16,17)*, regional *(10,18)*, or institutional *(19–21)* discharge and birth data, with reported VTE rates ranging from 0.6 to 1.3 episodes per 1000 deliveries, i.e., 5- to 10-fold that reported for nonpregnant women of reproductive age.

The majority of individuals with VTE during pregnancy are diagnosed with symptomatic DVT rather than PE, with DVT constituting approx 85% of confirmed thrombotic events (Table 2). This compares with a figure of approx 70% in nonpregnant patients with VTE, derived largely from clinical studies that did not include autopsy data *(22)*. As is the case in nonpregnant patients, it is likely that a large percentage of pregnant patients with

Table 1
Incidence of Nonfatal Pregnancy-Related VTE[a]

Study	Number of pregnancies (n)	Incidence/1000 pregnancies
Lindqvist (17)	479,422	1.3
Anderson (18)	63,319	0.85
Gherman (20)	268,525	0.6
McColl (19)	72,201	0.86
Simpson (21)	395,335	0.85
Samuelsson (10)	13,723	0.95

[a]All studies were retrospective, with the figures shown representing the combined incidence of DVT and PE.

Table 2
Incidence of Antepartum DVT and PE

Study	Deliveries (n)	Episodes DVT n (%)[a]	Episodes PE n (%)[a]	Incidence DVT/1000 deliveries	Incidence PE/1000 deliveries
Lindqvist (17)	479,422	518 (85.2)	90 (14.8)	1.1	0.2
Anderson (18)	63,319	52 (96.3)	2 (3.7)	0.8	0.03
Gherman (20)	268,525	127 (78.1)	38 (21.9)	0.5	0.1
McColl (19)	72,201	51 (82.3)	11 (17.7)	0.7	0.2
Simpson (21)	395,335	317 (88.3)	42 (11.7)	0.8	0.1
Total	1,278,802	1,065 (85.3)	183 (14.7)	0.8	0.1

[a]Represents percentage of total episodes of antepartum VTE. DVT, deep vein thrombosis; PE, pulmonary embolism.

symptomatic DVT have asymptomatic PE (23). It is possible that younger age and, therefore, improved cardiorespiratory reserve may account for the reduced frequency of symptomatic PE in patients with pregnancy-related thrombotic events.

Timing of Presentation of Pregnancy-Related VTE

The distribution of episodes of DVT throughout pregnancy and the puerperium has been examined in a meta-analysis (24), which found that 65.5% of events occurred antepartum and 34.5% postpartum, with the antepartum events distributed throughout all three trimesters. In contrast, 43 to 60% of pregnancy-related episodes of PE appear to occur after delivery (19–21). As the antepartum period is substantially longer than the 6-wk postpartum period, the *daily risk* of PE, as well as DVT, is substantially higher following delivery than during the antepartum period.

Clinical Risk Factors for Pregnancy-Related VTE

The evidence for an association between maternal clinical factors and an increased risk of VTE during pregnancy is almost entirely derived from case-control studies. Although the existing data for individual risk factors are conflicting, increased maternal age (usually defined as > 35 yr) (13,16,25), increased maternal body mass index (BMI) (21), a history of smoking (17,26), and, for postpartum VTE, delivery by caesarian section (13,17,20, 25), have been most consistently identified as risk factors for VTE (17,26). Other reported markers of increased risk include prior superficial thrombophlebitis (26), a family history of VTE *(19)*, blood group A *(21,27)*, and postpartum hemorrhage *(26)*. Contradictory results have been reported for increased parity *(21,26)* and preeclampsia *(17,21,26)*. However, with the possible exception of delivery by caesarian section, none of the individual risk factors (predictors of VTE) mentioned previously can be considered strong enough to influence management decisions about anticoagulant prophylaxis during pregnancy and the puerperium. The influence of a past personal history of VTE on the risk of further thrombotic events in subsequent pregnancies and, therefore, the need for prophylactic therapy in this setting will be discussed below in the section "Risk of Pregnancy-Related VTE in Women With Prior VTE".

PATHOGENESIS

VTE is a multifactorial disease, with thrombosis normally resulting from the interplay of separate predisposing conditions *(28)*. The same is likely to be true for pregnancy-related VTE, in which all three of Virchow's triad of risk factors, namely hypercoagulability, venous stasis, and vascular damage, are potentially present. Hemostatic changes that occur during normal pregnancy in preparation for delivery result in a prothrombotic state *(29)*. Increased levels of procoagulant factors, such as factor VIII, fibrinogen, and von Willebrand factor *(30,31)*; decreased levels of anticoagulant proteins such as protein S *(31,32)*; and a reduction in fibrinolytic activity, at least in part due to increased levels of the plasminogen activator inhibitors PAI-1 and PAI-2 *(33,34)*, all contribute to the hypercoagulable state. Venous stasis is also thought to be a significant contributing factor to the development of pregnancy-related VTE. Direct mechanical obstruction of the pelvic veins, by both the gravid uterus and fetal head, is likely to be the main contributing cause to the reduction in flow, and it has been demonstrated that the inferior vena cava may be almost completely compressed by the gravid uterus in late pregnancy *(35)*. Compression of the left common iliac vein where it crosses the right common iliac artery is exaggerated during pregnancy *(36)*. Finally, vascular injury to the pelvic veins may occur as a direct result of trauma during normal vaginal or operative delivery *(7)*, and it has been suggested that the venous distension associated with pregnancy may also lead to endothelial injury *(37)*, resulting in prothrombotic changes on the endothelial surface.

THROMBOPHILIA AND PREGNANCY-RELATED VTE

Thrombophilia (*see* Chapter 15) is defined as an increased tendency to develop thrombosis, which may be either acquired or inherited. Thrombophilic conditions predisposing to venous thrombosis vary in prevalence and in the magnitude of the associated increase in risk of VTE.

Antithrombin (AT), Protein C (PC), and Protein S (PS) Deficiency

There is significant variation in estimates of the risk of pregnancy-related VTE in women with inherited deficiencies of the natural anticoagulants, likely due to differences in study inclusion criteria (Table 3). Early family cohort studies suggested that the risk of developing VTE during pregnancy and the puerperium ranged from 35 to 70% for women with AT deficiency, 13 to 20% for PC deficiency, and 13 to 27% for PS deficiency *(38–41)*. However, the inclusion of propositi and individuals with VTE prior to pregnancy, along with the failure to confirm VTE using accurate testing, makes it likely that the risk of VTE was overestimated. This is supported by a subsequent study, which reported rates of pregnancy-related VTE of 3, 2, and 7%, for women with AT, PC, and PS deficiency,

Table 3
Cohort Studies Examining Risk of Pregnancy-Related VTE
in Women With Inherited Natural Anticoagulant Deficiency States

| | | (VTE [n] / Pregnancies [n] [%], Antepartum VTE [n] / Postpartum VTE [n]) | | |
Study	Included subjects	Antithrombin deficiency	Protein C deficiency	Protein S deficiency
Hellgren (38)	Propositi and relatives Prior VTE included	32/47 (66%), 24/8	–	–
Conard (39)	Propositi and relatives Prior VTE included	18/50 (36%), 7/11	15/74 (20%), 3/12	4/31 (13%), 0/4
De Stefano (40)	Propositi and relatives Prior VTE included	21/54 (39%), 6/13[a]	6/48 (13%), 1/5	3/22 (14%), 0/3
Pabinger (41)	Propositi and relatives Prior VTE included	21/45 (46%), 18/3	9/60 (15%), 6/3	19/71 (27%), 4/15
Friederich (42)	Relatives only No prior VTE 1/33	1/33 (3.0%), 1/0	1/60 (2.0%), 1/0	5/76 (7%), 0/5
Van Boven (43)	Relatives only No prior event	4/28 (14%), 0/4	–	–
	Prior event	6/10 (60%), 2/4	–	–

[a]The timing of two episodes of VTE in this study was unknown. VTE, venous thromboembolism.

respectively (42). In another study, the rate of pregnancy-related VTE in women with AT deficiency and no previous thrombosis was 14% (all postpartum), in comparison to a rate of 60% in those with a prior episode of VTE (43). It is likely, therefore, that women with a natural coagulation inhibitor deficiency and a personal history of VTE have a high risk of developing VTE during pregnancy. On the other hand, the increase in VTE risk in women without a past history of thrombosis is less well defined because of the low population prevalence of these thrombophilias. In a case-control study enrolling unselected patients (including individuals with VTE prior to pregnancy), Martinelli found the relative risk of a first episode of VTE during pregnancy for women with AT, PC, or PS deficiency grouped together to be 13.1 (95% confidence interval [CI] 5.0–34.2) (44). When examined specifically in case-control studies, AT deficiency has been associated with a 10- to 282-fold increase in the risk of pregnancy-related VTE (45–47).

Factor V Leiden (FVL) Mutation

An early study of individuals with a history of pregnancy-related VTE found 59% of women to have abnormal activated protein C (APC) resistance (48). Subsequent case-series, which used genotyping to confirm the diagnosis, found the prevalence of FVL heterozygosity to range from 20 to 78% (49–51). Estimates of the magnitude of the increase in risk of pregnancy-related VTE associated with FVL heterozygosity come from case–control studies. Most studies used age-matched women with a history of uneventful pregnancies as controls (44,52,53), although nulliparous women were included as controls in one study (47), and the odds ratio was calculated from the known population prevalence of the FVL mutation in another (45). In general, the odds ratios ranged from 4.5 to 16.3 (Table 4). Given the assumed incidence of 1 episode of VTE in 1000 pregnancies in the general population, these estimates correlate well with the observed incidence (1–3%) of pregnancy-related VTE in FVL heterozygotes in retrospective population

Table 4
Case–Control Studies Examining the Risk of Pregnancy-Related
VTE in Women With the Factor V Leiden or Prothrombin Gene Mutations

Thrombophilia study	Cases Carriers [n]/ Total [n] (%)	Controls Carriers [n]/ Total [n] (%)	Odds ratio OR (95% CI)
Factor V Leiden			
Grandone (52)	10/42 (23.8%)	4/213 (1.9%)	16.3 (4.8–54.9)
Gerhardt (47)	52/119 (43.7%)	18/233 (7.7%)	9.0 (4.7–17.4)
McColl (45)	7/75 (9.3%)	5/224 (2.2%)	4.5 (2.1–14.5)
Martinelli (44)	22/119 (18.5%)	6/232 (2.6%)	10.6 (5.6–20.4)
Yilmazer (53)	7/35 (20%)	0/32	–
Prothrombin Gene			
Grandone (52)	13/42 (31.0%)	9/213 (4.2%)	10.2 (4.0–25.9)
Gerhardt (47)	20/118 (16.9%)	3/226 (1.3%)	10.8 (2.9–40.3)
McColl (45)	5/55 (9.1%)	5/224 (2.2%)	4.4 (1.2–16)
Martinelli (44)	7/119 (5.9%)	7/232 (3.0)	2.9 (1.0–8.6)
Yilmazer (53)	2/35 (5.7%)	0/32	–

or family cohort studies (Table 5) (54–57). To date, prospective studies of FVL heterozygotes have included only small numbers of pregnancies and report incidences of pregnancy-related VTE ranging from 0 to 17% (Table 5) (58–60).

Fewer studies have examined the risk of pregnancy-related VTE in women homozygous for the FVL mutation (Table 5). In studies in which individuals were identified as a result of either a family or personal history of thrombosis, the incidence of pregnancy-related VTE ranged from 7 to 17% (58,61–63), although the CIs surrounding these estimates were wide. In a single prospective study of 18 homozygotes identified by population screening, no episodes of VTE were documented during pregnancy or the postpartum period (64). Overall, the risk of pregnancy-related VTE in FVL homozygous women with a personal or family history of VTE appears to be approx 10%, whereas the risk is probably lower in women identified incidentally.

Prothrombin (G20210A) Gene Mutation

There have been no prospective studies examining the incidence of pregnancy-related VTE in women carrying the PGM mutation. Case-control studies, comparing prothrombin gene mutation (PGM) heterozygotes with healthy women, have reported odds ratios for pregnancy-related VTE ranging from 2.9 to 10.8 (Table 4) (44,47,52,53). Using these data and the incidence of pregnancy-related VTE in the general population of 1 per 1000 pregnancies, a conservative estimate of the incidence of pregnancy-related VTE in PGM heterozygotes would be in the magnitude of 0.5%.

FVL/PGM Compound Heterozygotes

Given the high community prevalence of both the FVL and PGM mutations, compound heterozygosity for both conditions is not uncommon, with an expected prevalence of 1 per 1000 in Caucasian populations (65). Two retrospective cohort studies reported the incidence of pregnancy-related VTE to be 4 and 13.5%, respectively, in double heterozygotes without prior VTE (61,66), whereas the estimated risk from a case–control study was 5% (67).

Table 5
Cohort Studies Examining VTE Risk
During Pregnancy in Patients With the Factor V Leiden Mutation

Study	Methodology/Population	FVL + women VTE [n] / Deliveries [n] (%)	FVL – women VTE [n] / Deliveries [n] (%)
Heterozygotes			
Middeldorp (55)	Retrospective, family cohort	5/235 (2.1%)	0/188 (0%)
Simioni (57)	Retrospective, family cohort	3/157 (1.9%)	0/93 (0%)
Tormene (56)	Retrospective, family cohort	6/242 (2.5%)	1/215 (0.46%)
Lindqvist (64)	Prospective, population-based	3/270 (1.1%)	3/2210 (0.14%)
Middeldorp (58)	Prospective, family cohort	0/17 (0.0%)	–
Simioni (59)	Prospective, family cohort	2/12 (17%)	0/3 (0%)
Murphy (60)	Prospective, population-based	0/16 (0%)	0/572 (0%)
Homozygotes			
Lindqvist (64)	Prospective, population-based	0/18 (0%)	3/2210 (0.14%)
Middeldorp (62)	Retrospective, family cohort	4/24 (17%)	–
Martinelli (61)	Retrospective, family cohort	3/19 (16%)	1/182 (0.5%)
Tormene (56)	Retrospective, family cohort	1/14 (7.1%)	–
Procare group (63)	Retrospective cohort	(12%)	–

Acquired Thrombophilia

The antiphospholipid antibody syndrome is defined by the presence of persistent anti-phospholipid antibodies (APLA; either a lupus anticoagulant, also termed a nonspecific inhibitor, or anticardiolipin antibody) in combination with a characteristic clinical feature, such as venous thrombosis (68). Approximately 1 to 5% of healthy control subjects will have APLA (68), and the prevalence of APLA positivity during pregnancy is similar (69–71). The risk of an initial thrombotic event in APLA-positive individuals, either during or outside of pregnancy, is unknown, but it is probably low. Therefore, primary prophylaxis is not routinely recommended in this population. In contrast, the presence of APLA is felt to be associated with a high risk of recurrent VTE after an initial event and is usually an indication for long-term anticoagulation (72). Therefore, despite the lack of data on the absolute risk of recurrent VTE during pregnancy in the absence of prophylaxis, most women receive prophylaxis during the antepartum and postpartum period.

RISK OF PREGNANCY-RELATED VTE IN WOMEN WITH PRIOR VTE

Individuals with a prior history of VTE are at increased risk of future episodes of venous thrombosis in comparison to individuals lacking such a history, with the magnitude of the increase influenced by whether the initial episode was unprovoked or associated with an identifiable transient or permanent risk factor (73). Controversy has existed with regard to the magnitude of risk during pregnancy in women with a prior episode of VTE, with estimates from early studies ranging 0 to 13% (74–77). These studies, however, had methodological limitations, including patient selection, a lack of objective diagnosis of thrombotic events, and small sample sizes.

To provide a more accurate estimate of risk, Brill-Edwards and colleagues performed a prospective trial that enrolled 125 pregnant women with a prior single episode of VTE.

All women had antepartum prophylaxis withheld and received postpartum prophylaxis for 4 to 6 wk *(78)*. Three women had a recurrent event antepartum (2.4%, 95% CI 0.2 to 6.9%) and three were diagnosed with recurrent VTE postpartum. Of the women enrolled in the study, 95 underwent thrombophilia testing, and when the subgroup data were analyzed, it was found that no recurrent events in occurred in the 44 women with negative thrombophilia testing and a temporary risk factor (including pregnancy) at the time of the initial event. In comparison, women with abnormal thrombophilia testing or a prior idiopathic event had an antepartum risk of recurrentce of 5.9% (95% CI, 1.2 to 16%). In a subsequently published retrospective series of women with prior VTE and various thrombophilic conditions, antepartum recurrence was reported in 25% of pregnancies during which anticoagulant prophylaxis was not given *(79)*. Thus, although women with prior VTE have a higher risk of recurrence during pregnancy than outside of pregnancy *(80)*, the magnitude of the risk in women with a temporary risk factor and no thrombophilia does not appear to justify routine antepartum prophylaxis.

DIAGNOSIS OF PE DURING PREGNANCY

In both pregnant and nonpregnant patients, the diagnosis of PE is complicated by the fact that no individual symptom or sign is unique to either disorder or invariably found in the presence of confirmed disease *(81)* *(see also* Chapter 1). This is reflected by the low incidence (10%) of objectively confirmed VTE in patients in whom it is clinically suspected *(82)*. In a cohort study of pregnant women with suspected PE, the prevalence of confirmed disease was even lower, with only 5% of women having the diagnosis of PE objectively documented *(15)*. A possible explanation is that symptoms of chest pain and shortness of breath are common during pregnancy.

Because of the previously described problems with the clinical diagnosis of VTE, accurate diagnostic testing is required to confirm or refute a suspected diagnosis. To date, diagnostic strategies that incorporate clinical assessment, diagnostic imaging, and laboratory testing have not yet been validated in pregnant women. Therefore, the recommendations in the following section remain largely empirical.

Fetal Risk Associated With Diagnostic Imaging

The potential risk associated with exposure of the fetus ionizing radiation is an additional concern when performing diagnostic tests in pregnant women. Ginsberg and colleagues calculated that, if maximal precautions are taken, fetal radiation exposure is less than 500 µGy for pulmonary angiography by the brachial route, and less than 120 µGy with low-dose perfusion lung scanning *(83)*. The same authors concluded that radiation exposure *in utero* of up to 5 rads (0.05 Gy) was associated with, at maximum, a twofold increase in risk of childhood malignancy and a slight increase in minor congenital eye abnormalities. Further evidence for the safety of diagnostic imaging for PE in pregnant women comes from a prospective study of women undergoing ventilation-perfusion (V/Q) scan during pregnancy, in which no increase of congenital or developmental anomalies was observed in the 110 live offspring delivered *(15)*. Therefore, with appropriate precautions, the fetal risk associated with the previously described diagnostic imaging tests appears to be minimal. Against this risk should be balanced the possibility of significant maternal and fetal morbidity or mortality from a missed diagnosis of venous thrombosis, and the potential side effects of unnecessary anticoagulant therapy if empiric treatment is given in the absence of PE.

Spiral computerized tomography (CT) is increasingly being used in the diagnosis of PE *(84)*. Although fetal dose exposure with a modern helical CT (HCT) scanner appears to be less than with lung scanning *(85)*, maternal radiation exposure with this technique is likely to be greater. It has been suggested that the maternal radiation dose with thoracic CT scanning may be equivalent to between 40 and 400 chest X-rays, depending on patient size, type of CT scanner, and the imaging protocol used *(86)*.

Nonspecificity of D-Dimer Testing During Pregnancy

D-dimer levels rise progressively during normal pregnancy from the second trimester onwards, with higher levels seen in patients with complications of pregnancy, such as placental abruption and preeclampsia *(87,88)*. Therefore, although a negative D-dimer result during pregnancy may still be helpful in excluding acute PE, an increased rate of false-positive results will limit the clinical utility of D-dimer testing during pregnancy. It is possible that establishment of different cut-off values specific for pregnancy may reduce this problem *(89)*. At present, D-dimer testing has not been validated for use in the pregnant population.

Confirmation of Suspected PE in Pregnancy

As is the case in nonpregnant patients, acute onset or progressive shortness of breath, hemoptysis, or pleuritic chest pain should lead to a clinical suspicion of PE. Shortness of breath and chest pain, however, are common symptoms in pregnant women *(90)*. Clinical prediction rules for stratifying the pretest probability (PTP) of PE have been validated in nonpregnant individuals *(82,91)* (*see* Chapter 1), but the accuracy of empirical or structured assessment of PTP has not yet been evaluated in pregnant women.

V/Q Lung Scanning

V/Q lung scan remains widely used in the diagnosis of PE in nonpregnant patients, although use of spiral CT as the primary diagnostic test is increasing *(92)*. In a retrospective cohort study, high probability scans were seen in less than 2% of pregnant women (compared with 10–15% of the nonpregnant population), nondiagnostic scans in 20% (vs 50–70% in nonpregnant patients), and normal scans in nearly 75% of cases (as opposed to 10–30% in nonpregnant individuals) *(15,93,94)*. In this study, no woman with either normal or nondiagnostic scan results was reported to have VTE events during a mean follow-up period of 26 mo.

CT

The introduction of HCT has resulted in widespread use of CT pulmonary angiography (CTPA) as the primary diagnostic test for PE. Pregnant women were excluded from studies validating the use of CTPA. Therefore, in the absence of supportive data, CTPA should only be used to diagnose PE during pregnancy in the context of a clinical trial or when alternative diagnostic tests are either not available or have been inconclusive.

Imaging for DVT

In nonpregnant patients with acute PE, venographic evidence of DVT is found in approx 70% of cases, and 50% of patients will have proximal DVT detectable by compression ultrasound (CUS) *(95)*. Limited data exist on the accuracy and safety of CUS for diagnosis of DVT during pregnancy. In a small pilot study of pregnant women with suspected DVT, negative serial CUS appeared to safely exclude DVT *(96)*, and as CUS does not

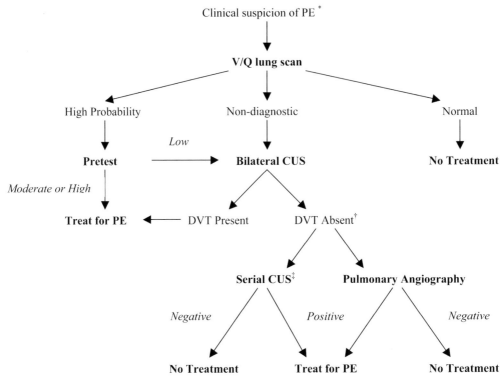

Fig. 1. Proposed diagnostic algorithm for suspected PE during pregnancy. V/Q denotes ventilation-perfusion lung scan; CUS, compression ultrasound. *Pretest probability of PE should be determined at presentation. [†]*See* text for discussion regarding the choice of serial CUS vs pulmonary angiography. [‡]Spiral CT may be performed prior to serial CUS in patients with a nondiagnostic V/Q scan.

involve exposure to ionizing radiation, some experts have advocated its use as the initial test in pregnant patients presenting with suspected PE.

Proposed Algorithm for Diagnosis of PE in Pregnancy

A proposed algorithm for diagnosis of PE during pregnancy is presented in Fig. 1. Careful clinical assessment and a chest X-ray should be initially performed to help exclude alternative diagnoses. Although structured clinical prediction rules have not been validated in pregnant populations, it is likely that experienced clinicians' gestalt provides a reasonable assessment of clinical probability in pregnant subjects, as is the case in nonpregnant individuals *(97)*.

It is recommended that V/Q scanning be performed as the initial imaging test, as a high percentage of women will have a normal perfusion lung scan, allowing PE to be safely excluded. Women with a high-probability lung scan and high or moderate clinical (pretest) probability should be treated for PE. Because the frequency of proven PE in nonpregnant women with a low clinical probability and a high-probability scan is modest, when this combination of findings occurs, further investigation is suggested. In women with a nondiagnostic V/Q scan, bilateral CUS should be performed and treatment commenced if DVT is found. If the initial CUS is normal, serial CUS repeated on days 6–8 and 12–14 (an approach that has been validated in nonpregnant subjects), CT angiography, or conventional pulmonary angiography is recommended.

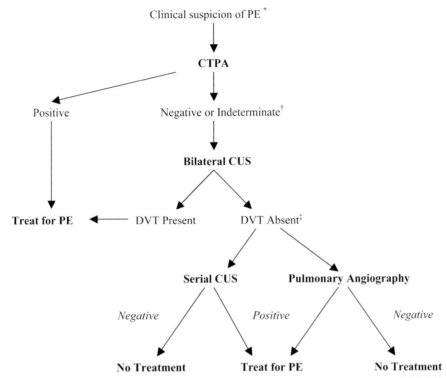

Fig. 2. Proposed diagnostic algorithm for suspected PE in pregnancy using CT as the initial diagnostic test. CTPA denotes computed tomographic pulmonary angiography; CUS, compression ultrasound. *Pretest probability of PE should be determined at presentation. [†]Additional testing should be considered if isolated subsegmental embolus is found in low pretest probability patients, as the positive predictive value of this finding is low. [‡]*See* text for discussion regarding choice of serial CUS vs pulmonary angiography. [¶]Ventilation-perfusion scan can be performed prior to serial CUS.

As many centers are currently using CTPA as the initial diagnostic test for suspected PE during pregnancy, an algorithm using this approach is presented in Fig. 2. Alternatively, some physicians have suggested that bilateral CUS be performed as the initial diagnostic test, with V/Q scanning or CTPA performed only if CUS is negative. This latter approach has the advantage of avoiding radiation exposure in several cases.

ANTICOAGULATION
FOR VTE DURING PREGNANCY

Randomized controlled trials examining the efficacy and safety of anticoagulants for the treatment and prevention of VTE have, as a rule, excluded pregnant women. As a result, much of the information presented in the following section is either extrapolated from trials in nonpregnant patients or is derived from small observational studies in pregnant women. Drugs studied for the treatment of VTE include unfractionated heparin (UFH), low-molecular-weight heparins (LMWHs), and the pentasaccharide fondaparinux, the heparinoid danaparoid, warfarin and other coumarin derivatives, and, more recently, direct thrombin inhibitors. The direct thrombin inhibitors, which cross the placenta, and fondaparinux, for which limited data exist in pregnant patients and which may also cross the placenta in small amounts *(98)*, will not be discussed further.

Fetal Complications of Anticoagulant Therapy During Pregnancy

Studies have shown that neither UFH *(99)* nor LMWH *(100,101)* cross the placenta during pregnancy. Both a retrospective cohort study *(102)* and a comprehensive literature review *(103)* reported no significant increase in the risk of serious adverse fetal outcomes following maternal treatment with UFH during pregnancy. Observational studies, in which treatment with either prophylactic- or therapeutic-dose LMWH did not appear to increase the rate of adverse fetal outcomes, further support the safety of LMWH during pregnancy *(104–110)*. Danaparoid is a glycosaminoglycan antithrombotic agent often used as an alternative anticoagulant in patients with heparin-induced thrombocytopenia (*see* "Non-Hemorrhagic Complications of Maternal Anticoagulation) *(111)*. Limited data suggest that danaparoid does not cross the placenta and appears to be a safe anticoagulant for use during pregnancy *(112)*. In contrast, warfarin and other coumarin derivatives cross the placenta and are known to be teratogenic *(113)*. Warfarin exposure in the first trimester of pregnancy can result in a characteristic embryopathy with clinical features of nasal hypoplasia, stippled epiphyses, and extremity shortening *(114)*. A recent systematic review reported the prevalence of congenital fetal anomalies in live births to be 11.1% when warfarin exposure had occurred between week 6 and 12 of pregnancy, in comparison to 0% if exposure was outside this time period, suggesting that the risk of embropathy is minimal if warfarin is not given between weeks 6 to 12 of gestation *(115)*. Central nervous system abnormalities, although rare, have been reported to occur with warfarin exposure in the second and third trimesters *(114)*. Increased rates of spontaneous abortion have also been reported with warfarin *(114,115)*, and neonatal hemorrhage may complicate warfarin exposure close to the time of delivery *(116)*.

Because of these safety issues, UFH or LMWH are preferred to coumarin derivatives for treatment and prevention of VTE during pregnancy *(117)*. On the other hand, neither warfarin nor heparin-related anticoagulants appear to be secreted in breast milk in significant amounts; therefore, these agents can be safely given to nursing mothers *(117–119)*.

Maternal Complications of Anticoagulant Therapy During Pregnancy

HEMORRHAGIC COMPLICATIONS

In a retrospective study of 100 pregnant women receiving UFH in prophylactic or therapeutic dosage, the reported rate of significant bleeding was 2% *(102)*, similar to that observed in nonpregnant patients receiving long-term UFH *(120)*. In a review of 486 pregnancies during which therapy with LMWH was given predominantly in prophylactic doses, no episodes of clinically important bleeding were recorded *(104)*. In a subsequent study, 11 episodes of serious bleeding occurred in 624 pregnancies during which either prophylactic or therapeutic dosages of enoxaparin were used (1.8%), although only 1 episode was judged to be related to anticoagulant therapy *(110)*. Therefore, from the limited data available, the risk of heparin-related maternal bleeding during pregnancy appears to be low *(121)*.

NONHEMORRHAGIC COMPLICATIONS

Long-term UFH may result in loss of bone density when administered for longer than 1 mo because of decreased rates of bone formation accompanied by increased bone resorption *(122)*. In prospective studies, 30% of women receiving long-term UFH during pregnancy had a significant reduction in lumbar spine bone mineral density (BMD) *(123, 124)*, and symptomatic vertebral fracture occurred in 2.2% of a series of 184 women receiv-

Table 6
Therapeutic and Prophylactic
Low-Molecular-Weight Heparin Regimens

Drug	Dosing regime[a]
Therapeutic	
Dalteparin	100 U/kg every 12 h; or 200 U/kg once daily
Enoxaparin	1 mg/kg every 12 h; or 1.5 mg/kg once daily
Tinzaparin	175 U/kg once daily
Prophylactic	
Dalteparin	5000 U once daily
Enoxaparin	40 mg once daily; or 30 mg twice daily
Tinzaparin	4500 U once daily

[a]All dosing regimens are administered by subcutaneous injection.

ing UFH twice daily throughout pregnancy (125). Importantly, evidence is accumulating that the risk of osteoporosis is much lower with prolonged LMWH than with UFH therapy (126,127). A prospective study of 55 patients treated with low-dose LMWH throughout pregnancy found bone loss was not significantly different from the physiological losses seen in normal pregnancy (128).

Heparin-induced thrombocytopenia (HIT) is a rare but potentially fatal syndrome, consisting of characteristic clinical events and concurrent detection of antibodies to heparin and platelet factor 4 in the setting of recent heparin therapy (129). The incidence of HIT with LMWH therapy appears to be less than with UFH (130), but accurate estimates of the frequency of HIT in pregnant women receiving either UFH or LMWH are not available at present. Use of danaparoid sodium is recommended for treatment of HIT during pregnancy, as it is an effective antithrombotic that does not cross the placenta (117,131) and, unlike LMWH, has low crossreactivity with UFH.

Recommended Treatment of Acute VTE During Pregnancy

Either LMWH or UFH should be used for treatment of VTE during pregnancy. Evidence for the efficacy of either agent for treatment of VTE during pregnancy is largely extrapolated from studies involving nonpregnant patients. LMWH is the preferred anticoagulant in most patients with PE during pregnancy (117) because of a more predictable anticoagulant response to weight-based therapy (132) and lower rates of associated HIT and osteoporosis. Although there has been some debate (133), the data presented previously support, in our opinion, LMWH therapy as being safe for both mother and fetus. A number of LMWH preparations are available, and although insufficient data exist to compare their efficacy and safety (121), use of any of the weight-adjusted regimens shown in Table 6 is reasonable. Although once-daily dosing has been found to be effective in nonpregnant patients, twice-daily dosing is recommended for treatment of acute VTE in pregnant women because of increased clearance of LMWH during pregnancy (117,134). Many women will gain weight throughout pregnancy, and the increased volume of drug distribution may alter plasma LMWH levels. Although some pharmacokinetic studies have shown LMWH activity, as measured by antifactor Xa assays, to decrease during pregnancy with fixed-dose LMWH therapy (135), the clinical importance of this observation is unclear. Nonetheless, it has been suggested that, when therapeutic doses of LMWH are given during pregnancy, either: (1) intermittent dose adjustment according to weight;

or (2) regular (monthly) antifactor Xa level monitoring should be performed, with the sample taken 4 h after the morning dose. The dose of LMWH should be adjusted to maintain an anti-Xa level of 0.5–1.2 U/mL if a twice-daily dosing regimen is being used, or 1.0–2.0 U/mL if a once-daily regimen is adopted (117). However, the data currently available cannot support firm recommendations with regard to dose adjustment of LMWH during pregnancy (105,136).

In individuals with extensive iliofemoral DVT, or extensive PE accompanied by right ventricular dysfunction, and in those at high risk of bleeding complications, initial use of adjusted-dose intravenous UFH may be preferred. The response of the activated partial thromboplastin time (APTT) to UFH in pregnancy is often attenuated because of increased factor VIII and heparin-binding protein levels; therefore, higher plasma heparin levels are required to obtain APTT results within the therapeutic range (137). If high doses of UFH are required to obtain "therapeutic" APTT results, adjustment of UFH dose according to anti-Xa heparin levels, rather than APTT, is appropriate. When either short- or long-term subcutaneous UFH is given, a starting regimen of at least 17,500 U every 12 h is recommended. The APTT should be checked 6 h after dose at least every 1 to 2 wk, and the heparin dose should be adjusted to maintain the levels within the therapeutic range (117).

MANAGEMENT OF PE DURING PREGNANCY: SPECIFIC ASPECTS

Thrombolysis in Pregnancy

No data exist on the use of thrombolytic therapy during pregnancy and concern exists with regards to the risk of fetal and maternal bleeding during the antepartum and immediate postpartum period. A small number of case reports have reported successful outcomes following thrombolytic therapy in women presenting with circulatory compromise due to massive PE either during pregnancy (138–140) or in the immediate postpartum period (141).

Management of Pregnant Women With an Increased Risk of VTE

As discussed, it is possible to identify women with an increased risk of pregnancy-related VTE due to either a personal history of venous thrombosis or the presence of an inherited or acquired thrombophilia. The threshold for recommending postpartum prophylaxis is lower than that for antepartum therapy because of the shorter length of required treatment, the increased average daily risk of VTE during the postpartum period, and the ability to use oral warfarin therapy during this period. LMWH is usually used for antepartum prophylaxis, and suggested regimens that have been associated with low rates of thrombosis in uncontrolled trials are shown in Table 6. Postpartum prophylaxis is given for 4 to 6 wk and consists of either LMWH or warfarin with a target international normalized ratio of 2.0 to 3.0. The following recommendations for prophylaxis during pregnancy are in accordance with the recent American College of Chest Physicians guidelines (117).

WOMEN WITH A PRIOR EPISODE OF VTE

In case of prior VTE related to a *transient risk factor* and without inherited thrombophilia, antepartum clinical surveillance will suffice, but it should be followed by postpartum anticoagulation. Consider antepartum prophylaxis if the transient risk factor was pregnancy or an estrogen-containing medication, or if additional risk factors (such as obesity) are present.

In case of *prior unprovoked VTE*, and/or if *inherited thrombophilia* is present, both antepartum prophylaxis with LMWH and postpartum prophylaxis are recommended. Some authors have suggested that women with AT deficiency, FVL homozygotes, FVL/ prothrombin gene mutation compound heterozygotes, or women with a history of multiple episodes of VTE should receive an intermediate-dose LMWH regimen (e.g., dalteparin 5000 U subcutaneously every 12 h or enoxaparin 40 mg subcutaneously every 12 h).

If there is a history of prior VTE in the setting of the *antiphospholipid antibody* syndrome, most of these women will be on long-term anticoagulation anyway, and they should be treated with full-dose anticoagulation during both the antepartum and the postpartum period.

WOMEN WITH INHERITED THROMBOPHILIA BUT NO PRIOR HISTORY OF VTE

The risk of pregnancy-related VTE is dependent on the type of thrombophilia and whether the patient is heterozygous or homozygous for the underlying condition. A history of prior adverse pregnancy outcomes (e.g., pregnancy loss, placental abruption, preeclampsia) may also influence the decision to administer antepartum prophylactic anticoagulation.

In *AT-deficient women, FVL/prothrombin gene mutation compound heterozygotes*, or *FVL homozygotes*, antepartum prophylaxis with LMWH and postpartum prophylaxis are recommended. In FVL homozygotes who lack a personal or family history of VTE, postpartum prophylaxis alone may be reasonable *(64)* after consideration of other individual risk factors and patient preference.

In *FVL heterozygotes*, and in women with *(isolated) prothrombin gene mutation, PC deficiency, or PS deficiency*, antepartum clinical surveillance will suffice, but it should be followed by postpartum anticoagulation. This recommendation is based on a low risk of antepartum VTE without prophylaxis weighed against the risks and inconvenience of antepartum prophylaxis.

Management of Women
on Long-Term Anticoagulant Therapy Prior to Pregnancy

As previously discussed, the risk of fetal complications is minimal with warfarin exposure prior to 6 wk gestation. Therefore, continued use of warfarin during attempted conception, until the pregnancy test becomes positive, is reasonable, provided that the patient is reliable and frequent pregnancy testing is indeed performed. On the other hand, some women will be unwilling to accept any risk of embryopathy and will prefer to switch from warfarin to LMWH prior to attempting conception. The benefits and risks of either approach should be discussed openly with the patients.

Anticoagulant Therapy at the Time of Delivery

Ideally, women who are receiving anticoagulant therapy should undergo elective induction of labor to minimize both the risk of spontaneous delivery (including that associated with neuroaxial anesthesia) and the duration of time during which recurrent VTE may occur while anticoagulation is interrupted. Extended prolongation of the APTT can occur with use of subcutaneous UFH in pregnancy, and it is recommended that therapeutic subcutaneous UFH be discontinued at least 24 h prior to induction of labor. The same approach should be followed women receiving therapeutic LMWH.

In women who develop VTE within 2 to 4 wk of expected delivery, the risk of recurrent VTE off anticoagulant therapy is high. In these cases, it is recommended that therapeutic intravenous UFH be commenced in place of LMWH and ceased 4–6 h prior to the expected time of delivery, and consideration should be given to the insertion of a temporary inferior vena cava filter. If the delivery is uncomplicated, UFH or LMWH can be restarted in prophylactic doses, along with warfarin, in the same evening or on the day following delivery. Anticoagulation should not be restarted within 3 h of epidural removal. Anticoagulant therapy is normally continued for at least 4 to 6 wk following delivery, or for a total duration of at least 3 mo when VTE occurs late in pregnancy.

FUTURE DIRECTIONS

Prevention of pregnancy-related VTE is an issue that requires continued effort. There is a need for properly designed prospective trials to determine optimum management of both previously symptomatic and asymptomatic women with thrombophilia, and because of the number of patients required, international collaboration will be necessary to make such trials feasible. Improvements in diagnostic tools such as CT and magnetic resonance venography are likely to have an impact on the diagnosis of VTE, and will require adequate assessment in the pregnant population. Finally, alternative anticoagulant agents are likely to become available over the next 10 yr, and evaluation of the efficacy and safety of these agents for treatment during pregnancy will be required.

REFERENCES

1. Weindling AM. The confidential enquiry into maternal and child health (CEMACH). Arch Dis Child 2003;88:1034–1037.
2. Confidential Enquiry into Maternal and Child Health. Why Mothers Die 2000–2002: The Sixth Report of the Confidential Enquiries into Maternal Death in the United Kingdom. RCOG Press, London, 2004.
3. Franks AL, Atrash HK, Lawson HW, Colberg KS. Obstetrical pulmonary embolism mortality, United States, 1970-85. Am J Public Health 1990;80:720–722.
4. Atrash HK, Koonin LM, Lawson HW, et al. Maternal mortality in the United States, 1979–1986. Obstet Gynecol 1990;76:1055–1060.
5. Berg CJ, Atrash HK, Koonin LM, Tucker M. Pregnancy-related mortality in the United States, 1987–1990. Obstet Gynecol 1996;88:161–167.
6. Chang J, Elam-Evans LD, Berg CJ, et al. Pregnancy-related mortality surveillance—United States, 1991–1999. MMWR Surveill Summ 2003;52:1–8.
7. Greer IA. Thrombosis in pregnancy: maternal and fetal issues. Lancet 1999;353:1258–1265.
8. Anderson FA Jr, Wheeler HB, Goldberg RJ, et al. A population-based perspective of the hospital incidence and case-fatality rates of deep vein thrombosis and pulmonary embolism. The Worcester DVT Study. Arch Intern Med 1991;151:933–938.
9. Nordstrom M, Lindblad B, Bergqvist D, Kjellstrom T. A prospective study of the incidence of deep-vein thrombosis within a defined urban population. J Intern Med 1992;232:155–160.
10. Samuelsson E, Hagg S. Incidence of venous thromboembolism in young Swedish women and possibly preventable cases among combined oral contraceptive users. Acta Obstet Gynecol Scand 2004;83: 674–681.
11. Aaro LA, Johnson TR, Juergens JL. Acute deep venous thrombosis associated with pregnancy. Obstet Gynecol 1966;28:553–558.
12. Solomons E. Puerperal thrombophlebitis: prevention and treatment. Postgrad Med 1963;34:105–111.
13. Treffers PE, Huidekoper BL, Weenink GH, Kloosterman GJ. Epidemiological observations of thromboembolic disease during pregnancy and in the puerperium, in 56,022 women. Int J Gynaecol Obstet 1983; 21:327–331.
14. Hull RD, Raskob GE, Carter CJ. Serial impedance plethysmography in pregnant patients with clinically suspected deep-vein thrombosis. Clinical validity of negative findings. Ann Intern Med 1990;112: 663–667.
15. Chan WS, Ray JG, Murray S, et al. Suspected pulmonary embolism in pregnancy: clinical presentation, results of lung scanning, and subsequent maternal and pediatric outcomes. Arch Intern Med 2002;162: 1170–1175.

16. Macklon NS, Greer IA. Venous thromboembolic disease in obstetrics and gynaecology: the Scottish experience. Scott Med J 1996;41:83–86.
17. Lindqvist P, Dahlback B, Marsal K. Thrombotic risk during pregnancy: a population study. Obstet Gynecol 1999;94:595–599.
18. Andersen BS, Steffensen FH, Sorensen HT, et al. The cumulative incidence of venous thromboembolism during pregnancy and puerperium—an 11 year Danish population-based study of 63,300 pregnancies. Acta Obstet Gynecol Scand 1998;77:170–173.
19. McColl MD, Ramsay JE, Tait RC, et al. Risk factors for pregnancy associated venous thromboembolism. Thromb Haemost 1997;78:1183–1188.
20. Gherman RB, Goodwin TM, Leung B, et al. Incidence, clinical characteristics, and timing of objectively diagnosed venous thromboembolism during pregnancy. Obstet Gynecol 1999;94:730–734.
21. Simpson EL, Lawrenson RA, Nightingale AL, Farmer RD. Venous thromboembolism in pregnancy and the puerperium: incidence and additional risk factors from a London perinatal database. BJOG 2001;108:56–60.
22. White RH. The epidemiology of venous thromboembolism. Circulation 2003;107:I4–18.
23. Huisman MV, Buller HR, ten Cate JW, et al. Unexpected high prevalence of silent pulmonary embolism in patients with deep venous thrombosis. Chest 1989;95:498–502.
24. Ray JG, Chan WS. Deep vein thrombosis during pregnancy and the puerperium: a meta-analysis of the period of risk and the leg of presentation. Obstet Gynecol Surv 1999;54:265–271.
25. Stein PD, Hull RD, Kayali F, et al. Venous thromboembolism in pregnancy: 21-year trends. Am J Med 2004;117:121–125.
26. Danilenko-Dixon DR, Heit JA, Silverstein MD, et al. Risk factors for deep vein thrombosis and pulmonary embolism during pregnancy or post partum: a population-based, case-control study. Am J Obstet Gynecol 2001;184:104–110.
27. Bergqvist A, Bergqvist D, Hallbook T. Deep vein thrombosis during pregnancy. A prospective study. Acta Obstet Gynecol Scand 1983;62:443–448.
28. Rosendaal FR. Venous thrombosis: a multicausal disease. Lancet 1999;353:1167–1173.
29. Hellgren M. Hemostasis during normal pregnancy and puerperium. Semin Thromb Hemost 2003;29:125–130.
30. Cerneca F, Ricci G, Simeone R, et al. Coagulation and fibrinolysis changes in normal pregnancy. Increased levels of procoagulants and reduced levels of inhibitors during pregnancy induce a hypercoagulable state, combined with a reactive fibrinolysis. Eur J Obstet Gynecol Reprod Biol 1997;73:31–36.
31. Clark P, Brennand J, Conkie JA, et al. Activated protein C sensitivity, protein C, protein S and coagulation in normal pregnancy. Thromb Haemost 1998;79:1166–1170.
32. Comp PC, Thurnau GR, Welsh J, Esmon CT. Functional and immunologic protein S levels are decreased during pregnancy. Blood 1986;68:881–885.
33. Wright JG, Cooper P, Astedt B, et al. Fibrinolysis during normal human pregnancy: complex interrelationships between plasma levels of tissue plasminogen activator and inhibitors and the euglobulin clot lysis time. Br J Haematol 1988;69:253–258.
34. Kruithof EK, Tran-Thang C, Gudinchet A, et al. Fibrinolysis in pregnancy: a study of plasminogen activator inhibitors. Blood 1987;69:460–466.
35. Kerr MG, Scott DB, Samuel E. Studies of the inferior vena cava in late pregnancy. Br Med J 1964;5382:532–533.
36. Ginsberg JS, Brill-Edwards P, Burrows RF, et al. Venous thrombosis during pregnancy: leg and trimester of presentation. Thromb Haemost 1992;67:519–520.
37. Stewart GJ, Lachman JW, Alburger PD, et al. Venodilation and development of deep vein thrombosis in total hip and knee replacement patients. Thromb Haemost 1987;58:242–245.
38. Hellgren M, Tengborn L, Abildgaard U. Pregnancy in women with congenital antithrombin III deficiency: experience of treatment with heparin and antithrombin. Gynecol Obstet Invest 1982;14:127–141.
39. Conard J, Horellou MH, Van Dreden P, et al. Thrombosis and pregnancy in congenital deficiencies in AT III, protein C or protein S: study of 78 women. Thromb Haemost 1990;63:319–320.
40. De Stefano V, Leone G, Mastrangelo S, et al. Thrombosis during pregnancy and surgery in patients with congenital deficiency of antithrombin III, protein C, protein S. Thromb Haemost 1994;71:799–800.
41. Pabinger I, Schneider B. Thrombotic risk in hereditary antithrombin III, protein C, or protein S deficiency. A cooperative, retrospective study. Gesellschaft fur Thrombose- und Hamostaseforschung (GTH) Study Group on Natural Inhibitors. Arterioscler Thromb Vasc Biol 1996;16:742–748.

42. Friederich PW, Sanson BJ, Simioni P, et al. Frequency of pregnancy-related venous thromboembolism in anticoagulant factor-deficient women: implications for prophylaxis. Ann Intern Med 1996;125:955–960.

43. van Boven HH, Vandenbroucke JP, Briet E, Rosendaal FR. Gene-gene and gene-environment interactions determine risk of thrombosis in families with inherited antithrombin deficiency. Blood 1999;94:2590–2594.

44. Martinelli I, De Stefano V, Taioli E, et al. Inherited thrombophilia and first venous thromboembolism during pregnancy and puerperium. Thromb Haemost 2002;87:791–795.

45. McColl MD, Ellison J, Reid F, et al. Prothrombin 20210 G→A, MTHFR C677T mutations in women with venous thromboembolism associated with pregnancy. BJOG 2000;107:565–569.

46. Greer IA. Inherited thrombophilia and venous thromboembolism. Best Pract Res Clin Obstet Gynaecol 2003;17:413–425.

47. Gerhardt A, Scharf RE, Beckmann MW, et al. Prothrombin and factor V mutations in women with a history of thrombosis during pregnancy and the puerperium. N Engl J Med 2000;342:374–380.

48. Hellgren M, Svensson PJ, Dahlback B. Resistance to activated protein C as a basis for venous thromboembolism associated with pregnancy and oral contraceptives. Am J Obstet Gynecol 1995;173:210–213.

49. Hirsch DR, Mikkola KM, Marks PW, et al. Pulmonary embolism and deep venous thrombosis during pregnancy or oral contraceptive use: prevalence of factor V Leiden. Am Heart J 1996;131:1145–1148.

50. Bokarewa MI, Bremme K, Blomback M. Arg506-Gln mutation in factor V and risk of thrombosis during pregnancy. Br J Haematol 1996;92:473–478.

51. Hallak M, Senderowicz J, Cassel A, et al. Activated protein C resistance (factor V Leiden) associated with thrombosis in pregnancy. Am J Obstet Gynecol 1997;176:889–893.

52. Grandone E, Margaglione M, Colaizzo D, et al. Genetic susceptibility to pregnancy-related venous thromboembolism: roles of factor V Leiden, prothrombin G20210A, and methylenetetrahydrofolate reductase C677T mutations. Am J Obstet Gynecol 1998;179:1324–1328.

53. Yilmazer M, Kurtay G, Sonmezer M, Akar N. Factor V Leiden and prothrombin 20210 G-A mutations in controls and in patients with thromboembolic events during pregnancy or the puerperium. Arch Gynecol Obstet 2003;268:304–308.

54. Lensen RP, Bertina RM, de Ronde H, et al. Venous thrombotic risk in family members of unselected individuals with factor V Leiden. Thromb Haemost 2000;83:817–821.

55. Middeldorp S, Henkens CM, Koopman MM, et al. The incidence of venous thromboembolism in family members of patients with factor V Leiden mutation and venous thrombosis. Ann Intern Med 1998;128:15–20.

56. Tormene D, Simioni P, Prandoni P, et al. Factor V Leiden mutation and the risk of venous thromboembolism in pregnant women. Haematologica 2001;86:1305–1309.

57. Simioni P, Sanson BJ, Prandoni P, et al. Incidence of venous thromboembolism in families with inherited thrombophilia. Thromb Haemost 1999;81:198–202.

58. Middeldorp S, Meinardi JR, Koopman MM, et al. A prospective study of asymptomatic carriers of the factor V Leiden mutation to determine the incidence of venous thromboembolism. Ann Intern Med 2001;135:322–327.

59. Simioni P, Tormene D, Prandoni P, et al. Incidence of venous thromboembolism in asymptomatic family members who are carriers of factor V Leiden: a prospective cohort study. Blood 2002;99:1938–1942.

60. Murphy RP, Donoghue C, Nallen RJ, et al. Prospective evaluation of the risk conferred by factor V Leiden and thermolabile methylenetetrahydrofolate reductase polymorphisms in pregnancy. Arterioscler Thromb Vasc Biol 2000;20:266–270.

61. Martinelli I, Legnani C, Bucciarelli P, et al. Risk of pregnancy-related venous thrombosis in carriers of severe inherited thrombophilia. Thromb Haemost 2001;86:800–803.

62. Middeldorp S, Libourel EJ, Hamulyak K, et al. The risk of pregnancy-related venous thromboembolism in women who are homozygous for factor V Leiden. Br J Haematol 2001;113:553–555.

63. The Procare Group. Risk of venous thromboembolism during pregnancy in homozygous carriers of the factor V Leiden mutation: are there any predictive factors? J Thromb Haemost 2004;2:359–360.

64. Lindqvist PG, Svensson PJ, Marsaal K, et al. Activated protein C resistance (FV:Q506) and pregnancy. Thromb Haemost 1999;81:532–537.

65. Emmerich J, Rosendaal FR, Cattaneo M, et al. Combined effect of factor V Leiden and prothrombin 20210A on the risk of venous thromboembolism—pooled analysis of 8 case-control studies including 2310 cases and 3204 controls. Study Group for Pooled-Analysis in Venous Thromboembolism. Thromb Haemost 2001;86:809–816.

66. Samama MM, Rached RA, Horellou MH, et al. Pregnancy-associated venous thromboembolism (VTE) in combined heterozygous factor V Leiden (FVL) and prothrombin (FII) 20210 A mutation and in heterozygous FII single gene mutation alone. Br J Haematol 2003;123:327–334.

67. Gerhardt A, Scharf RE, Zotz RB. Effect of hemostatic risk factors on the individual probability of thrombosis during pregnancy and the puerperium. Thromb Haemost 2003;90:77–85.

68. Levine JS, Branch DW, Rauch J. The antiphospholipid syndrome. N Engl J Med 2002;346:752–763.

69. Lockwood CJ, Romero R, Feinberg RF, et al. The prevalence and biologic significance of lupus anticoagulant and anticardiolipin antibodies in a general obstetric population. Am J Obstet Gynecol 1989;161:369–373.

70. Perez MC, Wilson WA, Brown HL, Scopelitis E. Anticardiolipin antibodies in unselected pregnant women. Relationship to fetal outcome. J Perinatol 1991;11:33–36.

71. Harris EN, Spinnato JA. Should anticardiolipin tests be performed in otherwise healthy pregnant women? Am J Obstet Gynecol 1991;165:1272–1277.

72. Crowther MA. Anticoagulant therapy for the thrombotic complications of the antiphospholipid antibody syndrome. Thromb Res 2004;114:443–446.

73. Kearon C. Long-term management of patients after venous thromboembolism. Circulation 2004;110:I10–I18.

74. de Swiet M, Floyd E, Letsky E. Low risk of recurrent thromboembolism in pregnancy. Br J Hosp Med 1987;38:264.

75. Badaracco MA, Vessey MP. Recurrence of venous thromboembolic disease and use of oral contraceptives. Br Med J 1974;1:215–217.

76. Howell R, Fidler J, Letsky E, de Swiet M. The risks of antenatal subcutaneous heparin prophylaxis: a controlled trial. Br J Obstet Gynaecol 1983;90:1124–118.

77. Tengborn L, Bergqvist D, Matzsch T, et al. Recurrent thromboembolism in pregnancy and puerperium. Is there a need for thromboprophylaxis? Am J Obstet Gynecol 1989;160:90–94.

78. Brill-Edwards P, Ginsberg JS, Gent M, et al. Safety of withholding heparin in pregnant women with a history of venous thromboembolism. Recurrence of Clot in This Pregnancy Study Group. N Engl J Med 2000;343:1439–1444.

79. Simioni P, Tormene D, Prandoni P, Girolami A. Pregnancy-related recurrent events in thrombophilic women with previous venous thromboembolism. Thromb Haemost 2001;86:929.

80. Pabinger I, Grafenhofer H, Kyrle PA, et al. Temporary increase in the risk for recurrence during pregnancy in women with a history of venous thromboembolism. Blood 2002;100:1060–1062.

81. Bell WR, Simon TL, DeMets DL. The clinical features of submassive and massive pulmonary emboli. Am J Med 1977;62:355–360.

82. Wells PS, Anderson DR, Rodger M, et al. Excluding pulmonary embolism at the bedside without diagnostic imaging: management of patients with suspected pulmonary embolism presenting to the emergency department by using a simple clinical model and d-dimer. Ann Intern Med 2001;135:98–107.

83. Ginsberg JS, Hirsh J, Rainbow AJ, Coates G. Risks to the fetus of radiologic procedures used in the diagnosis of maternal venous thromboembolic disease. Thromb Haemost 1989;61:189–196.

84. Kearon C. Excluding pulmonary embolism with helical (spiral) computed tomography: evidence is catching up with enthusiasm. CMAJ 2003;168:1430–1431.

85. Winer-Muram HT, Boone JM, Brown HL, et al. Pulmonary embolism in pregnant patients: fetal radiation dose with helical CT. Radiology 2002;224:487–492.

86. Diederich S, Lenzen H. Radiation exposure associated with imaging of the chest: comparison of different radiographic and computed tomography techniques. Cancer 2000;89:2457–2460.

87. Bremme K, Ostlund E, Almqvist I, et al. Enhanced thrombin generation and fibrinolytic activity in normal pregnancy and the puerperium. Obstet Gynecol 1992;80:132–137.

88. Nolan TE, Smith RP, Devoe LD. Maternal plasma D-dimer levels in normal and complicated pregnancies. Obstet Gynecol 1993;81:235–238.

89. Morse M. Establishing a normal range for D-dimer levels through pregnancy to aid in the diagnosis of pulmonary embolism and deep vein thrombosis. J Thromb Haemost 2004;2:1202–1204.

90. Milne JA, Howie AD, Pack AI. Dyspnoea during normal pregnancy. Br J Obstet Gynaecol 1978;85:260–263.

91. Kruip MJ, Slob MJ, Schijen JH, et al. Use of a clinical decision rule in combination with D-dimer concentration in diagnostic workup of patients with suspected pulmonary embolism: a prospective management study. Arch Intern Med 2002;162:1631–1635.

92. Stein PD, Hull RD, Ghali WA, et al. Tracking the uptake of evidence: two decades of hospital practice trends for diagnosing deep vein thrombosis and pulmonary embolism. Arch Intern Med 2003;163: 1213–1219.

93. Hull RD, Hirsh J, Carter CJ, et al. Diagnostic value of ventilation-perfusion lung scanning in patients with suspected pulmonary embolism. Chest 1985;88:819–828.

94. The PIOPED Investigators. Value of the ventilation/perfusion scan in acute pulmonary embolism. Results of the prospective investigation of pulmonary embolism diagnosis (PIOPED). The PIOPED Investigators. JAMA 1990;263:2753–2759.

95. Kearon C. Natural history of venous thromboembolism. Circulation 2003;107:I22–I30.

96. Chan WS, Chunilal SD, Lee AY, et al. Diagnosis of deep vein thrombosis during pregnancy: a pilot study evaluating the role of d-dimer and compression leg ultrasound during pregnancy. Blood 2002; 100:275A (abstract).

97. Chunilal SD, Eikelboom JW, Attia J, et al. Does this patient have pulmonary embolism? JAMA 2003; 290:2849–2858.

98. Dempfle CE. Minor transplacental passage of fondaparinux in vivo. N Engl J Med 2004;350:1914–1915.

99. Flessa HC, Kapstrom AB, Glueck HI, Will JJ. Placental transport of heparin. Am J Obstet Gynecol 1965;93:570–573.

100. Forestier F, Daffos F, Capella-Pavlovsky M. Low molecular weight heparin (PK 10169) does not cross the placenta during the second trimester of pregnancy study by direct fetal blood sampling under ultrasound. Thromb Res 1984;34:557–560.

101. Forestier F, Daffos F, Rainaut M, Toulemonde F. Low molecular weight heparin (CY 216) does not cross the placenta during the third trimester of pregnancy. Thromb Haemost 1987;57:234.

102. Ginsberg JS, Kowalchuk G, Hirsh J, et al. Heparin therapy during pregnancy. Risks to the fetus and mother. Arch Intern Med 1989;149:2233–2236.

103. Ginsberg JS, Hirsh J, Turner DC, et al. Risks to the fetus of anticoagulant therapy during pregnancy. Thromb Haemost 1989;61:197–203.

104. Sanson BJ, Lensing AW, Prins MH, et al. Safety of low-molecular-weight heparin in pregnancy: a systematic review. Thromb Haemost 1999;81:668–672.

105. Rodie VA, Thomson AJ, Stewart FM, et al. Low molecular weight heparin for the treatment of venous thromboembolism in pregnancy: a case series. BJOG 2002;109:1020–1024.

106. Sorensen HT, Johnsen SP, Larsen H, et al. Birth outcomes in pregnant women treated with low-molecular-weight heparin. Acta Obstet Gynecol Scand 2000;79:655–659.

107. Ulander VM, Stenqvist P, Kaaja R. Treatment of deep venous thrombosis with low-molecular-weight heparin during pregnancy. Thromb Res 2002;106:13–17.

108. Smith MP, Norris LA, Steer PJ, et al. Tinzaparin sodium for thrombosis treatment and prevention during pregnancy. Am J Obstet Gynecol 2004;190:495–501.

109. Rowan JA, McLintock C, Taylor RS, North RA. Prophylactic and therapeutic enoxaparin during pregnancy: indications, outcomes and monitoring. Aust N Z J Obstet Gynaecol 2003;43:123–128.

110. Lepercq J, Conard J, Borel-Derlon A, et al. Venous thromboembolism during pregnancy: a retrospective study of enoxaparin safety in 624 pregnancies. BJOG 2001;108:1134–1140.

111. Ibbotson T, Perry CM. Danaparoid: a review of its use in thromboembolic and coagulation disorders. Drugs 2002;62:2283–2314.

112. Lindhoff-Last E, Kreutzenbeck HJ, Magnani HN. Treatment of 51 pregnancies with danaparoid because of heparin intolerance. Thromb Haemost 2005;93:63–69.

113. Quick AJ. Experimentally induced changes in the prothrombin level of the blood: III. Prothrombin concentrations of newborn pups of a mother given Dicoumarol before parturition. J Biol Chem 1946; 164:371–376.

114. Hall JG, Pauli RM, Wilson KM. Maternal and fetal sequelae of anticoagulation during pregnancy. Am J Med 1980;68:122–140.

115. Chan WS, Anand S, Ginsberg JS. Anticoagulation of pregnant women with mechanical heart valves: a systematic review of the literature. Arch Intern Med 2000;160:191–196.

116. Hirsh J, Cade JF, Gallus AS. Fetal effects of coumadin administered during pregnancy. Blood 1970;36: 623–627.

117. Bates SM, Greer IA, Hirsh J, Ginsberg JS. Use of antithrombotic agents during pregnancy: the Seventh ACCP Conference on Antithrombotic and Thrombolytic Therapy. Chest 2004;126:627S–644S.

118. Orme ML, Lewis PJ, de Swiet M, et al. May mothers given warfarin breast-feed their infants? Br Med J 1977;1:1564–1565.

119. McKenna R, Cole ER, Vasan U. Is warfarin sodium contraindicated in the lactating mother? J Pediatr 1983;103:325–327.
120. Hull R, Delmore T, Carter C, et al. Adjusted subcutaneous heparin versus warfarin sodium in the long-term treatment of venous thrombosis. N Engl J Med 1982;306:189–194.
121. Dolovich LR, Ginsberg JS, Douketis JD, et al. A meta-analysis comparing low-molecular-weight heparins with unfractionated heparin in the treatment of venous thromboembolism: examining some unanswered questions regarding location of treatment, product type, and dosing frequency. Arch Intern Med 2000;160:181–188.
122. Shaughnessy SG, Hirsh J, Bhandari M, et al. A histomorphometric evaluation of heparin-induced bone loss after discontinuation of heparin treatment in rats. Blood 1999;93:1231–1236.
123. Douketis JD, Ginsberg JS, Burrows RF, et al. The effects of long-term heparin therapy during pregnancy on bone density. A prospective matched cohort study. Thromb Haemost 1996;75:254–257.
124. Barbour LA, Kick SD, Steiner JF, et al. A prospective study of heparin-induced osteoporosis in pregnancy using bone densitometry. Am J Obstet Gynecol 1994;170:862–869.
125. Dahlman TC. Osteoporotic fractures and the recurrence of thromboembolism during pregnancy and the puerperium in 184 women undergoing thromboprophylaxis with heparin. Am J Obstet Gynecol 1993;168:1265–1270.
126. Monreal M, Lafoz E, Olive A, et al. Comparison of subcutaneous unfractionated heparin with a low molecular weight heparin (Fragmin) in patients with venous thromboembolism and contraindications to coumarin. Thromb Haemost 1994;71:7–11.
127. Pettila V, Kaaja R, Leinonen P, et al. Thromboprophylaxis with low molecular weight heparin (dalteparin) in pregnancy. Thromb Res 1999;96:275–282.
128. Carlin AJ, Farquharson RG, Quenby SM, et al. Prospective observational study of bone mineral density during pregnancy: low molecular weight heparin versus control. Hum Reprod 2004;19:1211–1214.
129. Warkentin TE. Heparin-induced thrombocytopenia: pathogenesis and management. Br J Haematol 2003;121:535–555.
130. Lindhoff-Last E, Nakov R, Misselwitz F, et al. Incidence and clinical relevance of heparin-induced antibodies in patients with deep vein thrombosis treated with unfractionated or low-molecular-weight heparin. Br J Haematol 2002;118:1137–1142.
131. Schindewolf M, Mosch G, Bauersachs RM, Lindhoff-Last E. Safe anticoagulation with danaparoid in pregnancy and lactation. Thromb Haemost 2004;92:211.
132. Hirsh J, Raschke R. Heparin and low-molecular-weight heparin: the Seventh ACCP Conference on Antithrombotic and Thrombolytic Therapy. Chest 2004;126:188S–203S.
133. Ginsberg JS, Chan WS, Bates SM, Kaatz S. Anticoagulation of pregnant women with mechanical heart valves. Arch Intern Med 2003;163:694–698.
134. Casele HL, Laifer SA, Woelkers DA, Venkataramanan R. Changes in the pharmacokinetics of the low-molecular-weight heparin enoxaparin sodium during pregnancy. Am J Obstet Gynecol 1999;181:1113–1117.
135. Shiach CR. Monitoring of low molecular weight heparin in pregnancy. Hematology 2003;8:47–52.
136. Barbour LA, Oja JL, Schultz LK. A prospective trial that demonstrates that dalteparin requirements increase in pregnancy to maintain therapeutic levels of anticoagulation. Am J Obstet Gynecol 2004; 191:1024–1029.
137. Chunilal SD, Young E, Johnston MA, et al. The APTT response of pregnant plasma to unfractionated heparin. Thromb Haemost 2002;87:92–97.
138. Ahearn GS, Hadjiliadis D, Govert JA, Tapson VF. Massive pulmonary embolism during pregnancy successfully treated with recombinant tissue plasminogen activator: a case report and review of treatment options. Arch Intern Med 2002;162:1221–1227.
139. Patel RK, Fasan O, Arya R. Thrombolysis in pregnancy. Thromb Haemost 2003;90:1216–1217.
140. Yap LB, Alp NJ, Forfar JC. Thrombolysis for acute massive pulmonary embolism during pregnancy. Int J Cardiol 2002;82:193–194.
141. Aya AG, Saissi G, Eledjam JJ. In situ pulmonary thrombolysis using recombinant tissue plasminogen activator after cesarean delivery. Anesthesiology 1999;91:578–579.

18

Venous Thromboembolism in the Era of Air Travel

Frédéric Lapostolle, MD,
Jean Catineau, MD, Claude Lapandry, MD,
and Frédéric Adnet, MD, PhD

CONTENTS

SUMMARY

The relationship between pulmonary embolism (PE) and air travel remained questionable for a long time, despite the increasing number of passengers on long-distance flights suffering from PE. It was proposed by some authors that the observed occurrence of PE in some individuals after air travel was caused by chance alone. We recently reviewed all documented cases of PE requiring medical care upon arrival at Roissy-Charles-de-Galle, the busiest airport in France. All patients requiring medical care and transport to a hospital because of suspected PE were included, if the diagnosis of PE was confirmed. Between November 1993 and December 2000, 56 patients with confirmed PE were included. All patients had traveled at least 4000 km. The incience of PE increased with the distance traveled, and the risk of PE increased as much as 11-fold after 5000 km. The total incidence of PE reached 4.8 cases per million passengers who traveled distances longer than 7500 km. A similar incidence of PE was found in a cohort of patients arriving at Madrid airport. As the role of other predisposing (risk) factors remains uncertain, the risk of suffering PE cannot be directly determined for each passenger. We therefore believe that risk assessment with regard to air-travel-related PE should take into account the usual predisposing conditions for PE in the general population. Given the risk associated with long-duration air travel, prophylactic measures should always be considered. Behavioral and mechanical prophylaxis, including use of graduated compression stockings and minor physical activity, are currently recommended, because they are safe, easy to apply, and inexpensive. Pharmacological prophylaxis also has been discussed.

From: *Contemporary Cardiology: Management of Acute Pulmonary Embolism*
Edited by: S. Konstantinides © Humana Press Inc., Totowa, NJ

The indications should be individualized, taking into account travel duration, circumstances of travel, and the passenger's preexisting risk factors for PE.

Key Words: Air travel; pulmonary embolism; prophylaxis; economy class; risk factors.

HISTORICAL REVIEW

The history of the relation between air travel and venous thromboembolism (VTE) can be summarized in three important dates. In 1954, Homans reported on five patients with thromboembolic events; deep venous thrombosis (DVT) occurred after travel in four cases, including air travel in two *(1)*. In 1967, Beighton was the first to report pulmonary embolism (PE) after air travel *(2)*. Finally, in 1977, Symington proposed the term "economy-class syndrome" to describe these events *(3)*. In this study of 182 patients with PE, recent prolonged air travel in the economy class was the (possible) cause in three cases.

Conditions of travel in the economy class clearly decrease mobility and may thus be responsible for an increased incidence of thromboembolic events. In fact, approx 100 cases of PE occurring after air travel have been reported during the last three decades. However, most of these reports included small numbers of patients with either DVT or PE, or they were based on poorly documented cases. As a result, the relationship between PE and air travel remained questionable for a long time, despite the increasing number of passengers on long-distance flights who suffered from PE. In fact, apparently contradicting reports contributed to the uncertainty and ongoing debate. For example, in a case control study, Kraajihagen et al. investigated the history of recent (within the past 4 wk) prolonged (i.e., of more than 3 h duration) air travel in a group of patients with DVT, as opposed to a control group of patients with similar symptoms but no DVT *(4)*. They found no significant differences between air travellers and nontravellers with regard to the incidence of DVT. In contrast, in an other case-control study, Ferrari et al. reported an increased risk (odds ratio [OR], 3.98; 95% confidence interval, 1.9 to 8.4) of thromboembolic events after recent (within 4 wk) and prolonged (more than 4 h duration) air travel *(5)*.

Further studies provided ultrasonographic evidence of (deep) venous thrombosis after prolonged air travel *(6,7)*. In fact, in the study by Scurr et al., this finding was present in 10% of the passengers *(7)*. In contrast, in an autopsy study of 14 patients who died of PE after air travel, 5 had evidence of preexisting pulmonary thromboembolic disease, and in 4 cases the fatal thrombus had embolized into the lung before the flight *(8)*, but fresh premortem thrombus was found in only 9 cases. Finally, the incidence of air-travel-related PE was estimated at only 0.5 cases per million passengers arriving at the Roissy-Charles-de-Gaulle (CDG) Airport in Paris, France *(9)*. This low estimate is, of course, insufficient to support a causative relation between air travel and the pathogenesis of PE. It was thus proposed by some authors that the observed occurrence of PE in some individuals after air travel was due to chance alone *(10,11)*.

PATHOPHYSIOLOGY
OF THROMBOEMBOLISM ASSOCIATED WITH AIR TRAVEL

The three factors of Virchow's triad, venous stasis, vessel wall injury, and systemic hypercoagulability, may all be present during air travel, increasing the risk of venous thrombosis *(12)*. The sitting position, even for 1 h, is associated with venous stasis, a significant decrease in blood flow, an increase in hematocrit, and the concentration of blood protein in the legs

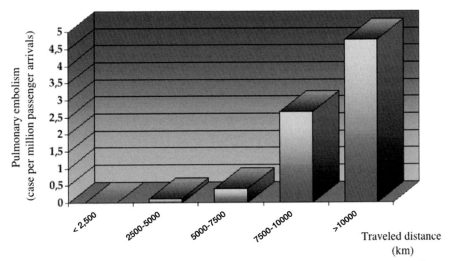

Fig. 1. Incidence of pulmonary embolism (cases per million passengers arriving) according to distance traveled (km).

(13,14). Moreover, immobility predisposes to thrombus formation. Landgraf and colleagues simulated a flight of 12 h and demonstrated that blood viscosity increased in relation to the individual's immobility. Finally, vascular injury due to mechanical compression by the seat itself has been implicated as a pathogenetic factor *(14)*.

RELATION BETWEEN PROLONGED AIR TRAVEL AND PE

In a recent study *(15)*, we systematically reviewed all documented cases of PE requiring medical care upon arrival at CDG, the busiest airport of France. All patients requiring medical care and transport to a hospital by a prehospital medical team (SAMU 93) because of suspected PE were included if the diagnosis of PE was confirmed by high-probability ventilation-perfusion lung scan, pulmonary angiography, or high-resolution helical computed tomographic angiography. It should be noted that SAMU takes care of all patients requiring emergency transport from CDG airport. Suspicion of PE was based on the occurrence of clinical symptoms and signs within 1 h of arrival. Between November 1993 and December 2000, 56 patients with confirmed PE were included. Of these, 42 patients (75%) were female and 14 (25%) were male. The mean age was 57 ± 12 yr without significant differences between men and women. All patients with confirmed PE had traveled at least 4000 km. The incidence of PE as a function of distance traveled was calculated as cases per million passengers at 2500-kilometer increments (Fig. 1). We found that the incidence of PE increased with the distance traveled, and particularly that the risk of PE increased as much as 11-fold after 5000 km ($p < 0.0001$). The total incidence of PE reached 4.8 cases per million passengers for distances longer than 7500 km. It should further be noted that: (1) the first symptoms suggesting PE appeared on arrival in 48 cases (86%) and during air travel itself in 8 cases (14%), but in no case after leaving the airplane; (2) findings suggesting severe PE were present in all patients; and (3) three patients (6%) with PE complicated by an ischemic stroke caused by paradoxical embolism (*see* Chapter 6) had a poor outcome with persistent neurological deficit, and another patient ultimately died of this complication *(16)*.

In a recently published study, Perez-Rodriguez et al. reported a similar incidence of PE (0.39 cases per million passengers) in a cohort of patients arriving at Madrid airport *(17)*. They also reported a dramatic increase in the incidence of PE for travels of more than 6 to 8 h duration. In our opinion, however, the incidence of air-travel-related PE was seriously underestimated in both studies. One reason is that patients presenting with cardiac arrest during flight, after landing, or in the airport were not included in either study. It is unknown, at present, what proportion of cardiac arrests occurring during flight or immediately after landing is attributable to PE. Furthermore, patients pronounced dead before arrival of the prehospital medical team (SAMU 93) were excluded, and this may be responsible for the low mortality rate, at least in our study. Another possible reason for underestimation is the failure to detect less severe cases of PE. In our study, at least one of the following criteria suggesting or directly indicating severe PE was found in every patient with confirmation of the thromboembolic event: tachycardia in 15 cases (27%), syncope in 27 (48%), acute right-ventricular dysfunction in 30 (54%), Miller index greater than 50% in 9 (16%), cardiogenic shock in 6 (11%), and cardiac arrest in 1 (2%). Severe (massive or submassive) PE accounts for approx 20% of all cases of PE, and therefore, based on the data of our study, one might expect 1 severe PE episode per 25 per million passengers after flights of at least 7500 km. However, it is likely that, at least in our study, passengers with minor clinical symptoms such as mild to moderate chest or calf pain left the airport without medical consultation and thus without confirmation of PE diagnosis. Several reports have indeed suggested that passengers may develop PE several weeks after air travel *(5,18)*. Therefore, we speculate that the incidence of VTE is likely to be higher after long-distance air travel. As mentioned previously, thromboembolic events were reported in almost 5 to 10% of passengers in previously published studies *(6,7)*.

RISK FACTORS FOR THROMBOEMBOLIC EVENTS IN AIR TRAVEL

Prolonged travel appears to be the important determinant of air-travel-related PE, so that "long-distance-travel syndrome" could be more appropriate than the current term "economy-class syndrome." On the other hand, the role of other risk factors and, particularly, the exact role of flight itself remains uncertain, as prolonged sitting occurs more frequently during flight compared to other ways of traveling *(19)*. This ongoing debate has recently been summarized as "too much flying or too much sitting?" *(20)*.

The relation between PE and air-travel conditions such as hypoxemia and/or hypobaria remains debated. In a group of 20 healthy male volunteers who were exposed for 8 h to hypobaric atmosphere simulating cabin conditions, Bendz et al. reported activation of coagulation *(21)*. In contrast to these results, Crosby et al., using a slightly different method, studied eight healthy male volunteers also exposed for 8 h to hypobaric atmosphere and reported no effects in comparison to a control group *(22)*. Thus, the exact role of air-travel conditions in the pathogenesis of thromboembolic events remains uncertain. This makes it particularly difficult to estimate the risk of PE during flight and optimize prophylactic measures.

The role of other particular circumstances related to air travel, such as traveling in the "economy class" as opposed to business or first class, also has not been directly demonstrated. The same is true for increased immobility due to alcohol or sedative drug consumption by some passengers during flight. Because of the relative rarity of thromboembolic events in this setting, it is unrealistic to expect that prospective studies can be performed to dissect the roles of various risk factors. Thus, the risk of suffering PE cannot be directly

Table 1
Risk Factors for Venous Thrombosis

Age > 40 yr
History of venous thrombosis
Surgery requiring > 30 min of anesthesia
Prolonged immobilization
Cerebrovascular accident
Congestive heart failure
Cancer
Fracture of pelvis, femur, or tibia
Obesity
Pregnancy or recent delivery
Estrogen therapy
Inflammatory bowel disease
Genetic or acquired thrombophilia

Data from ref. *23.*

determined for each passenger. We therefore believe that risk assessment with regard to air travel-related PE should take into account the usual predisposing conditions for PE in the general population *(23)* (Table 1).

PROPHYLACTIC MEASURES

Given the risk associated with long-duration air travel, prophylactic measures should always be considered. Behavioral and mechanical prophylaxis is easy to perform and includes consumption of nonalcoholic beverages, refraining from smoking, avoidance of tight clothing that may limit blood flow, use of graduated compression stockings, avoidance of leg-crossing, frequent changes of posture while seated, and minor physical activity, such as walking or at least moving the limbs. Of all these measures, only the use of compression stockings has clearly been demonstrated to be beneficial. In the Lonflit II study, DVT diagnosed by ultrasonography performed after prolonged air travel decreased from 4.5 to 0.24% in high-risk patients wearing stockings *(6)*. However, even if not scientifically validated, all of the previous measures are currently recommended, because they are safe, easy to apply, and inexpensive.

Pharmacological prophylaxis also has been discussed. The Lonflit III study showed the absence of benefit of aspirin. On the other hand, in the same study, DVT diagnosed by ultrasonography performed after prolonged air travel decreased from 4.8 to 0% in high-risk patients receiving prophylactic low-molecular-weight heparin *(24)*. Nevertheless, because of the lack of data allowing optimal risk stratification, the use of pharmacological treatment to prevent thromboembolic events during or after air travel is generally not recommended. The indications should be individualized, taking into account travel duration, circumstances of travel, and the passenger's preexisting risk factors for PE *(25,26)*.

CONCLUSION

The duration of flight appears to be the most important risk factor for symptomatic PE associated with air travel. The relative importance of other risk factors remains unknown, as control groups are unavailable because of the low incidence of this complication and the (assumed) large number of undiagnosed events. Thus, optimal prophylaxis is particularly difficult to standardize. Prophylactic behavioral and mechanical measures, which are safe, easy to apply, and inexpensive should generally be recommended. In contrast, pharmacological measures should be considered on an individual basis.

REFERENCES

1. Homans J. Thrombosis of the leg veins due to prolonged sitting. N Engl J Med 1954;250:148–149.
2. Beighton PH, Richards PR. Cardiovascular disease in air travelers. Br Heart J 1968;30:367–372.
3. Symington IS, Stack BH. Pulmonary thromboembolism after travel. Br J Dis Chest 1977;71:138–140.
4. Kraaijenhagen RA, Haverkamp D, Koopman MM, Prandoni P, Piovella F, Buller HR. Travel and risk of venous thrombosis. Lancet 2000;356:1492–1493.
5. Ferrari E, Chevallier T, Chapelier A, Baudouy M. Travel as a risk factor for venous thromboembolic disease. A case control study. Chest 1999;115:440–444.
6. Belcaro G, Geroulakos G, Nicolaides AN, Myers KA, Winford M. Venous thromboembolism from air travel: the LONFLIT study. Angiology 2001;52:369–374.
7. Scurr JH, Machin SJ, Bailey-King S, Mackie IJ, McDonald S, Smith PD. Frequency and prevention of symptomless deep-vein thrombosis in long-haul flights: a randomised trial. Lancet 2001;357:1485–1489.
8. Cheung B, Duflou J. Pre-existing pulmonary thromboembolic disease in passengers with the "economy class syndrome." Aviat Space Environ Med 2001;72:747–749.
9. Clerel M, Caillard G. Thromboembolic syndrome from prolonged sitting and flights of long duration: experience of the Emergency Medical Service of the Paris Airports. Bull Acad Natl Med 1999;183:985–997.
10. Geroulakos G. The risk of venous thromboembolism from air travel. The evidence is only circumstantial. Br Med J 2001;322:188.
11. Davis RM. Air travel and risk of venous thromboembolism. Pulmonary embolism after air travel may occur by chance alone. Br Med J 2001;322:1184.
12. Virchow RLK. Gesammelte Abhandlungen zur Wissenschaftlichen Medicin. Frankfurt am Main, Von Meidinger & Sohn, 1856, p. 227.
13. Landgraf H, Vanselow B, Schulte-Huermann D, Mulmann MV, Bergau L. Economy class syndrome: rheology, fluid balance, and lower leg edema during a simulated 12-hour long distance flight. Aviat Space Environ Med 1994;65:930–935.
14. Moyses C, Cederholm-Williams SA, Michel CC. Haemoconcentration and accumulation of white cells in the feet during venous stasis. Int J Microcirc Clin Exp 1987;5:311–320.
15. Lapostolle F, Surget V, Borron SW, et al. Severe pulmonary embolism associated with air travel. N Engl J Med 2001;345:779–783.
16. Lapostolle F, Borron SW, Surget V, Sordelet D, Lapandry C, Adnet F. Stroke associated with pulmonary embolism after air travel. Neurology 2003;60:1983–1985.
17. Perez-Rodriguez E, Jimenez D, Diaz G, Perez-Walton I, Luque M, Guillen C, Manas E, Yusen RD. Incidence of air travel-related pulmonary embolism at the Madrid-Barajas airport. Arch Intern Med 2003;163:2766–2767.
18. Eklof B, Kistner RL, Masuda EM, Sonntag BV, Wong HP. Venous thromboembolism in association with prolonged air travel. Dermatol Surg 1996;22:637–641.
19. Lapostolle F, Catineau J, Lapandry C, Adnet F. Venous thromboembolism in long-distance air travellers. Lancet 2004;363:896.
20. Dalen JE. Too much flying or too much sitting? JAMA 2003;163:2674–2676.
21. Bendz B, Rostrup M, Sevre K, Andersen TO, Sandset PM. Association between acute hypobaric hypoxia and activation of coagulation in human beings. Lancet 2000;356:1657–1658.
22. Crosby A, Talbot NP, Harrison P, Keeling D, Robbins PA. Relation between acute hypoxia and activation of coagulation in human beings. Lancet 2003;361:2207–2208.
23. Fedullo PF, Tapson VF. Clinical practice. The evaluation of suspected pulmonary embolism. N Engl J Med 2003;349:1247–1256.
24. Cesarone MR, Belcaro G, Nicolaides AN, et al. Venous thrombosis from air travel: the Lonflit 3 study—prevention with aspirin vs low molecular heparin in hight risk subjects: a randomized trial. Angiology 2002;53:1–6.
25. Brenner B. Prophylaxis for travel-related thrombosis? Yes. J Thromb Haemost 2004;2:2089–2091.
26. Lubetsky A. Prophylaxis for travel-related thrombosis? No. J Thromb Haemost 2004;2:2092–2093.

19

Chronic Thromboembolic Pulmonary Hypertension

Irene M. Lang, MD *and Walter Klepetko,* MD

CONTENTS

SUMMARY

Chronic thromboembolic pulmonary hypertension (CTEPH) is a poorly understood disorder. It is characterized by pulmonary hypertension associated with an apparent failure to resolve extensive, typically major-vessel pulmonary thromboemboli. Although CTEPH is believed to be a thromboembolic disease, the typical risk factors for venous thromboembolism are absent. According to the 2003 Venice classification of pulmonary hypertension, CTEPH represents group IV of pulmonary hypertensive diseases and thus does not rank as a subgroup of pulmonary arterial hypertension. Since 2003, however, it is well recognized that CTEPH predominantly results in changes in the major pulmonary arteries, in combination with significant pulmonary vascular disease, which is indistinguishable from classic idiopathic pulmonary hypertension. The present review provides an update on our current knowledge of the pathophysiology, diagnosis, and treatment options for CTEPH.

Key Words: Pulmonary hypertension; venous thromboembolism; thrombus organization; in situ thrombosis; vascular obstruction.

DEFINITION

Chronic thromboembolic pulmonary hypertension (CTEPH) is the result of a single or of recurrent pulmonary thromboemboli arising from sites of venous thrombosis. It is thought to occur in 0.1–5% of cases of acute pulmonary thromboembolism *(1,2)*. The natural history of pulmonary thromboemboli is to undergo total resolution, or resolution leaving minimal residua, with restoration of normal pulmonary hemodynamics. For reasons

From: *Contemporary Cardiology: Management of Acute Pulmonary Embolism*
Edited by: S. Konstantinides © Humana Press Inc., Totowa, NJ

still unclear, however, thromboemboli in patients with CTEPH fail to resolve and form endothelialized obstructions of the pulmonary vascular bed, including the major branches. Although CTEPH is understood as a rare outlier disease in the spectrum of venous thromboembolism (VTE) (Fig. 1), the disease does not share important characteristics of VTE such as systemic thrombotic tendency *(3,4)* or evidence of deep vein thrombosis (DVT) during the course of the disease, which has led to alternative pathophysiologic theories *(5)*. On the other hand, plain histology shows a striking similarity between organized DVT and pulmonary vascular obstruction in CTEPH (Fig. 2).

PATHOPHYSIOLOGY

Epidemiology

Development of CTEPH after diagnosis of acute pulmonary embolism (PE) has been considered rare. A recent review has estimated CTEPH to occur in only 0.1–0.5% of acute nonfatal pulmonary thromboemboli *(2)*. The natural history of pulmonary thromboemboli is to undergo total resolution, or resolution leaving minimal residua, with restoration of normal pulmonary hemodynamics within 30 d in more than 90% of patients. Repeated catheterizations after acute PE have led to the observation that right heart pressures return to near-normal values in the majority of patients within 10 to 21 d.

Recent echocardiographic data suggest that there may be more patients with significant persistent pulmonary hypertension after acute PE than previously reported *(1)*. For example, Pengo et al. observed a cumulative incidence of 3.8% of CTEPH in a carefully conducted prospective multicenter cohort study with a median observation period of almost 8 yr *(6)*. However, preliminary data derived from a large series of patients with VTE *(7)* suggest that this number may be too high. Seen from another perspective, the initial thromboembolic event is asymptomatic in the majority of patients with CTEPH *(2)*. For example, 90 of 142 consecutive patients with CTEPH (63%) who were followed at our institution had not experienced symptomatic VTE (unpublished data). Therefore, the true incidence of CTEPH is still unknown and may differ from the cumulative incidence in a cohort of patients with symptomatic VTE *(6)*. A recent report further demonstrated that apparently unrelated conditions such as splenectomy, ventriculoatrial (VA) shunt, and chronic inflammatory states (osteomyelitis, inflammatory bowel disease) were independent risk factors for CTEPH *(8)*. These observations contradict the traditional concept of symptomatic pulmonary thromboembolism preceding the development of CTEPH.

Natural History

After an initial thromboembolic event that may or may not be symptomatic, patients experience a "honeymoon period" lasting months or years without any clinical symptoms. Gradually, however, dyspnea on exertion develops. Clinical deterioration parallels the deterioration of right ventricular function. While right ventricular hypertrophy develops, additional changes in the pulmonary vascular bed occur. These changes are histologically indistinguishable from pulmonary vascular lesions found in other kinds of pulmonary vascular hypertension *(9)* and further increase pulmonary vascular resistance (PVR). It is suspected that the degree of these "secondary" changes determines the potential for pressure normalization after successful pulmonary thromboendarterectomy. While the initial major vessel red thrombi transform into whitish adherent masses of granulation tissue, high PVR and slow flow through multiple irregular vascular channels lined with dysfunctional

DVT

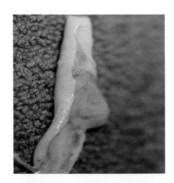

EMBOLUS IN TRANSIT

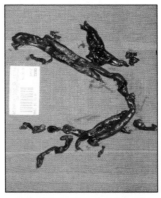

ACUTE PE

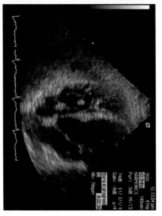

CTEPH

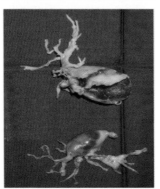

Fig. 1. Spectrum of venous thromboembolism (VTE). The arrow shows the course of VTE from the peripheral venous bed to the pulmonary arteries as the ultimate landing zone. DVT, deep vein thrombosis; PE, pulmonary embolism.

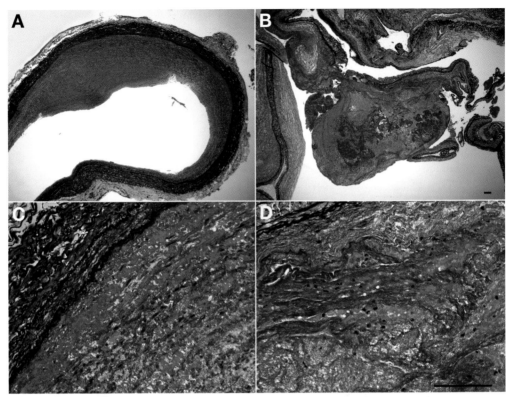

Fig. 2. Trichrome stain of a representative deep vein thrombosis (DVT) (**A,C**) and a pulmonary arterial thrombus (**B,D**) harvested at pulmonary thromboendarterectomy (PEA). The modified trichrome stain identifies elastic fibers as black, collagen as green, fibrin as red, erythrocytes as orange-yellow, and nuclei as blue-black. Panels **A** and **C** show a representative example of partly organized DVT, with Panel **C** (200X) representing a higher magnification of Panel **A** (40X). Panels **B** and **D** show a representative chronic thromboembolic pulmonary hypertension (CTEPH) thrombus, with Panel **D** representing a higher magnification of Panel **B** (200 vs 40X). Scale bars correspond to 100 μm.

endothelium cause further apposition of fresh red thrombus. Because of segmental under-perfusion, alveolar dead space increases. Finally, right ventricular failure ensues. Hypoxemia becomes exaggerated by a combination of factors, including a decline in cardiac output with a fall in mixed venous oxygen saturation, worsening ventilation-perfusion (V/Q) relations, reopening of the foramen ovale, and development of small pulmonary arteriovenous fistulas in the lungs. The complexity of these interactions possibly accounts for the findings of a study utilizing the inert gas technique, in which the magnitude of V/Q mismatch correlated poorly with PVR, mean pulmonary arterial pressure, or the magnitude of vascular obstruction *(10)*.

Cardiac Hemodynamics

As PVR rises, left ventricular diastolic function deteriorates because of interventricular interdependence and diastolic forward movement of the ventricular septum *(11,12)*. In contrast to acute right ventricular pressure rise, pericardial constriction does not appear to play a role in this process *(13)*. Right ventricular impairment is reversible with a decrease of PVR *(14)*. Of note, hemodynamics at rest may be normal in patients with unilateral disease.

Coagulation and Fibrinolysis

No abnormalities of coagulation *(15)* or fibrinolysis *(16)* have been identified in patients with CTEPH. On the other hand, recent data suggest that lupus anticoagulant (LAC), high levels of anticardiolipin, and anti-β2-glycoprotein I antibodies are associated with CTEPH *(17)*. Approximately 10% of the patients have LAC, and a significant association exists between LAC and heparin-induced thrombocytopenia *(18)*. Studies demonstrated no increased prevalence of the factor V Leiden mutation in CTEPH *(4)*, but a 20–50% frequency of anticardiolipin antibodies could be found *(3,19)*. Combined coagulation defects are rare *(20,21)*.

A recent study *(22)* showed that factor VIII (FVIII) levels greater than 230 IU/dL were more prevalent in patients with CTEPH (39%) than in patients with pulmonary artery hypertension (20%) or controls (5%). Overall, mean FVIII (233 ± 83 IU/dL) and von Willebrand factor antigen (VWF:Ag; 261 ± 130 IU/dL) plasma levels were higher in CTEPH than in patients with nonthromboembolic pulmonary hypertension (FVIII, 158 ± 61 IU/dL; VWF:Ag, 204 ± 107 IU/dL) or in controls (FVIII, 123 ± 40 IU/dL; VWF:Ag, 132 ± 48 IU/dL) after adjusting for the covariates age and sex. Moreover, mean FVIII and VWF:Ag concentrations remained unchanged 1 yr after surgery when compared with preoperative values. In contrast to reports from patients with nonthromboembolic pulmonary hypertension *(23)*, high-molecular-weight multimers of VWF were preserved in pre- and postoperative plasma samples of patients with CTEPH, and multimeric distribution did not differ from healthy control samples assayed in parallel. Accordingly, VWF cleaving protease activity, which is responsible for multimeric distribution, was within the normal range (117 ± 48%) and remained unchanged after surgery.

Associated Conditions

The only existing epidemiological study on CTEPH, a prospective multicenter cohort study with a median observation period of almost 8 yr, demonstrated in 223 patients that the cumulative incidence of symptomatic CTEPH was 1.0% (95% confidence interval [CI], 0 to 2.4) at 6 mo, 3.1% (95% CI, 0.7 to 5.5) at 1 yr, and 3.8% (95% CI, 1.1 to 6.5) at 2 yr. Previous PE, younger age, larger perfusion defects, and idiopathic presentation were independently associated with an increased risk of CTEPH *(6)*.

Case reports have suggested a link between chronic thromboembolism and prior splenectomy *(24–26)*, VA shunt for the treatment of hydrocephalus *(27–33)*, or chronic inflammatory conditions *(34)*. We performed a prospective case-control study of 109 patients with CTEPH. No patient had a plasmatic risk factor for VTE or had been on long-term oral anticoagulation prior to diagnosis. The diagnosis of CTEPH was established by chest X-ray, transthoracic and transesophageal echocardiography, pulmonary function tests including arterial blood gas analysis at rest and exercise, right heart catheterization, pulmonary angiography, V/Q scan of the lungs, and multislice high-resolution computed tomography (CT). A panel of cardiologists, pulmonologists, radiologists, and cardiothoracic surgeons reviewed each case. CTEPH type *(35)* was classified according to imaging, and, if available, according to the surgical specimen. All patients were referred for exertional or resting dyspnea, with 10 patients in New York Heart Association functional class II, 67 in class III, and 32 in class IV. Because CTEPH is believed to be a thromboembolic disorder *(2)* and is suspected to result partly from inadequate anticoagulation after silent pulmonary thromboembolism, patients with proven PE, (in the absence of thrombophilic disorders requiring lifelong anticoagulation) were followed as controls. Physical examination of control patients was performed at 3-mo intervals during the first year after enrollment and every 6 mo thereafter. Dyspnea on exertion and/or rest, syncope, or chest pain were considered clinical signs of pulmonary hypertension. Echocardiography was performed in patients who developed any of these symptoms during the observation period. Splenectomy, VA shunt, and chronic inflammation, e.g., osteomyelitis or inflammatory bowel disease, remained independent risk factors for CTEPH by multivariate analysis, with splenectomy increasing the likelihood of CTEPH 13-fold ($p = 0.015$), VA shunt 13-fold ($p = 0.0014$), and chronic inflammation 67-fold ($p < 0.0001$). These data suggest that a number of conditions can be identified which increase an individual's risk to develop CTEPH. Hypothetically, thrombi originating from VA shunts, osteomyelitis, or Crohn's disease may be biologically different, rendering them resistant to plasmatic and cellular thrombus resolution. Thus, apparent limitations to the thromboembolic hypothesis of CTEPH find an explanation *(5)*.

Apart from these observations, association of CTEPH with pacemaker leads, sickle-cell disease *(36)*, hereditary stomatocytosis *(37)*, myeloproliferative disorders *(38)*, and Klippel-Trenaunay syndrome *(39)* has been suggested.

Genetics of CTEPH

Because of the finding of elevated VWF levels in CTEPH and the fact that blood group oligosaccharide structures on the VWF molecule account for the clearance and plasma levels of the FVIII/VWF complex *(40)*, the blood group distribution among patients with CTEPH was analyzed. Blood groups other than 0 were more prevalent in patients with CTEPH (82%) than in patients with pulmonary arterial hypertension (PAH) (56%), or in the Middle European population (approx 60%). Despite these data, evidence is lacking that CTEPH occurs in a familial pattern. The bone morphogenic protein receptor II (*BMPRII*) gene has been identified by linkage analysis as one causal gene defect underlying familiar pulmonary hypertension *(41)*, but, to date, no mutation of this gene has been described in patients with CTEPH.

A Japanese study recently reported increased frequency of the human leukocyte antigen (HLA) polymorphisms HLA-B*5201 (40 vs 24%) and DPB1*0202 (19 vs 6%) in patients with CTEPH compared with controls. HLA-B*5201-positive patients showed a significant female predominance. In the patients carrying HLA-B*5201 and/or -DPB1* 0202, the frequency of DVT was significantly lower than the other patients. These observations suggest that susceptibility and clinical characteristics of CTEPH are controlled in part by the HLA-B and -DPB1 loci *(42)*. However, they also raise the possibility that CTEPH comprises several subtypes that may be triggered by acquired and endemic diseases such as Takayasu arteritis *(43)* or histoplasmosis.

Polymorphisms of the promoter region of prostacyclin synthase gene *(44)*, or mutations on the serotonin transporter gene *(45)*, have not been found in association with CTEPH.

Animal Models

The difficulty to induce CTEPH in mongrel dogs by repeated release of preformed clots from the inferior vena cava *(46)* was resolved by a thorough biochemical dissection of factors contributing to increased vascular fibrinolytic activity in these animals *(47)*. In particular, it was found that high plasma levels and activity of urokinase-type plasminogen activator (u-PA), a protease associated with canine platelets and mediating rapid clot lysis, are present in this species and thus prevent thrombus persistence and organization *(48)*.

Molecular Biology of Pulmonary Arterial Thromboemboli

There is a striking difference between the macroscopic appearance of thromboembolic material harvested during pulmonary thromboendarterectomy (PEA) and that of acute PE retrieved during embolectomy (Fig. 1, compare the lower two panels). CTEPH thrombi comprise mostly of whitish, organized tissue tightly attached to the pulmonary arterial medial layer and replacing the normal intima. The organization status of CTEPH thrombus explains why it is largely unaccessible to therapeutic thrombolysis. In contrast, PEs are red, fragile thrombi that are loosely adherent to the pulmonary arterial wall.

Under the assumption that CTEPH thrombi result from the embolization of thrombi to the pulmonary vasculature, we designed experiments to understand the regulation of fibrinolytic genes in the first hours after massive PE. Because previous data suggested that the balance between plasminogen activators (PAs) and type 1 plasminogen activator inhibitor (PAI-1) plays a role in regulating cell migration within the extracellular matrix, we investigated the expression of these molecules by immunohistochemical and in situ hybridization analysis of pulmonary artery specimens from patients suffering fatal PE. The data were compared with the expression of these molecules in the patients' noninvolved pulmonary segments and in organ-donor pulmonary arteries. u-PA expression was detected in mononuclear cells within the thrombus in the initial phase of thromboembolism and within cells migrating into the thrombus during the later stages of organization. PAI-1 expression was elevated in the monolayer of endothelial cells underlying the fresh platelet-fibrin thromboembolus and in a proliferating cell nuclear antigen -positive cell population present between the pulmonary arterial intima and the thromboembolus that represents early organization. Thus, increased expression of PAI-1 may play a role in inhibiting proteolysis and fostering the localization of the acute fibrin-platelet thrombus to the vascular wall, which is followed by the upregulation of u-PA in migrating cells during the reorganization process *(49)*.

Recent research has focused on local gene expression within pulmonary arterial thromboemboli and pulmonary arteries from patients with CTEPH. By a candidate gene approach utilizing in situ techniques, increased expression of PAI-1 was found in small thrombus neovessels, potentially promoting small vessel thrombosis and thrombus growth from within *(49)*. On the other hand, elevated PAI-1 gene expression was also identified at a specific stage in the natural course of organization of acute pulmonary thromboemboli *(49)*. This analysis of patterns of gene expression during the vascular remodeling associated with organization of pulmonary thromboemboli has shed new light on the events leading to restoration of normal pulmonary blood flow after VTE. One hypothesis emerging from these studies is that, by a mechanism yet to be defined, DVT undergo extensive organization in the vascular compartment of the deep femoral and pelvic veins. When such thrombi embolize, even well-functioning mechanisms of fibrinolysis do not suffice to remove them, leading to CTEPH.

In further studies, the expression of a potent inhibitor of Factor IXa and Factor XIa (protease nexin-2/amyloid β-protein precursor [β-PP]) was demonstrated in the organized vascular occlusions harvested from patients with CTEPH *(50)*. Clot vessel hemorrhage is a feature of CTEPH thrombus histology and it is thought to be a powerful stimulator for angiogenesis. In fact, recent studies have correlated the expression of angiogenetic molecules with CTEPH severity *(51)*.

In summary, the pathogenesis of CTEPH is still unclear, but it is widely accepted that the disease is not caused by thromboembolic obliteration alone. Vascular remodeling due to a variety of factors, such as shear stress, pressure, inflammation *(52)*, endothelial dysfunction *(53)*, release of cytokines *(54)*, and vasculotrophic mediators *(55)*, is involved in the development of a pulmonary vasculopathy that is indistinguishable from pulmonary vascular lesions found in other types of chronic pulmonary hypertension.

DIAGNOSIS
Clinical Presentation

Exertional dyspnea is the leading complaint. The key to diagnosis is to consider CTEPH in patients complaining of exertional dyspnea in the presence of a normal lung function.

Physical Findings

In the absence of right ventricular failure, clinical findings are poor. Tricuspid regurgitation and pulmonary flow murmurs are the only findings.

Differential Diagnosis

Diagnosis and differential diagnosis of CTEPH require experienced clinicians *(57)*. Idiopathic pulmonary hypertension (IPH) must be ruled out. Female prevalence (men: women, 1:2), familial occurrence, past intake of appetite suppressant drugs, a normal or patchy nonsegmentally abnormal V/Q scan, and vascular pruning on the angiogram are strong evidence for idiopathic PAH. However, distal forms of CTEPH, and IPH with thrombi in the major pulmonary arteries, complicate the diagnosis *(58)*. Further diseases to be ruled out include fibrosing mediastinitis, pulmonary arterial tumor or tumoral invasion of the pulmonary arteries, tumor embolism *(59)*, or pulmonary arteritis *(60)* such as giant cell arteritis *(61)*. Because of excessive bronchopulmonary anastomoses *(62)*, vascular transformation of mediastinal lymph nodes may occur *(63)*. Finally, in the moderately symptomatic patient, left ventricular diastolic dysfunction with oxygen desaturation on exercise is a frequent differential diagnosis.

ECG

The ECG may reflect chronic right ventricular hypertrophy, and thus serve as an indirect sign of advanced pulmonary vascular disease. P waves are tall-peaked in leads II and aVF, and in the mid precordium. Right axis deviation, monophasic R waves in V1, and prominent S waves in V6 are also observed. Sinus tachycardia is an ominous sign of right heart failure, along with persistently negative precordial T waves, which indicate right ventricular strain. Initially, T waves may reverse, reflecting intermittent right ventricular ischemia. Atrial fibrillation is exceptional, and if present, major hemodynamic compromise may ensue. Finally, ECG signs of severe ischemia may be caused by compression of the left main coronary artery by the dilated proximal pulmonary arteries *(64,65)*.

Pulmonary Function Testing and Blood Gas Analysis

Pulmonary function tests are usually within normal limits. Approximately 20% of patients have a "restrictive defect" due to parenchymal scarring *(66)*. The transfer of carbon monox-

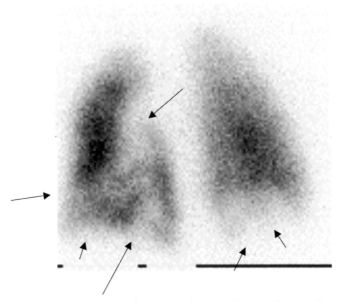

Fig. 3. Example of a perfusion scintigram of a patient with chronic thromboembolic pulmonary hypertension. The corresponding ventilation scan was normal. The perfusion scan shows multiple segmental triangular mismatched defects (arrows). An anterior-posterior view is shown.

ide (DLCO) can be impaired for the same reason, but does not reflect the degree of vascular obstruction. Although DLCO may be reduced, a normal DLCO does not exclude the diagnosis of CTEPH. Normalization of DLCO in the course of the disease probably reflects the extensive bronchial arterial collateral flow exceeding 10% of cardiac output in these patients *(67)*. Arterial blood gas studies at rest and on exercise are important for patient evaluation. A decline in arterial PO_2 and widening of the alveolar-arterial oxygen difference on exercise is a frequent finding, even in patients with normal blood gases at rest.

Chest X-ray

The lung fields will be clear in most patients with CETPH. On a closer look, areas of hypoperfusion may be seen, especially in combination with pleuritic changes *(68)*. The hilar structures may be prominent and may be interpreted as enlarged lymph nodes. In extreme cases, a reduction in vascular size may be mistaken for agenesis of the pulmonary artery(ies). In some patients, cavitary lesions may form at any time during the course of the disease in areas of past pulmonary infarctions.

V/Q Lung Scan

In CTEPH, a segmental V/Q mismatch is considered diagnostic (Fig. 3). In the absence of at least one segmental defect, the diagnosis of CTEPH cannot be made. However, the extent and severity of V/Q mismatches frequently underestimates the severity of vascular occlusions *(69)*. Importantly, although CTEPH is a vascular disorder, ventilation scan must always be performed, and patients with CTEPH and concomitant chronic obstructive pulmonary disease represent particular diagnostic challenges. In these patients, spiral CT and pulmonary angiography can yield important diagnostic clues.

Postoperatively, "reverse" V/Q scan patterns are observed because of a vascular steal of blood flow from the nonatherectomized segments *(70)*. Of note, as the disease progresses, segmental flow abnormalities appear to gradually decrease over time, paralleling the decline of right ventricular performance *(71)*.

Exercise Stress Test

Exercise stress test with arterial blood gas analysis is important for patients with normal resting pulmonary pressures and suspicion of unilateral disease. Frequently, desaturation on exercise is the first objective finding in patients who present early in the course of the disease. Exercise ECG may also unravel CTEPH when screening patients at risk. At this early stage, the possible development of left ventricular diastolic dysfunction on exercise may obscure exercise-induced pulmonary vascular disease and thus pose diagnostic challenges.

Echocardiography

Transthoracic echocardiography is an easily accessible and a very helpful tool for the diagnosis of CTEPH. Paradoxical interventricular septal motion, enlarged right ventricular cavity dimensions, increased thickness of the right ventricular free wall, and a high velocity of the tricuspid regurgitant jet allow making the diagnosis of pulmonary hypertension *(14)*. However, because cardiac output cannot be reliably estimated from echocardiography, the indication for surgery cannot be solely based on noninvasive pulmonary artery pressure measurement. In our experience, approx 20% of patients with CTEPH, and particularly the younger patients, present with normal or near-normal right ventricular cavity dimensions on echocardiography.

Transesophageal echocardiography is helpful for the exclusion of an open or functionally open foramen ovale (*see* Chapter 6) and may thus help explain severe hypoxemia in some patients. Furthermore, in approx 20% of the patients, a proximal pulmonary arterial thrombus can be seen. Unfortunately, however, wall irregularities, scars, and bands in the pulmonary artery cannot be visualized with this technique. In the majority of patients, these signs are the only proximal signs of the disease and can, at present, only be demonstrated by angioscopy, a method not belonging to routine diagnostic workup.

CT

Spiral CT with contrast medium is a valuable and indispensable diagnostic procedure for the diagnosis of CTEPH *(72)*. However, because of limitations in resolution beyond segmental arteries, distal vascular occlusions may not be seen. In these instances and in all other cases, a mosaic perfusion pattern reflecting perfusion inequalities offers indirect but important diagnostic clues. Recently, modern CT technologies such as multislice CT have revolutionized imaging in CTEPH, with images that get closer to the quality of pulmonary angiography *(73)* (Figs. 4 and 5). These techniques offer resolution comparable to that of magnetic resonance tomography.

Lung Biopsy

Because of a lack in specific pathological changes in CTEPH *(9)*, lung biopsy cannot provide differential diagnostic clues.

Right Heart Catheterization

Right heart catheterization must be performed in every case of suspected pulmonary hypertension. Measurement of pulmonary systolic, diastolic, and mean pressures, pul-

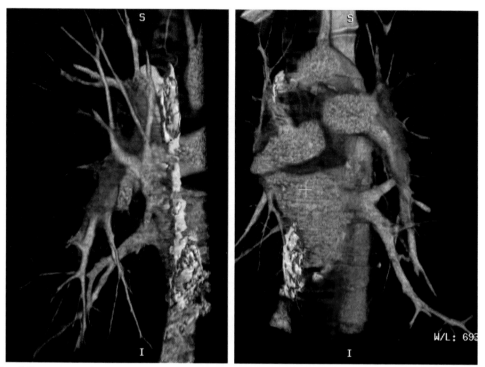

Fig. 4. Representative computed tomography images of a patient with type 2 chronic thromboembolic pulmonary hypertension. The three-dimensional reconstruction demonstrates thrombus in red. Pulmonary arteries and veins are visualized at the same time.

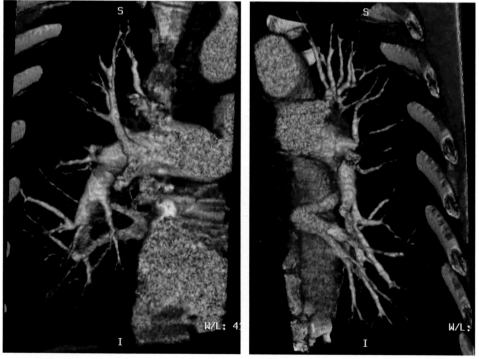

Fig. 5. Representative computed tomography images of a patient with type 4 chronic thromboembolic pulmonary hypertension. Imaging as in Fig. 4.

monary capillary wedge pressure, cardiac output, and oxygen saturation, is important for the calculation of PVR and shunting (if present). Central venous saturation, PVR, and cardiac output are the most important prognostic parameters.

The primary site of vasculopathy in CTEPH are the large elastic pulmonary arteries, although concomitant small vessel arteriopathy is also frequently present at varying degrees *(9)*. In these latter patients, pulmonary hypertension persists despite removal of proximal material. Persistent pulmonary hypertension after PEA remains a serious problem and is associated with high morbidity and mortality. More than one-third of perioperative deaths and nearly half of long-term deaths have been attributed to persistent pulmonary hypertension *(74–76)*. The current standard preoperative evaluation does not accurately assess the presence and degree of small vessel involvement in patients with CTEPH, nor is it suitable for predicting postoperative hemodynamic outcome. In a recent paper, Kim et al. evaluated a sophisticated pulmonary artery occlusion (Poccl) technique to estimate pressure in the precapillary small pulmonary arteries preoperatively *(77)*. With Poccl, the pulmonary arterial resistance can be partitioned into a larger arterial (upstream) and a small arterial plus venous (downstream) component *(78)*. The authors showed that a higher upstream resistance (Rup) was observed in patients with CTEPH who had predominantly proximal (large-vessel) disease, whereas patients with CTEPH who had a Rup less than 60% demonstrated significant concomitant small-vessel disease, had the highest postoperative pulmonary artery and total PVR, and suffered perioperative deaths more frequently *(79)*.

Pulmonary Angiography

Pulmonary angiography usually completes the diagnostic sequence. In general, it is an indispensable examination. Experience over the past decade has indicated that pulmonary angiography can be carried out safely in any patient with pulmonary hypertension when a rigorous protocol is followed *(80)*. Access may be from an arm, neck, or femoral vein if cavography is performed first to rule out vena caval thrombosis. Usually, diagnostic right heart catheterization is carried out prior to angiography. Selective injection of nonionic contrast medium and restrictive use of contrast medium in general guarantee that hemodynamic compromise will not occur. The pulmonary angiographic findings suggestive of chronic thromboembolic disease include "pouching" defects, webs or bands, intimal irregularities, abrupt vascular narrowing, and complete vascular obstruction *(81)* (Fig. 6). If bands, webs, and vessel breakoffs are found in the conventional pulmonary angiogram, and segmental defects in the digital angiogram, the procedure is concluded with the insertion of a vena caval filter when a lower extremity thromboembolic etiology is likely. However, several centers are starting to abandon caval filter placement because of the uncertainty of the thromboembolic nature of the disease.

RISK STRATIFICATION

Preoperative parameters can be utilized to assess postoperative mortality and hemodynamic improvement after PEA. Patient age, sex, and the relationship between severity of pulmonary hypertension *(82)* and location (proximal vs distal) of vascular occlusions determine hospital mortality. Preoperative PVR greater than 1000 dynes $\cdot$ s $\cdot$ cm^{-5} raises surgical mortality to 10%. Surgical classification of CTEPH is also useful *(35)* (Fig. 7), but it does not account for the degree of secondary vasuclar changes. In a multivariate analysis, right atrial pressure ($p = 0.002$) and female sex ($p = 0.007$) were risk factors predicting lack of hemodynamic improvement *(82)*. Recently, it was reported that *fractional*

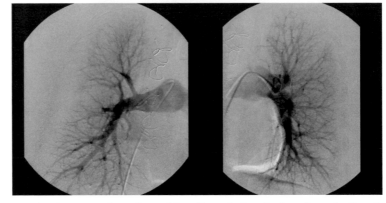

7-1999

3-2002

Fig. 6. Follow-up pulmonary angiograms of a patient with unilateral chronic thromboembolic pulmonary hypertension. The upper panel demonstrates a cine-angiogram showing total obstruction of the right pulmonary artery. The lower panel shows a follow-up digital angiogram 2 yr after successful unilateral PEA.

pulse pressure (defined as pulmonary arterial pulse pressure/mean pulmonary arterial pressure) was higher in CTEPH than in primary pulmonary hypertension, and that fractional pulse pressure in PEA survivors (1.26 ± 0.21) was significantly higher than in nonsurvivors (1.06 ± 0.16). Fractional pulse pressure is a significant predictor of mortality in patients with PVR greater than 1100 dynes $\cdot$ s $\cdot$ cm^{-5} *(83)*.

The prognosis of medically treated patients with CTEPH is determined by hemodynamics, coexistence of chronic obstructive pulmonary disease, and the degree of exercise tolerance *(84)*.

TREATMENT

PEA

Surgical treatment of CTEPH was proposed as early as three decades ago *(85)*. Once the diagnosis of CTEPH is established, the decision for surgical therapy is made based on: (1) the degree of functional impairment; (2) the severity of pulmonary arterial hypertension; and (3) the surgical accessibility of the thromboembolic lesions. A preoperative period of at least 3 mo of adequate anticoagulation is mandatory. Although the operation historically has been described as pulmonary thromboendarterectomy *(86)*, it is better termed *pulmonary endarterectomy* (PEA). Fewer than 3000 PEA operations have been performed worldwide, although it is a potentially curative treatment option even for very

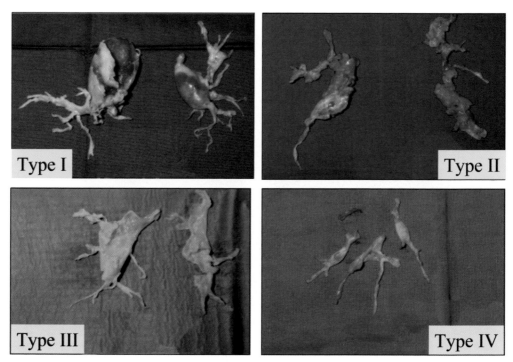

Fig. 7. Surgical classification of chronic thromboembolic pulmonary hypertension. The majority of patients (roughly two-thirds) present with type II disease. Type IV disease does not yield any thrombus at surgery in most cases. In the example shown, small amounts of thrombus were recovered.

sick patients with CTEPH. The surgical techniques and evolving modifications have been well described *(75,87–93)*. With rare exceptions, thromboembolic pulmonary hypertension is a bilateral disease, and therefore PEA is a bilateral procedure. Unilateral disease is rare *(94)*, with unpredictable postoperative outcome.

The operation is not an embolectomy but a true endarterectomy, removing the organized and incorporated fibrous obstructive tissue from the pulmonary arteries (Figs. 8 and 9). Because visibility in the distal pulmonary artery branches is essential and bronchial artery collateral flow is significant in CTEPH, extracorporeal circulation and periods of circulatory arrest under deep hypothermia are essential for successful endarterectomy. Following a proximal intrapericardial pulmonary artery incision, the correct endarterectomy plane is established and circumferentially followed down to the lobar segmental and sometimes subsegmental branches using special suction dissectors. The endarterectomy procedure on one side is usually possible within a 20-min period of circulatory arrest, followed by a period of reperfusion and another period of circulatory arrest for the endarterectomy on the contralateral side. After closure of the pulmonary artery incision, additional cardiac procedures (e.g., coronary artery bypass grafting) can be performed during the rewarming period, if necessary. As tricuspid valve competence usually returns after successful PEA, tricuspid valve repair is not necessary *(95)*. For a small subset of patients who present with concomitant coronary or valvular disease, combined surgical treatment is required *(96)*.

Jamieson et al. *(91)* proposed an intraoperative classification of CTEPH (Fig. 7): type I (central thrombus present) and type II (thickened intima, fibrous webs and bands) represent the typical condition of surgical patients; type III occlusions in the segmental and

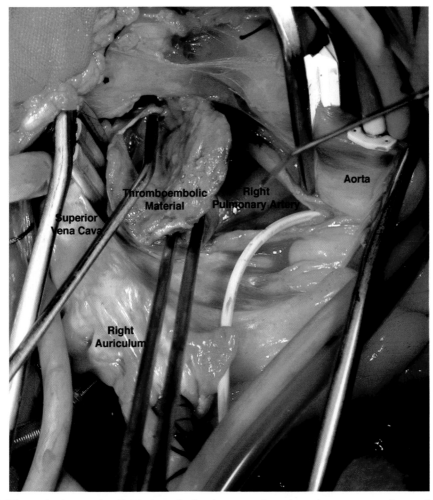

Fig. 8. The typical operative field of surgical pulmonary thromboendarterectomy shows a longitudinally incised pulmonary artery with a sizeable thrombus being removed.

subsegmental branches require adequate surgical experience with dissection within the peripheral pulmonary arteries; and type IV disease represents very distal disease that cannot be treated by PEA. In general, whenever surgically accessible thrombus is documented, PEA is the treatment of choice for CTEPH *(15,97)*. Recent clinical practice guidelines by the American College of Chest Physicians requested the referral of a patient with CTEPH to a center with the expertise for surgical therapy of this disorder *(98)*. In contrast to acute pulmonary embolectomy, which is discussed in Chapter 12 and is generally regarded as "easy" to perform *(99,100)*, this is a procedure that poses a great challenge for the surgeon *(101)*. As mentioned previously, indications for PEA are surgically accessible pulmonary thrombus (thrombi visible at least at the origin of the segmental arteries) and a resting PVR of more than 300 dynes · s · cm^{-5}) or inadequate pressure rise under exertion. Acute pulmonary arterial thrombosis after deendothelialization is not a realistic problem after PEA, yet meticulous postoperative care is demanded. A 24-h mechanical ventilation period and fluid restriction are designed to prevent pulmonary reperfusion edema *(102)*. This life-threatening complication of PEA is an acute lung injury pattern resulting

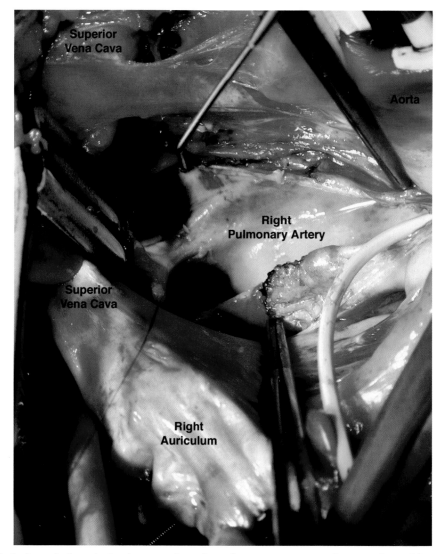

Fig. 9. At the end of surgical pulmonary thromboendarterectomy, a new inner surface of the pulmonary artery has been created that is devoid of fibrotic thrombus tissue. The most relevant anatomical structures are labeled in the photograph.

from perfusion of a dysfunctional capillary bed in a chronically underperfused lung segment. Recent pharmacological approaches block selectin-mediated adhesion of neutrophils to the endothelium with Cylexin® (CY-1503) and demonstrated a decreased incidence of reperfusion injury albeit with no impact on the total number of days on mechanical ventilation *(103)*.

Lung Transplantation

Lung transplantation is an established treatment *(93)* for patients who are not PEA candidates and deteriorate under medical therapy. The purpose of the pretransplantation assessment is to identify patients whose prognosis will be improved by transplantation and whose cardiopulmonary status or other medical problems will not unduly jeopardize the success of transplantation. The major specific goals of the evaluation for transplantation are to confirm the diagnosis, to assess the severity of the disease, and to optimize medical management. The potential benefit of transplantation (natural course of the disease vs prognosis after transplantation) has to be established, and suitable candidates for transplantation have to be selected together with the ideal transplantation procedure. The clinical status must be reexamined periodically, and the medical management and transplantation strategy adjusted accordingly. The threshold of irreversible right ventricular failure is unknown (if such a boundary exists), but severe right ventricular dysfunction has been reversed after isolated lung transplantation. However, although afterload is immediately reduced by lung transplantation, right ventricular function does not return to normal right away, and hemodynamic instability is a common problem in the early postoperative period.

In a study of cardiopulmonary exercise testing in patients with pulmonary arterial hypertension, peak oxygen uptake and peak systolic blood pressure both were prognostically important. A peak oxygen uptake of at least 10.4 mL/(kg · min) and a peak systolic blood pressure less than 120 mmHg were associated with 1-yr mortality rates of approx 50 and 70%, respectively, and among patients with both of these risk factors, only 23% survived for 1 yr *(104)*. Thus, transplantation might offer a survival benefit to patients with these risk factors, and this threshold may be useful for choosing the appropriate time for transplantation.

Medical and Interventional Treatment

Because of the favorable outcomes after PEA, medical treatment in the absence of surgery is currently only justified for: (1) distal, inaccessible disease; (2) hemodynamic instability; (3) comorbidities precluding PEA; (4) a PVR greater than 1000 dynes · s · cm^{-5} in the presence of distal clots; and (5) recurrent pulmonary hypertension after PEA. In our center, approx 50% of the patients with CTEPH are not suitable for surgery, and surgery fails, either over the short term or over the long term, in 10% of the patients.

Conventional (medical) therapy consists of diuretics, digitalis, anticoagulation and caval filters, chronic oxygen therapy, and low-dose calcium antagonists. The only randomized study including patients with CTEPH to date was the AIR study, which compared 33 iloprost-treated patients with 24 patients who received placebo. In this subgroup, no significant beneficial effect of iloprost could be found regarding the combined end point New York Heart Association class plus 6-min walking distance *(105)*. On the other hand, recent reports do suggest a benefit of prostacyclin therapy following surgical treatment of CTEPH *(106–109)*.

Recently, some European groups published uncontrolled patient series that evaluated the role of the endothelin receptor antagonist bosentan in CTEPH. A German multicenter study showed that, over a 3-mo follow-up period, 6-min walking distance improved under bosentan from 340 ± 102 to 413 ± 130 meters ($p = 0.009$) with unchanged dyspnea scores, and this effect was paralleled by a decrease in PVR from 914 ± 329 to 611 ± 220 dynes · s · cm^{-5} ($P < 0.001$) *(110)*. Series from the Vienna, Clamart, and Papworth hospital yielded similar findings *(111)*. Another uncontrolled study reported symptomatic and hemodynamic improvement under the treatment with the phosphodiesterase-5-inhibitor sildenafil *(112)*.

Finally, balloon pulmonary angioplasty has been proposed by few experienced investigators and centers as a treatment option for severely ill patients who are not candidates for PEA *(113,114)*.

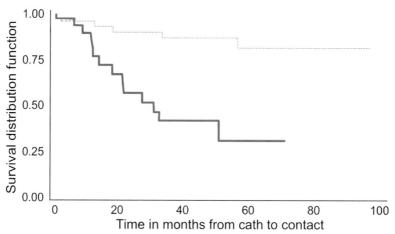

Fig. 10. Kaplan Meyer survival curves of patients undergoing pulmonary thromboendarterectomy in our center (dashed line), compared with patients on medical treatment (solid line).

OUTCOME

Prognosis of untreated CTEPH is poor and inversely correlated with the degree of pulmonary hypertension *(84)*. There is currently no doubt about the benefits of PEA surgery in CTEPH compared to conservative treatment *(115)*. For example, Fig. 10 shows survival curves obtained in patients from the Vienna PEA center over a period of 8 yr. On conservative treatment, 3-yr survival has been as low as 25–30%, which is in accordance with data from other centers *(84)*. In surgically treated patients, patient age, hemodynamics and clinical status, location of thrombus, and comorbidity determine postoperative outcome *(116)*. In particular, distal location of pulmonary thromboemboli doubles the operative risk. Perioperative mortality also depends on the surgeon's experience and on postoperative care, ranging from 4 to 25% *(75,89,117)*. To date, the most experienced PEA center at the University of California at San Diego has performed over 2000 PEAs, with a mortality rate as low as 4% in uncomplicated cases *(92,93)*. Other than coumadin, patients do not usually require specific postoperative medication. Favorable results have been reported for the perioperative use of nitric oxide *(118)*, epoprostenol *(107,109)*, or iloprost *(108)*. Recurrent thromboembolism is a rare event. It is, however, unexplained and presently unforeseeable why some patients (approx 10%) do not achieve or maintain hemodynamic improvement despite removal of significant amounts of thrombus.

REFERENCES

1. Ribeiro A, Lindmarker P, Johnsson H, Juhlin-Dannfelt A, Jorfeldt L. Pulmonary embolism: one-year follow-up with echocardiography doppler and five-year survival analysis. Circulation 1999;99(10): 1325–1330.
2. Fedullo PF, Auger WR, Kerr KM, Rubin LJ. Chronic thromboembolic pulmonary hypertension. N Engl J Med 2001;345(20):1465–1472.
3. Wolf M, Boyer-Neumann C, Parent F, et al. Thrombotic risk factors in pulmonary hypertension. Eur Respir J 2000;15(2):395–399.
4. Lang IM, Klepetko W, Pabinger I. No increased prevalence of the factor V Leiden mutation in chronic major vessel thromboembolic pulmonary hypertension (CTEPH). Thromb Haemost 1996;76(3):476–477.

5. Egermayer P, Peacock AJ. Is pulmonary embolism a common cause of chronic pulmonary hypertension? Limitations of the embolic hypothesis. Eur Respir J 2000;15(3):440–448.
6. Pengo V, Lensing AW, Prins MH, et al. Incidence of chronic thromboembolic pulmonary hypertension after pulmonary embolism. N Engl J Med 2004;350(22):2257–2264.
7. Kyrle PA, Eichinger S. The risk of recurrent venous thromboembolism: the Austrian Study on Recurrent Venous Thromboembolism. Wien Klin Wochenschr 2003;115(13–14):471–474.
8. Bonderman D, Jakowitsch J, Adlbrecht C, et al. Medical conditions increasing the risk of chronic thromboembolic pulmonary hypertension. Thromb Haemost 2005;93(3):512–516.
9. Moser KM, Bloor CM. Pulmonary vascular lesions occurring in patients with chronic major vessel thromboembolic pulmonary hypertension. Chest 1993;103(3):685–692.
10. Kapitan KS, Buchbinder M, Wagner PD, Moser KM. Mechanisms of hypoxemia in chronic thromboembolic pulmonary hypertension. Am Rev Respir Dis 1989;139(5):1149–1154.
11. Mahmud E, Raisinghani A, Hassankhani A, et al. Correlation of left ventricular diastolic filling characteristics with right ventricular overload and pulmonary artery pressure in chronic thromboembolic pulmonary hypertension. J Am Coll Cardiol 2002;40(2):318–324.
12. Menzel T, Wagner S, Kramm T, et al. Pathophysiology of impaired right and left ventricular function in chronic embolic pulmonary hypertension: changes after pulmonary thromboendarterectomy. Chest 2000; 118(4):897–903.
13. Blanchard DG, Dittrich HC. Pericardial adaptation in severe chronic pulmonary hypertension. An intraoperative transesophageal echocardiographic study. Circulation 1992;85(4):1414–1422.
14. Dittrich HC, Chow LC, Nicod PH. Early improvement in left ventricular diastolic function after relief of chronic right ventricular pressure overload. Circulation 1989;80(4):823–830.
15. Moser KM, Auger WR, Fedullo PF. Chronic major-vessel thromboembolic pulmonary hypertension. Circulation 1990;81(6):1735–1743.
16. Olman MA, Marsh JJ, Lang IM, Moser KM, Binder BR, Schleef RR. Endogenous fibrinolytic system in chronic large-vessel thromboembolic pulmonary hypertension. Circulation 1992;86(4):1241–1248.
17. Martinuzzo ME, Pombo G, Forastiero RR, Cerrato GS, Colorio CC, Carreras LO. Lupus anticoagulant, high levels of anticardiolipin, and anti-beta2-glycoprotein I antibodies are associated with chronic thromboembolic pulmonary hypertension. J Rheumatol 1998;25(7):1313–1319.
18. Auger WR, Permpikul P, Moser KM. Lupus anticoagulant, heparin use, and thrombocytopenia in patients with chronic thromboembolic pulmonary hypertension: a preliminary report. Am J Med 1995; 99(4):392–396.
19. Colorio CC, Martinuzzo ME, Forastiero RR, Pombo G, Adamczuk Y, Carreras LO. Thrombophilic factors in chronic thromboembolic pulmonary hypertension. Blood Coagul Fibrinolysis 2001;12(6): 427–432.
20. Brilakis ES, Manginas AN, Cokkinos DV. Chronic thromboembolic pulmonary hypertension in a patient heterozygous for both factor V Leiden and G20210 prothrombin mutation. Heart 2001;86(2):149.
21. Laczika K, Lang IM, Quehenberger P, et al. Unilateral chronic thromboembolic pulmonary disease associated with combined inherited thrombophilia. Chest 2002;121(1):286–289.
22. Bonderman D, Turecek PL, Jakowitsch J, et al. High prevalence of elevated clotting factor VIII in chronic thromboembolic pulmonary hypertension. Thromb Haemost 2003;90(3):372–376.
23. Veyradier A, Nishikubo T, Humbert M, et al. Improvement of von Willebrand factor proteolysis after prostacyclin infusion in severe pulmonary arterial hypertension. Circulation 2000;102(20):2460–2462.
24. Cappellini MD, Robbiolo L, Bottasso BM, Coppola R, Fiorelli G, Mannucci AP. Venous thromboembolism and hypercoagulability in splenectomized patients with thalassaemia intermedia. Br J Haematol 2000;111(2):467–473.
25. Stewart GW, Amess JA, Eber SW, et al. Thrombo-embolic disease after splenectomy for hereditary stomatocytosis. Br J Haematol 1996;93(2):303–310.
26. Chou R, DeLoughery TG. Recurrent thromboembolic disease following splenectomy for pyruvate kinase deficiency. Am J Hematol 2001;67(3):197–199.
27. Favara BE, Paul RN. Thromboembolism and cor pulmonale complicating ventriculovenous shunt. JAMA 1967;199(9):668–671.
28. Haasnoot K, van Vught AJ. Pulmonary hypertension complicating a ventriculo-atrial shunt. Eur J Pediatr 1992;151(10):748–750.
29. Unnithan RR, Bahuleyan CG, Sambasivan M, Roy VC. Ventriculo-atrial shunt producing pulmonary hypertension. J Assoc Physicians India 1984;32(11):1000–1001.
30. Rao PS, Molthan ME, Lipow HW. Cor pulmonale as a complication of ventriculoatrial shunts. Case report. J Neurosurg 1970;33(2):221–225.

31. Trowitzsch E, Ostrejz M, Evers D, Engert J, Brode P. Echocardiographic proof of pulmonary hypertension with irreversible increased resistance in the pulmonary circulation as a complication after place-ment of a ventriculo-atrial shunt for internal hydrocephalus. Eur J Pediatr Surg 1992;2(6):361–364.
32. Drucker MH, Vanek VW, Franco AA, Hanson M, Woods L. Thromboembolic complications of ventriculoatrial shunts. Surg Neurol 1984;22(5):444–448.
33. Pascual JM, Prakash UB. Development of pulmonary hypertension after placement of a ventriculoatrial shunt. Mayo Clin Proc 1993;68(12):1177–1182.
34. Ralston DR, St John RC. Progressive shortness of breath in a 50-year-old man with ulcerative colitis. Chest 1996;110(6):1608–1610.
35. Thistlethwaite PA, Mo M, Madani MM, et al. Operative classification of thromboembolic disease determines outcome after pulmonary endarterectomy. J Thorac Cardiovasc Surg 2002;124(6):1203–1211.
36. Yung GL, Channick RN, Fedullo PF, et al. Successful pulmonary thromboendarterectomy in two patients with sickle cell disease. Am J Respir Crit Care Med 1998;157(5 Pt 1):1690–1693.
37. Murali B, Drain A, Seller D, Dunning J, Vuylsteke A. Pulmonary thromboendarterectomy in a case of hereditary stomatocytosis. Br J Anaesth 2003;91(5):739–741.
38. Kadikoylu G, Onbasili A, Tekten T, Barutca S, Bolaman Z. Functional and morphological cardiac changes in myeloproliferative disorders (clinical study). Int J Cardiol 2004;97(2):213–220.
39. Walder B, Kapelanski DP, Auger WR, Fedullo PF. Successful pulmonary thromboendarterectomy in a patient with Klippel-Trenaunay syndrome. Chest 2000;117(5):1520–1522.
40. Kamphuisen PW, Eikenboom JC, Bertina RM. Elevated factor VIII levels and the risk of thrombosis. Arterioscler Thromb Vasc Biol 2001;21(5):731–738.
41. Deng Z, Morse JH, Slager SL, et al. Familial primary pulmonary hypertension (gene PPH1) is caused by mutations in the bone morphogenetic protein receptor-II gene. Am J Hum Genet 2000;67(3):737–744.
42. Tanabe N, Kimura A, Amano S, et al. Association of clinical features with HLA in chronic pulmonary thromboembolism. Eur Respir J 2005;25(1):131–138.
43. Kashiwabara K, Nakamura H, Sarashina G, et al. [Chronic thromboembolic pulmonary hypertension associated with initial pulmonary involvement in Takayasu arteritis]. Nihon Kokyuki Gakkai Zasshi 1998;36(7):633–637.
44. Amano S, Tatsumi K, Tanabe N, et al. Polymorphism of the promoter region of prostacyclin synthase gene in chronic thromboembolic pulmonary hypertension. Respirology 2004;9(2):184–189.
45. Eddahibi S, Humbert M, Fadel E, et al. Serotonin transporter overexpression is responsible for pulmonary artery smooth muscle hyperplasia in primary pulmonary hypertension. J Clin Invest 2001;108(8): 1141–1150.
46. Marsh JJ, Konopka RG, Lang IM, et al. Suppression of thrombolysis in a canine model of pulmonary embolism. Circulation 1994;90(6):3091–3097.
47. Lang IM, Marsh JJ, Konopka RG, et al. Factors contributing to increased vascular fibrinolytic activity in mongrel dogs. Circulation 1993;87(6):1990–2000.
48. Moser KM, Cantor JP, Olman M, et al. Chronic pulmonary thromboembolism in dogs treated with tranexamic acid. Circulation 1991;83(4):1371–1379.
49. Lang IM, Moser KM, Schleef RR. Elevated expression of urokinase-like plasminogen activator and plasminogen activator inhibitor type 1 during the vascular remodeling associated with pulmonary thromboembolism. Arterioscler Thromb Vasc Biol 1998;18(5):808–815.
50. Lang IM, Moser KM, Schleef RR. Expression of Kunitz protease inhibitor—containing forms of amyloid beta-protein precursor within vascular thrombi. Circulation 1996;94(11):2728–2734.
51. Du L, Sullivan CC, Chu D, et al. Signaling molecules in nonfamilial pulmonary hypertension. N Engl J Med 2003;348(6):500–509.
52. Kimura H, Okada O, Tanabe N, et al. Plasma monocyte chemoattractant protein-1 and pulmonary vascular resistance in chronic thromboembolic pulmonary hypertension. Am J Respir Crit Care Med 2001;164(2):319–324.
53. Sakamaki F, Kyotani S, Nagaya N, Sato N, Oya H, Nakanishi N. Increase in thrombomodulin concentrations after pulmonary thromboendarterectomy in chronic thromboembolic pulmonary hypertension. Chest 2003;124(4):1305–1311.
54. Damas JK, Otterdal K, Yndestad A, et al. Soluble CD40 ligand in pulmonary arterial hypertension: possible pathogenic role of the interaction between platelets and endothelial cells. Circulation 2004; 110(8):999–1005.
55. Humbert M, Sitbon O, Simonneau G. Treatment of pulmonary arterial hypertension. N Engl J Med 2004; 351(14):1425–1436.

56. Ignatescu M, Kostner K, Zorn G, et al. Plasma Lp(a) levels are increased in patients with chronic thrombo-embolic pulmonary hypertension. Thromb Haemost 1998;80(2):231–232.

57. Auger WR, Channick RN, Kerr KM, Fedullo PF. Evaluation of patients with suspected chronic thromboembolic pulmonary hypertension. Semin Thorac Cardiovasc Surg 1999;11(2):179–190.

58. Moser KM, Fedullo PF, Finkbeiner WE, Golden J. Do patients with primary pulmonary hypertension develop extensive central thrombi? Circulation 1995;91(3):741–745.

59. Paw P, Jamieson SW, Ueno Y, Koike H, Annoh S, Nishio S. Pulmonary thromboendarterectomy for the treatment of pulmonary embolism caused by renal cell carcinoma anti-inflammatory effects of beraprost sodium, a stable analogue of PGI2, and its mechanisms. J Thorac Cardiovasc Surg 1997;114(2): 295–297.

60. Kerr KM, Auger WR, Fedullo PF, Channick RH, Yi ES, Moser KM. Large vessel pulmonary arteritis mimicking chronic thromboembolic disease. Am J Respir Crit Care Med 1995;152(1):367–373.

61. Brister SJ, Wilson-Yang K, Lobo FV, Yang H, Skala R. Pulmonary thromboendarterectomy in a patient with giant cell arteritis. Ann Thorac Surg 2002;73(6):1977–1979.

62. Ley S, Kauczor HU, Heussel CP, et al. Value of contrast-enhanced MR angiography and helical CT angiography in chronic thromboembolic pulmonary hypertension. Eur Radiol 2003;13(10):2365–2371.

63. Meysman M, Diltoer M, Raeve HD, Monsieur I, Huyghens L. Chronic thromboembolic pulmonary hypertension and vascular transformation of the lymph node sinuses. Eur Respir J 1997;10(5):1191–1193.

64. Bonderman D, Fleischmann D, Prokop M, Klepetko W, Lang IM. Images in cardiovascular medicine. Left main coronary artery compression by the pulmonary trunk in pulmonary hypertension. Circulation 2002;105(2):265.

65. Ngaage DL, Lapeyre AC, McGregor CG. Left main coronary artery compression in chronic thromboembolic pulmonary hypertension. Eur J Cardiothorac Surg 2005;27(3):512.

66. Morris TA, Auger WR, Ysrael MZ, et al. Parenchymal scarring is associated with restrictive spirometric defects in patients with chronic thromboembolic pulmonary hypertension. Chest 1996;110(2):399–403.

67. Endrys J, Hayat N, Cherian G. Comparison of bronchopulmonary collaterals and collateral blood flow in patients with chronic thromboembolic and primary pulmonary hypertension. Heart 1997;78(2):171–176.

68. Satoh T, Kyotani S, Okano Y, Nakanishi N, Kunieda T. Descriptive patterns of severe chronic pulmonary hypertension by chest radiography. Respir Med 2005;99(3):329–336.

69. Ryan KL, Fedullo PF, Davis GB, Vasquez TE, Moser KM. Perfusion scan findings understate the severity of angiographic and hemodynamic compromise in chronic thromboembolic pulmonary hypertension. Chest 1988;93(6):1180–1185.

70. Olman MA, Auger WR, Fedullo PF, Moser KM. Pulmonary vascular steal in chronic thromboembolic pulmonary hypertension. Chest 1990;98(6):1430–1434.

71. Skoro-Sajer N, Becherer A, Klepetko W, Kneussl MP, Maurer G, Lang IM. Longitudinal analysis of perfusion lung scintigrams of patients with unoperated chronic thromboembolic pulmonary hypertension. Thromb Haemost 2004;92(1):201–207.

72. Bergin CJ, Rios G, King MA, Belezzuoli E, Luna J, Auger WR. Accuracy of high-resolution CT in identifying chronic pulmonary thromboembolic disease. AJR Am J Roentgenol 1996;166(6):1371–1377.

73. Fleischmann D, Scholten C, Klepetko W, Lang IM. Three-dimensional visualization of pulmonary thromboemboli in chronic thromboembolic pulmonary hypertension with multiple detector-row spiral computed tomography. Circulation 2001;103(24):2993.

74. Archibald CJ, Auger WR, Fedullo PF, et al. Long-term outcome after pulmonary thromboendarterectomy. Am J Respir Crit Care Med 1999;160(2):523–528.

75. Jamieson SW, Nomura K. Indications for and the results of pulmonary thromboendarterectomy for thromboembolic pulmonary hypertension. Semin Vasc Surg 2000;13(3):236–244.

76. Kramm T, Mayer E, Dahm M, et al. Long-term results after thromboendarterectomy for chronic pulmonary embolism. Eur J Cardiothorac Surg 1999;15(5):579–583; discussion 83–84.

77. Fesler P, Pagnamenta A, Vachiery JL, et al. Single arterial occlusion to locate resistance in patients with pulmonary hypertension. Eur Respir J 2003;21(1):31–36.

78. Hakim TS, Michel RP, Chang HK. Partitioning of pulmonary vascular resistance in dogs by arterial and venous occlusion. J Appl Physiol 1982;52(3):710–715.

79. Kim NH, Fesler P, Channick RN, et al. Preoperative partitioning of pulmonary vascular resistance correlates with early outcome after thromboendarterectomy for chronic thromboembolic pulmonary hypertension. Circulation 2004;109(1):18–22.

80. Nicod P, Peterson K, Levine M, et al. Pulmonary angiography in severe chronic pulmonary hypertension. Ann Intern Med 1987;107(4):565–568.

81. Auger WR, Fedullo PF, Moser KM, Buchbinder M, Peterson KL. Chronic major-vessel thromboembolic pulmonary artery obstruction: appearance at angiography. Radiology 1992;182(2):393–398.

82. Tscholl D, Langer F, Wendler O, Wilkens H, Georg T, Schafers HJ. Pulmonary thromboendarterectomy—risk factors for early survival and hemodynamic improvement. Eur J Cardiothorac Surg 2001;19(6): 771–776.

83. Tanabe N, Okada O, Abe Y, Masuda M, Nakajima N, Kuriyama T. The influence of fractional pulse pressure on the outcome of pulmonary thromboendarterectomy. Eur Respir J 2001;17(4):653–659.

84. Lewczuk J, Piszko P, Jagas J, et al. Prognostic factors in medically treated patients with chronic pulmonary embolism. Chest 2001;119(3):818–823.

85. Moser KM, Houk VN, Jones RC, Hufnagel CC. Chronic, massive thrombotic obstruction of the pulmonary arteries. Analysis of four operated cases. Circulation 1965;32(3):377–385.

86. Moser KM, Braunwald NS. Successful surgical intervention in severe chronic thromboembolic pulmonary hypertension. Chest 1973;64(1):29–35.

87. Daily PO, Dembitsky WP, Iversen S. Technique of pulmonary thromboendarterectomy for chronic pulmonary embolism. J Card Surg 1989;4(1):10–24.

88. Mayer E, Dahm M, Hake U, et al. Mid-term results of pulmonary thromboendarterectomy for chronic thromboembolic pulmonary hypertension. Ann Thorac Surg 1996;61(6):1788–1792.

89. Dartevelle P, Fadel E, Chapelier A, et al. [Pulmonary thromboendarterectomy with video-angioscopy and circulatory arrest: an alternative to cardiopulmonary transplantation and post-embolism pulmonary artery hypertension]. Chirurgie 1998;123(1):32–40.

90. Dartevelle P, Fadel E, Mussot S, et al. Chronic thromboembolic pulmonary hypertension. Eur Respir J 2004;23(4):637–648.

91. Jamieson SW, Kapelanski DP. Pulmonary endarterectomy. Curr Probl Surg 2000;37(3):165–252.

92. Jamieson SW, Kapelanski DP, Sakakibara N, et al. Pulmonary endarterectomy: experience and lessons learned in 1,500 cases. Ann Thorac Surg 2003;76(5):1457–1462; discussion 62–64.

93. Klepetko W, Mayer E, Sandoval J, et al. Interventional and surgical modalities of treatment for pulmonary arterial hypertension. J Am Coll Cardiol 2004;43(12 Suppl):73S–80S.

94. Hirsch AM, Moser KM, Auger WR, Channick RN, Fedullo PF. Unilateral pulmonary artery thrombotic occlusion: is distal arteriopathy a consequence? Am J Respir Crit Care Med 1996;154(2 Pt 1):491–496.

95. Thistlethwaite PA, Jamieson SW. Tricuspid valvular disease in the patient with chronic pulmonary thromboembolic disease. Curr Opin Cardiol 2003;18(2):111–116.

96. Thistlethwaite PA, Auger WR, Madani MM, Pradhan S, Kapelanski DP, Jamieson SW. Pulmonary thromboendarterectomy combined with other cardiac operations: indications, surgical approach, and outcome. Ann Thorac Surg 2001;72(1):13–17; discussion 7–9.

97. Zoia MC, D'Armini AM, Beccaria M, et al. Mid term effects of pulmonary thromboendarterectomy on clinical and cardiopulmonary function status. Thorax 2002;57(7):608–612.

98. Badesch DB, Abman SH, Ahearn GS, et al. Medical therapy for pulmonary arterial hypertension: ACCP evidence-based clinical practice guidelines. Chest 2004;126(1 Suppl):35S–62S.

99. Augustinos P, Ouriel K. Invasive approaches to treatment of venous thromboembolism. Circulation 2004;110(9 Suppl 1):I27–134.

100. Yalamanchili K, Fleisher AG, Lehrman SG, et al. Open pulmonary embolectomy for treatment of major pulmonary embolism. Ann Thorac Surg 2004;77(3):819–823; discussion 23.

101. Hagl C, Khaladj N, Peters T, et al. Technical advances of pulmonary thromboendarterectomy for chronic thromboembolic pulmonary hypertension. Eur J Cardiothorac Surg 2003;23(5):776–781; discussion 81.

102. Levinson RM, Shure D, Moser KM. Reperfusion pulmonary edema after pulmonary artery thromboendarterectomy. Am Rev Respir Dis 1986;134(6):1241–1245.

103. Kerr KM, Auger WR, Marsh JJ, et al. The use of cylexin (CY-1503) in prevention of reperfusion lung injury in patients undergoing pulmonary thromboendarterectomy. Am J Respir Crit Care Med 2000; 162(1):14–20.

104. Wensel R, Opitz CF, Anker SD, et al. Assessment of survival in patients with primary pulmonary hypertension: importance of cardiopulmonary exercise testing. Circulation 2002;106(3):319–324.

105. Olschewski H, Simonneau G, Galie N, et al. Inhaled iloprost for severe pulmonary hypertension. N Engl J Med 2002;347(5):322–329.

106. Kerr KM, Rubin LJ. Epoprostenol therapy as a bridge to pulmonary thromboendarterectomy for chronic thromboembolic pulmonary hypertension. Chest 2003;123(2):319–320.

107. Nagaya N, Sasaki N, Ando M, et al. Prostacyclin therapy before pulmonary thromboendarterectomy in patients with chronic thromboembolic pulmonary hypertension. Chest 2003;123(2):338–343.

108. Kramm T, Eberle B, Krummenauer F, Guth S, Oelert H, Mayer E. Inhaled iloprost in patients with chronic thromboembolic pulmonary hypertension: effects before and after pulmonary thromboendarterectomy. Ann Thorac Surg 2003;76(3):711–718.

109. Bresser P, Fedullo PF, Auger WR, et al. Continuous intravenous epoprostenol for chronic thromboembolic pulmonary hypertension. Eur Respir J 2004;23(4):595–600.

110. Hoeper MM, Kramm T, Wilkens H, et al. Bosentan therapy for inoperable chronic thromboembolic pulmonary hypertension. Chest 2005;128(4):2363–2367.

111. Bonderman D, Nowotny R, Skoro-Sajer N, et al. Bosentan therapy for inoperable chronic thromboembolic pulmonary hypertension. Chest 2005;128(4):2599–2603.

112. Ghofrani HA, Schermuly RT, Rose F, et al. Sildenafil for long-term treatment of nonoperable chronic thromboembolic pulmonary hypertension. Am J Respir Crit Care Med 2003;167(8):1139–1141.

113. Feinstein JA, Goldhaber SZ, Lock JE, Ferndandes SM, Landzberg MJ. Balloon pulmonary angioplasty for treatment of chronic thromboembolic pulmonary hypertension. Circulation 2001;103(1):10–13.

114. Pitton MB, Herber S, Mayer E, Thelen M. Pulmonary balloon angioplasty of chronic thromboembolic pulmonary hypertension (CTEPH) in surgically inaccessible cases. Rofo 2003;175(5):631–634.

115. Cerveri I, D'Armini AM, Vigano M. Pulmonary thromboendarterectomy almost 50 years after the first surgical attempts. Heart 2003;89(4):369–370.

116. Hartz RS, Byrne JG, Levitsky S, Park J, Rich S. Predictors of mortality in pulmonary thromboendarterectomy. Ann Thorac Surg 1996;62(5):1255–1259; discussion 1259–1260.

117. Klepetko W, Moritz A, Burghuber OC, et al. [Chronic thromboembolic pulmonary hypertension and its treatment with pulmonary thrombendarterectomy]. Wien Klin Wochenschr 1995;107(13):396–402.

118. Imanaka H, Miyano H, Takeuchi M, Kumon K, Ando M. Effects of nitric oxide inhalation after pulmonary thromboendarterectomy for chronic pulmonary thromboembolism. Chest 2000;118(1):39–46.

INDEX